CLINICAL PATHOLOGY, HEMATOLOGY AND BLOOD BANKING

(For DMLT Students)

CLINICAL PATHOLOGY, HEMATOLOGY AND BLOOD BANKING

(For DMLT Students)

(Fourth Edition)

Nanda Maheshwari MSc BEd
Lecturer
Suburban College of Paramedical Education (SCOPE)
Mumbai, Maharashtra, India

Foreword
SM Arora

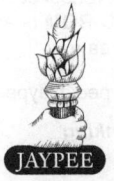

JAYPEE BROTHERS MEDICAL PUBLISHERS
The Health Sciences Publisher
New Delhi | London

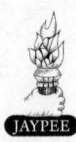

Jaypee Brothers Medical Publishers (P) Ltd

Headquarter
Jaypee Brothers Medical Publishers (P) Ltd
EMCA House, 23/23-B
Ansari Road, Daryaganj
New Delhi 110 002, India
Landline: +91-11-23272143, +91-11-23272703
+91-11-23282021, +91-11-23245672
Email: jaypee@jaypeebrothers.com

Corporate Office
Jaypee Brothers Medical Publishers (P) Ltd
4838/24, Ansari Road, Daryaganj
New Delhi 110 002, India
Phone: +91-11-43574357
Fax: +91-11-43574314
Email: jaypee@jaypeebrothers.com

Overseas Office
J.P. Medical Ltd
83 Victoria Street, London
SW1H 0HW (UK)
Phone: +44 20 3170 8910
Fax: +44 (0)20 3008 6180
Email: info@jpmedpub.com

Website: www.jaypeebrothers.com
Website: www.jaypeedigital.com

© 2021, Jaypee Brothers Medical Publishers

The views and opinions expressed in this book are solely those of the original contributor(s)/author(s) and do not necessarily represent those of editor(s) of the book.

All rights reserved. No part of this publication may be reproduced, stored or transmitted in any form or by any means, electronic, mechanical, photocopying, recording or otherwise, without the prior permission in writing of the publishers.

All brand names and product names used in this book are trade names, service marks, trademarks or registered trademarks of their respective owners. The publisher is not associated with any product or vendor mentioned in this book.

Medical knowledge and practice change constantly. This book is designed to provide accurate, authoritative information about the subject matter in question. However, readers are advised to check the most current information available on procedures included and check information from the manufacturer of each product to be administered, to verify the recommended dose, formula, method and duration of administration, adverse effects and contraindications. It is the responsibility of the practitioner to take all appropriate safety precautions. Neither the publisher nor the author(s)/editor(s) assume any liability for any injury and/or damage to persons or property arising from or related to use of material in this book.

This book is sold on the understanding that the publisher is not engaged in providing professional medical services. If such advice or services are required, the services of a competent medical professional should be sought.

Every effort has been made where necessary to contact holders of copyright to obtain permission to reproduce copyright material. If any have been inadvertently overlooked, the publisher will be pleased to make the necessary arrangements at the first opportunity. The **CD/DVD-ROM** (if any) provided in the sealed envelope with this book is complimentary and free of cost. **Not meant for sale.**

Inquiries for bulk sales may be solicited at: jaypee@jaypeebrothers.com

Clinical Pathology, Hematology and Blood Banking

First Edition: 2005

Second Edition: 2008

Third Edition: 2017

Fourth Edition: 2021, *Reprint*: **2025**

ISBN: 978-93-90595-76-1

Printed at: Samrat Offset Pvt. Ltd.

Affectionately Dedicated to

*Yogendra, Arushi and Kabir
for their
Unconditional Love
and
Unwavering Support*

Foreword

It is a privilege to write a Foreword for fourth edition of *Clinical Pathology, Hematology and Blood Banking* written by Nanda Maheshwari, faculty member of SCOPE. Being associated with the paramedical education for a decade, I can acknowledge that this can serve every purpose for paramedical students. The contents are divided into three sections: Pathology, Hematology and Blood Banking. This represents perfect blend of her rich practical experience and keen academic interest.

The author has taken tremendous pain in preparing this book, focusing attention to cover various aspects of the subject. She has maintained simplicity and readability that would help reading and understanding for any beginner and expert alike. The reference diagrams and flowcharts make it easier to relate with tests/practical by students and laboratory professionals. The book has maintained balance between theoretical manual methods and practical world of automation.

I congratulate the author for writing fourth edition of Clinical Pathology, Hematology and Blood Banking. I am sure this book will go a long way in filling the void between academics and industry. May almighty give her courage and achievements she deserves. I wish her great success in all her endeavors.

SM Arora
Founder
Suburban College of Paramedical Education (SCOPE)
Mumbai, Maharashtra, India
info@suburbancollege.com

Preface to the Fourth Edition

To improve is to change; to be perfect is to change often.

Journey of this book was started in 2005. With continuous adaptation of latest technology, and improved documentation, *Clinical Pathology, Hematology and Blood Banking* is ready to launch its fourth edition in 2021.

In this era of robotics and automation, diagnostic science has made a tremendous progress. With the aim to introduce latest technologies to students, I have added latest topics: Urilyzer, Multistix Urinalysis Strips and Polymerase Chain Reaction in Chapter—Automation in Pathology Laboratory. To bridge the gap between theory and practical world, some of the tests which are regular for today's diagnostic world like bone marrow test and hemoglobinopathies have also been added in this edition. The primary objective of this book is to meet the requirements of Diploma in Medical Laboratory Technology (DMLT) and undergraduate students. This book is successfully serving as a reference book for Laboratory Technicians and Paramedical professionals.

In addition to the new chapters, I have succinctly explained various concepts in simple language. As each topic is covered in a small chapter, it makes it easy for the students to assimilate the concept in totality.

The order and style of presentation of this book is similar to the first edition. The orientation of this book is to provide simple yet advanced content such that the book suffices the needs of not only DMLT/MLT/BSc students but also students of diverse backgrounds who require an exposure to this field. I hope that the simple language and illustrative images of this edition will boost your interest in the field of Clinical Pathology and Hematology.

I welcome constructive criticism and suggestions from teachers, colleagues, students and interested readers for the next revised edition.

Nanda Maheshwari

nandabaheti@hotmail.com

Preface to the First Edition

It gives me a great pleasure to introduce this book on *Clinical Pathology and Haematology*. In this book, I have tried to solve the difficulty of students to understand the tests and getting the exact data. The aims and objects of this book are primarily to meet the requirements of DMLT and undergraduate courses.

Clinical Pathology and Haematology is an important subject of DMLT courses, but there is non-availability of good books on this subject. The books available are vast and mainly written for MBBS students. I have tried to overcome this problem by writing in easy language and providing exact data. I hope that this book will satisfy the needs of DMLT students.

I welcome constructive criticism and suggestions from teachers, colleagues and students for the next revised edition.

Nanda Maheshwari

Acknowledgments

It is a feeling of pride for me to introduce the fourth edition of *Clinical Pathology, Hematology and Blood Banking* to my readers. I owe this incredible journey of 16 years to many souls around.

Special thanks to all past and present students and teachers for reading and recommending this book. Feedback from avid readers provided valuable support for me during the course of writing this edition.

In order to learn about the latest technological developments and current lab practices in the field, I visited Central Processing Laboratory of Suburban Diagnostics in Mumbai. During my visit, Dr Anupa Dixit, Lab Director and all her staff members were extremely helpful. I could write the chapter about Automation only because of their help and guidance. Staff members of different departments introduced me a variety of latest techniques in Pathology and patiently answered all my queries. I am immensely grateful to all for their kind cooperation.

Dr SM Arora, Founder of Suburban College of Paramedical Education (SCOPE), Mumbai, took great effort to write the Foreword of this book. I am sincerely thankful to him.

It took me more than a year to finish writing and compiling this work. During this period of research, writing the manuscript, editing, proofreading, etc., my husband Mr Yogendra Maheshwari and my little angels Arushi and Kabir patiently cooperated with me. I would like to express deepest thanks to my parents, Mr Ramesh Ji Baheti and Ms Kusumlata Baheti; whatever I am today, is a result of their blessings and confidence in my abilities. I am fortunate to have good friends and close kin who continuously encouraged me to pursue my work.

Lastly, my acknowledgment would remain incomplete without mentioning M/s Jaypee Brothers Medical Publishers and their team. My special thanks to them for walking the extra mile and putting in great efforts in publishing this book.

Contents

SECTION 1 Pathology

1. **Introduction to Clinical Pathology** 3
   Terminology in Pathology 3
   Branches of Pathology 4

2. **Cellular Pathology** 7
   Cell Organelles 7
   Functions of Cell 9
   Cell Pathology 10
   Overview of Cell Injury 10
   Types of Cell Death 17

3. **Inflammation** 22
   Causes of Inflammation 22
   Effects of Inflammation 23
   Types of Inflammation 24
   Repair—Cell Growth and Regeneration 29

4. **Pathology Laboratory** 33
   Levels of Laboratories 33
   Infrastructure 34
   Safety in Laboratories 35
   Handling Biomedical Waste 36

5. **Tumor Markers** 42
   Types of Tumor Markers 42
   Uses of Tumor Markers 43
   Limitations of Tumor Markers 44
   List of Tumor Markers 44
   Testing of Tumor Markers 49

6. **Electrolytes** 50
   Introduction and Classification 50
   Serum Sodium and Potassium 51

Urine Sodium and Potassium 54
Serum and Urine Chloride 55
Serum and Urine Phosphorus 56
Serum and Urine Calcium 57

7. Body Fluid 59
Seminal Fluid 59
Amniotic Fluid 62
Cerebrospinal Fluid 64
Pericardial Fluid 65
Pleural Fluid 69
Peritoneal Fluid 73
Synovial Fluid 76

8. Urine Analysis 79
Collection and Preservation 79
Physical Examination 79
Chemical Examination 81
Microscopic Examination 82

9. Stool Analysis 87
Macrosopic Examination 87
Chemical Examination 88
Microscopic Examination 88

10. Sputum Examination 91
Clinical Significance 91
Macroscopic Assessment 93
Sputum Microscopy 93
Sputum Culture 96

11. Automation in Pathology Laboratory 98
Automation Objective 98
Urilyzer 102
Multistix Urinalysis Strips 103
Polymerase Chain Reaction 105

SECTION 2 Hematology

12. The Blood 111
Blood 111
Blood Cells 111

Plasma 114
Functions of Blood 115

13. Hemopoiesis ... 116
Erythropoiesis 117
Leukopoiesis 118
Thrombopoiesis 120

14. Collection of Blood ... 122
Arterial Blood Collection 122
Capillary Blood Collection 122
Venous Blood Collection 123
Use of Evacuated Tube for Vein Punctures 126

15. Anticoagulants ... 129
Chemical Anticoagulants 129
Biological Anticoagulant: Heparine 130

16. Total RBC Count ... 131
Hemocytometer 132
Procedure 132
Calculations 133
Clinical Significance 133

17. Total White Cell Count ... 135
Hemocytometer 136
Procedure 136
Calculations 137
Clinical Significance 137

18. Differential Leukocyte Count ... 138
Preparation of Blood Smear 138
Staining of Blood Smear 139
Microscopic Examination 139
Clinical Significance 141

19. Absolute Eosinophil Count ... 143
Indirect Method 143
Direct Method 143
Clinical Significance 144

20. Erythrocyte Sedimentation Rate ... 145
Westergren Method 145
Wintrobe Method 146

Possible Errors in ESR 147
Factors Affecting ESR 147

21. Packed Cell Volume 148
Macrohematocrit 148
Microhematocrit 149

22. Hemoglobin Estimation 151
Sahli's Acid Hematin Method 151
Colorimetric Method 152
Specific Gravity Method 153
Gasometric Method 153
Chemical Method 153
Clinical Importance 153

23. Hemoglobinopathies 154
Structure of Hemoglobin 154
Hemoglobinopathies 154
Diagnosis 155

24. Red Cell Indices 158
Mean Cell Volume 158
Mean Cell Hemoglobin 158
Mean Cell Hemoglobin Concentration 159
Clinical Significance 159

25. Special Blood Cell Tests 160
Lupus Erythematosus 160
Osmotic Fragility 162
Fetal Hemoglobin 164
Heinz Bodies 167

26. Reticulocyte Count 169
Principle 169
Procedure 169
Clinical Significance 170

27. Sickle Cells Preparation 171
Sickle Cell Trait 171
Principle 172
Procedure 172

28. Morphology of Normal and Abnormal RBCs … 173
Normal Morphology 173
Color Reaction 173
Size Variations 174
Shape Variation 174
Other Conditions 176
Abnormalities in Normal Content of RBC 176

29. Bone Marrow … 178
Structure and Function 178
Sample Collection 179
Preparation of Bone Marrow Film 180
Staining of Bone Marrow Aspirate Slides 180
Importance of Detection of Sideroblast 182
Sample Report 184

30. Blood Coagulation … 185
Coagulation Factors 185
Mechanism of Coagulation 186
Hemostasis 187

31. Hemorrhagic Disorders … 189
Bleeding Time 190
Whole Blood Coagulation Time 191
Clot Retraction 192
Prothrombin Time 192
Platelet Count 193
Tourniquet Test 194
Activated Partial Thromboplastin Time 194
Purpura 195

32. Hemophilia and Polycythemia … 196
Hemophilia 196
Polycythemia 198

33. Anemia … 200
Classification 200
Thalassemia (Cooley's anemia) 202
Schilling Test 202

34. Leukemia 203

Classification on the Basis of Course of Disease 203
Classification on the Basis of Cell of Origin 203

35. Hemoparasites 206

Plasmodium (Malaria) 206
Leishmania (Kala-Azar) 216
Trypanosoma (Sleeping Sickness) 221
Wuchereria Bancrofti (Filariasis) 224

36. Analyzers in Hematology 230

Hematology Analyzer (Cell Counter) Technology 230
Factors to Consider when Buying a Hematology Analyzer 232
Automation in ESR 235

SECTION 3   Blood Banking
---

37. Historical Aspect 241

Definition 241
History 241

38. Organization and Operation of Blood Bank 245

Objectives of the Blood Bank 245
Main Functions of the Department 246
Operation of Blood Bank 249
Documentation and Record Maintenance 252

39. Immunohematology and Serum Immunoglobulin 254

Antigens 254
Antibodies 255
General Functions of Immunoglobulins 257

40. ABO Blood Group System 259

Biochemistry of the ABO System 261
Production of A, B, and H Antigens 261
Subgroups 262

41. Rhesus Blood Group System 264

Rhesus Factor 264
Universal Donor and Universal Acceptor 265
Rhesus System Inheritance 267

42. Other Blood Group System — 269
Other Types of Blood Grouping 269
Bombay Blood Group 272

43. Preparation and Preservation of Antisera — 273
Antisera 273
Hybridomas 274

44. Technique of Blood Grouping and Crossmatching — 275
ABO Blood Grouping 275
Rh Blood Typing 277
Crossmatching 278

45. Coombs' Test — 281
Direct Coombs' Test 281
Indirect Coombs' test 283
Determination of D^u 284
Antibody Titration 284

46. Blood Transfusion Technique — 286
Preparation and Properties of Anticoagulant 286
Donor Selection 288
Blood Collection (Phlebotomy) 290
Care of Collected Blood Unit 292

47. Transfusion Reactions — 294
Types of Transfusion Reactions 294
Transfusion Transmitted Diseases 298

48. Hemolytic Disease of Newborn — 299
Causes 299
Clinical Features 300
Diagnosis 301

49. Exchange Transfusion — 303
Selection of Blood for Exchange Transfusion 303
Types of Exchange Transfusion 304
Exchange Transfusion Techniques 304
Risks Associated with Exchange Transfusion 305

50. Transfusion-Transmitted Diseases — 306
Viruses 307
Bacterial Contamination 308
Parasitic Infection 309

51. Blood Component Transfusion 311

Whole Blood 313
Red Cell 313
Platelet Transfusion 315
Granulocytes 317

52. Hemapheresis 319

Plasmapheresis 319
Cytapheresis 321

53. Recent Advances in Blood Banking 323

Stem Cells 323
Artificial Blood 325
Molecular Typing 329
Pathogen Inactivation Methods 333
Recent Crossmatch Techniques 335

Index 343

Plate 1

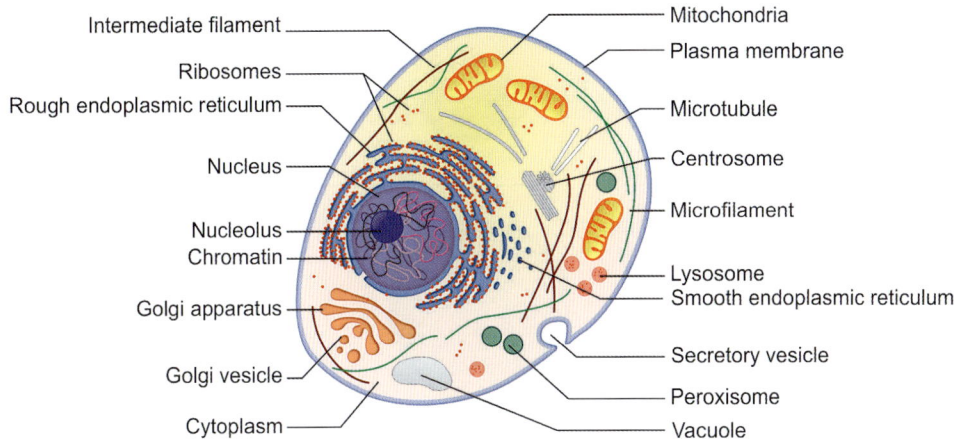

Fig. 2.1: Typical human cell.

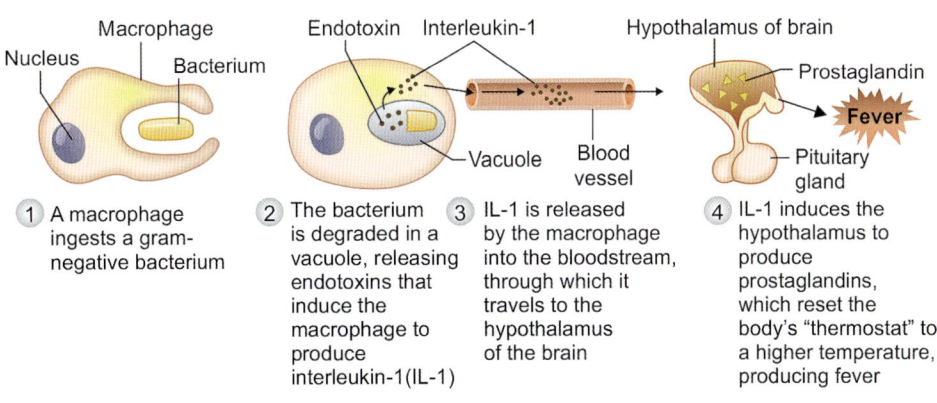

Fig. 3.1: Fever due to bacterial infection.

Plate 2

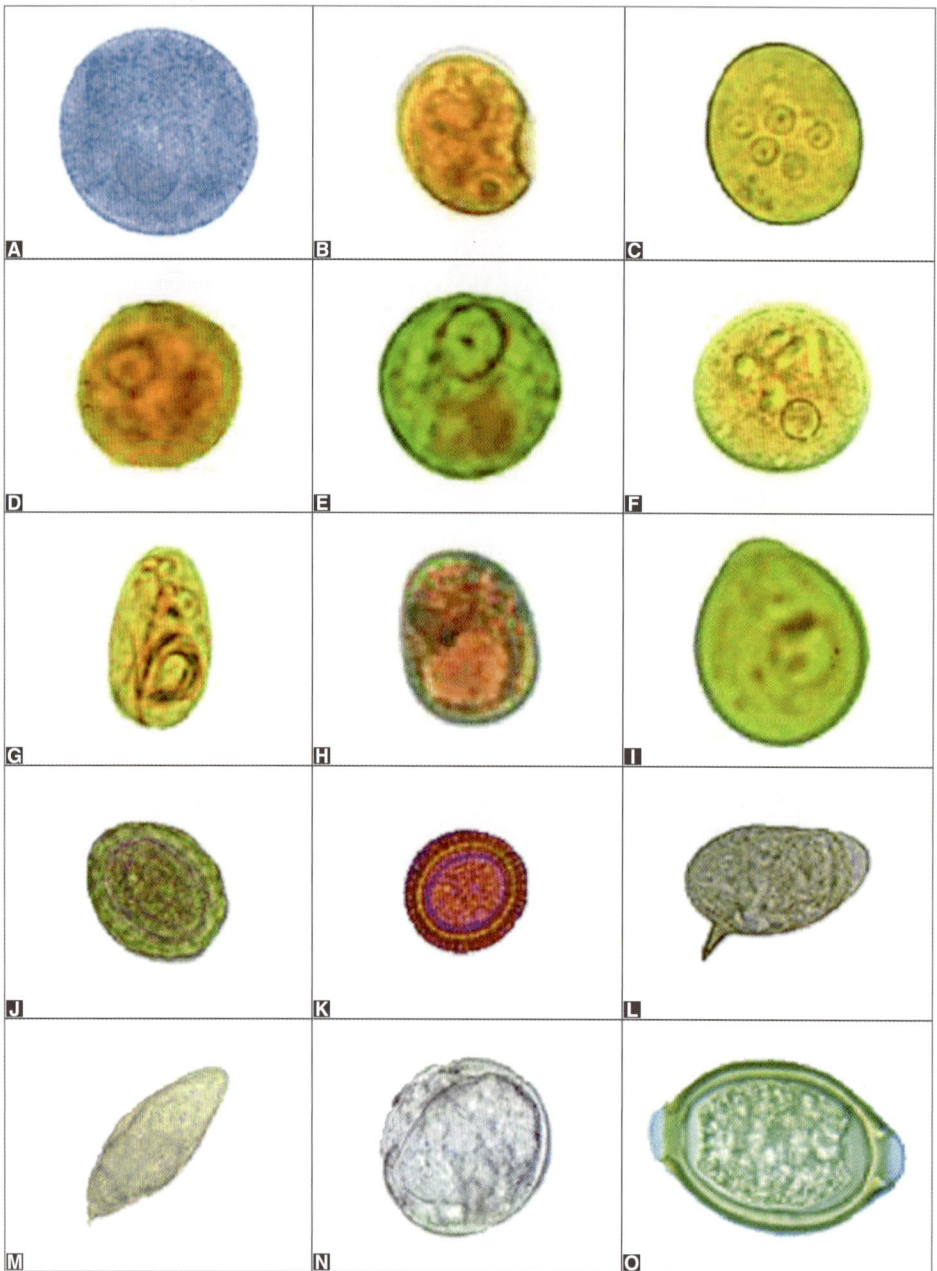

Figs. 9.1A to O: Microscopic images of each of the 15 types of parasites to recognize. (A) *Balantidium coli* cyst; (B) *Endolimax nana* cyst; (C) *Entamoeba coli* cyst; (D) *Entamoeba hartmanni* cyst; (E) *Entamoeba histolytica* cyst; (F) *Entamoeba polecki* cyst; (G) *Giardia lamblia* cyst; (H) *Iodamoeba butschlii* cyst; (I) *Chilomastix mesnili* cyst; (J) *Ascaris* egg; (K) Tapeworm egg; (L) *Schistosoma mansoni* egg; (M) *Schistosoma intercalatum* egg; (N) *Schistosoma japonicum* egg; (O) Whipworm egg.

Plate 3

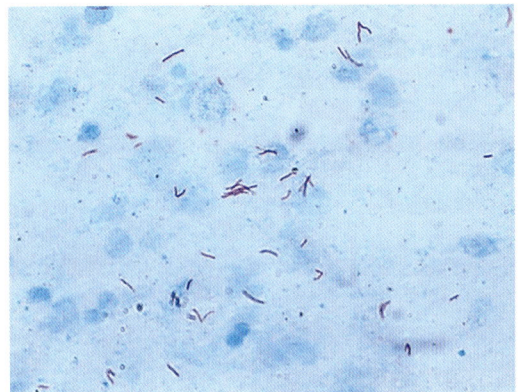

Fig. 10.1: 3+ slide of AFB stained with ZN stain.

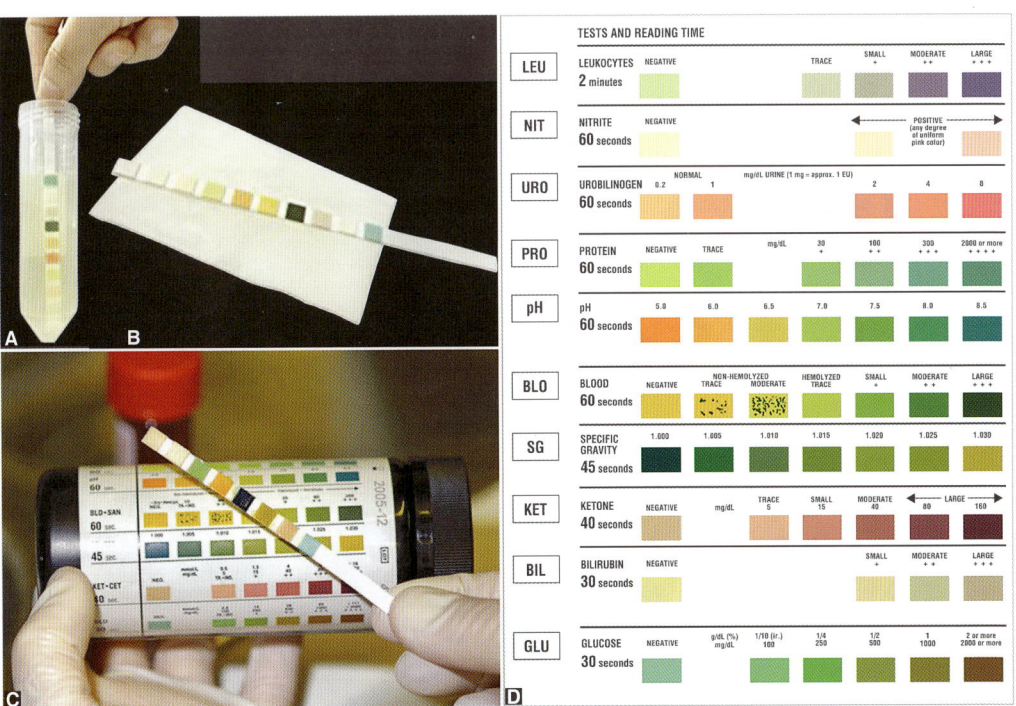

Figs. 11.2A to D: (A) Stick dipped in urine; (B) Wait for few seconds; (C) Match with the color code provided; (D) Color code for different tests with reading time.

Plate 4

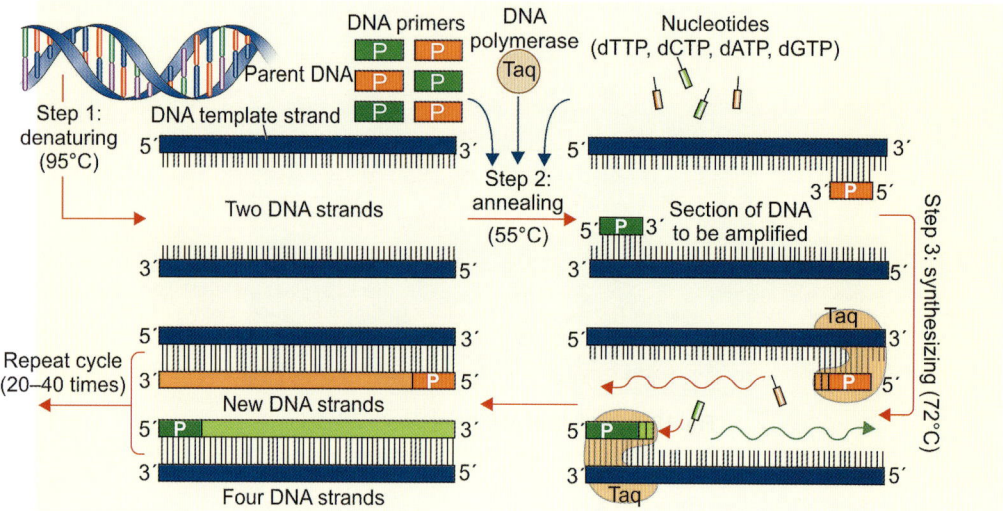

Fig. 11.3: PCR mechanism.

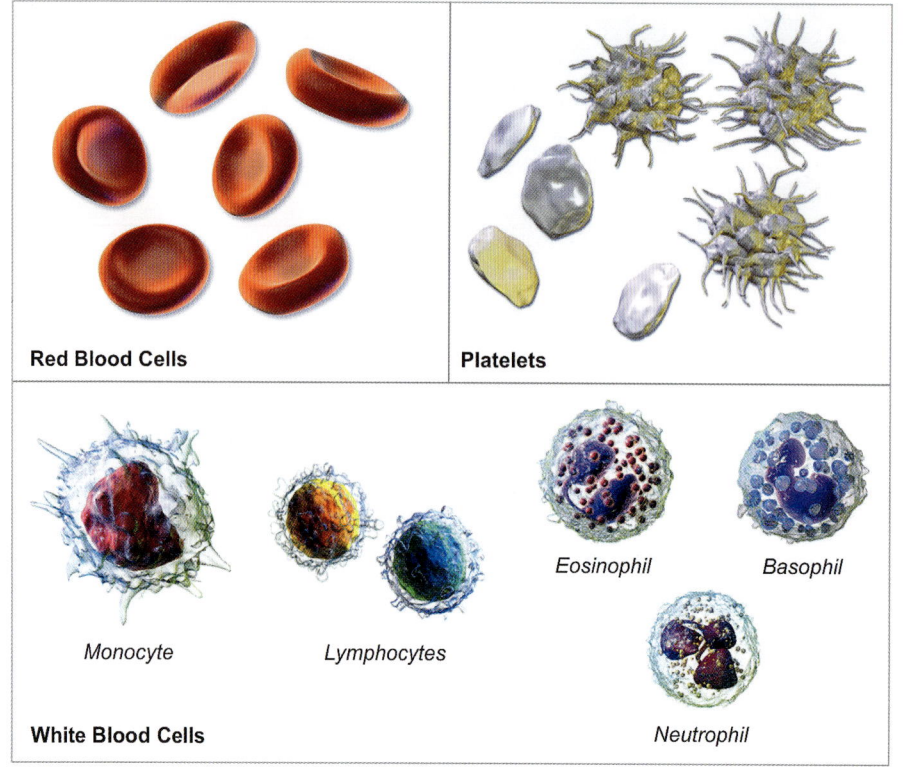

Fig. 12.8: Elements of blood.

Plate 5

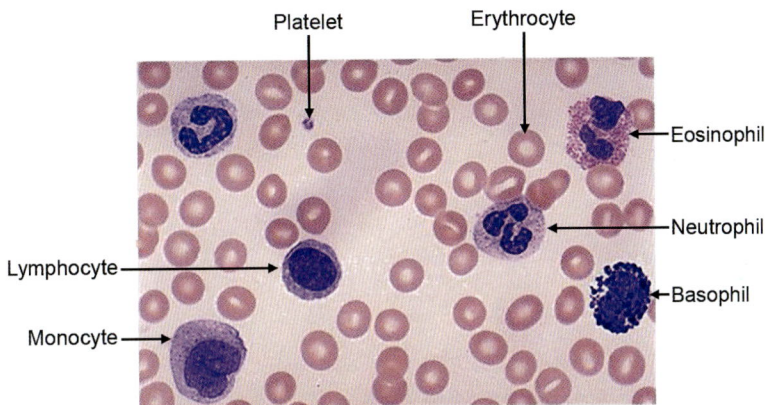

Fig. 18.3: Peripheral blood smear.

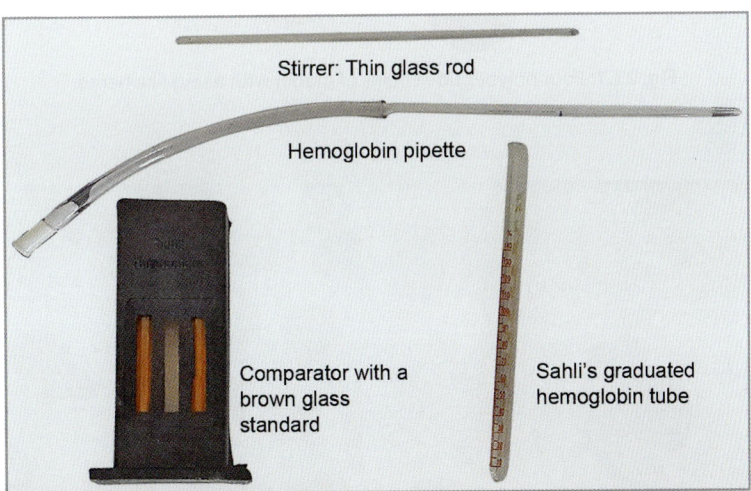

Actual anemia				Suggestive Anemia		Normal	
Men and women blow 70%				Men - 70 to 85% Women - 70 to 80%		Men - Above 85% Women - Above 80%	
30%	40%	50%	60%	70%	80%	90%	100%
4.7 gms.	6.3 gms.	7.8 gms.	9.4 gms.	10.9 gms.	12.5 gms.	14.1 gms.	15.6 gms.

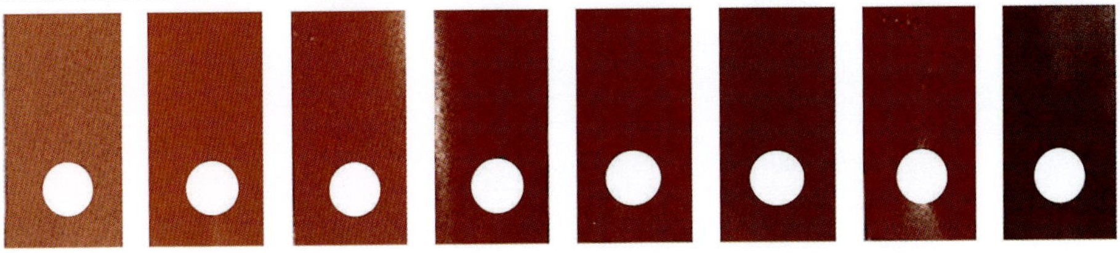

Fig. 22.1: Hemoglobin estimation by Sahli's acid hematin method.

Plate 6

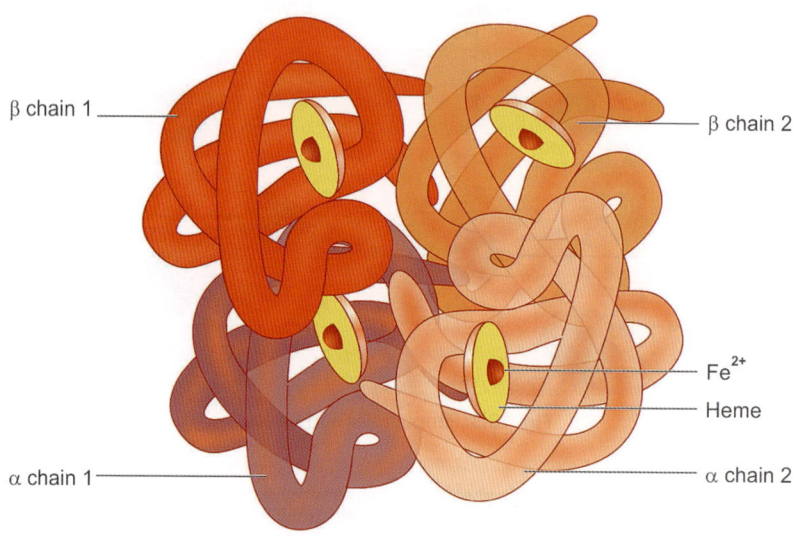

Fig. 23.1: Four polypeptide chains of globin with a ring like heme.

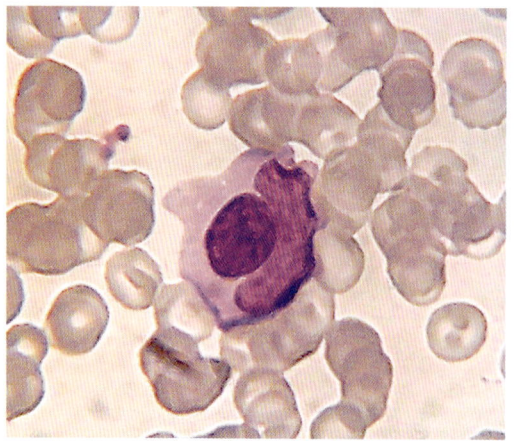

Fig. 25.1: Blood film showing LE bodies.

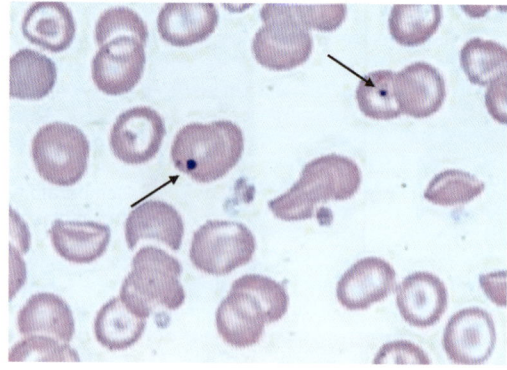

Fig. 25.3: Heinz bodies.

Plate 7

RBC Normal and Abnormal Morphology

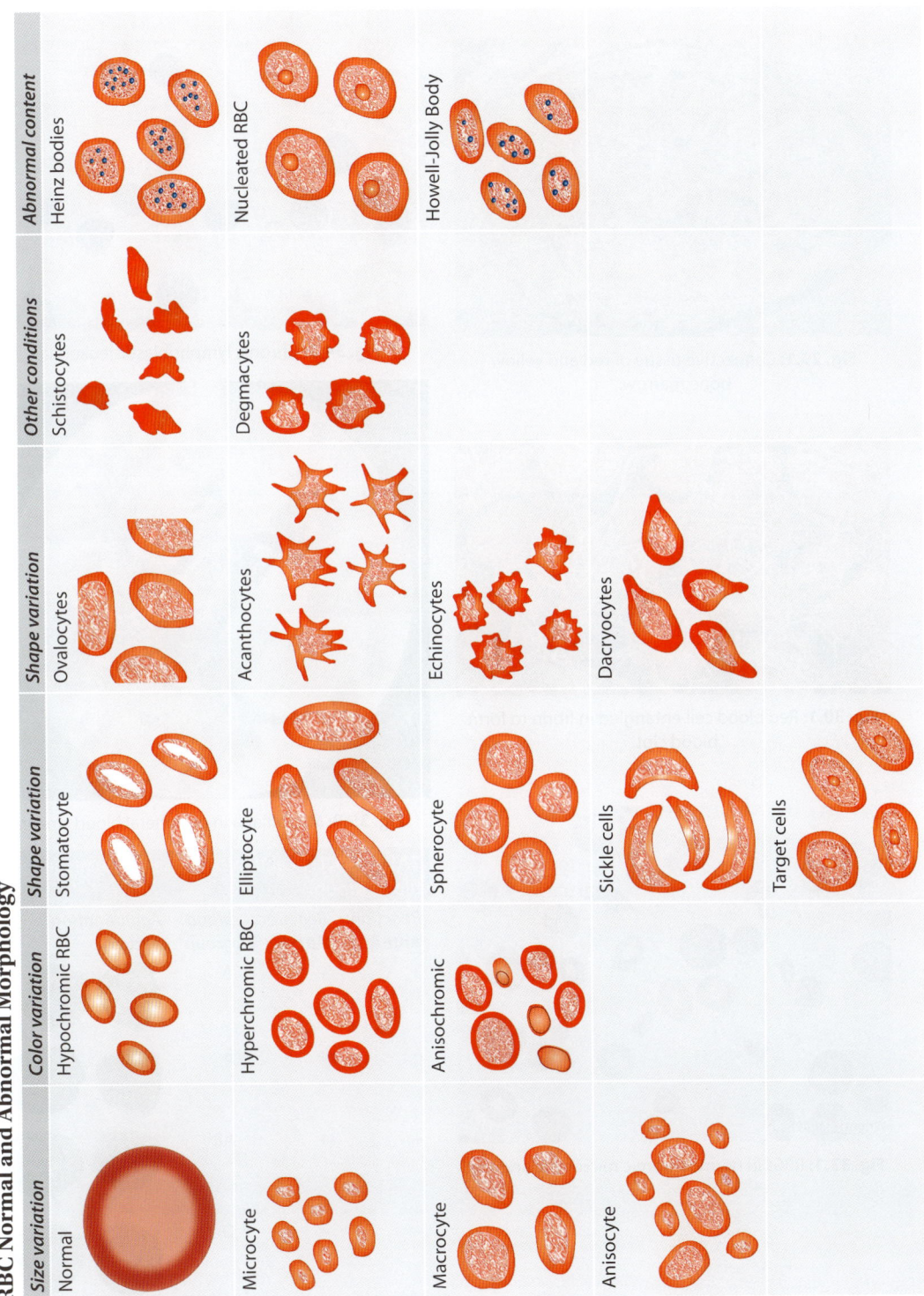

Plate 8

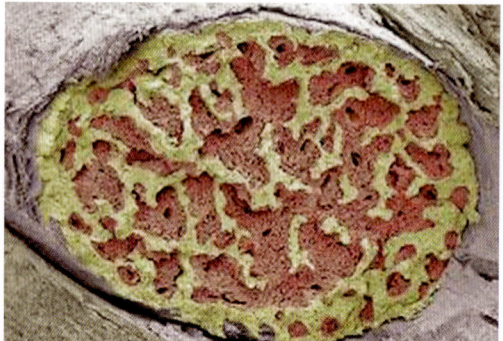

Fig. 29.1: Connective tissue of red and yellow bone marrow.

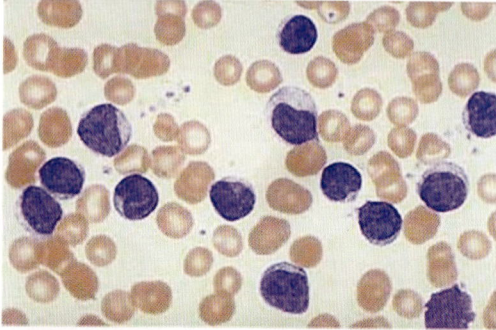

Fig. 34.2: Chronic lymphoblastic leukemia.

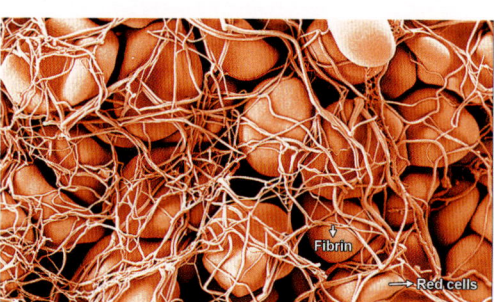

Fig. 30.1: Red blood cell entangled in fibrin to form blood clot.

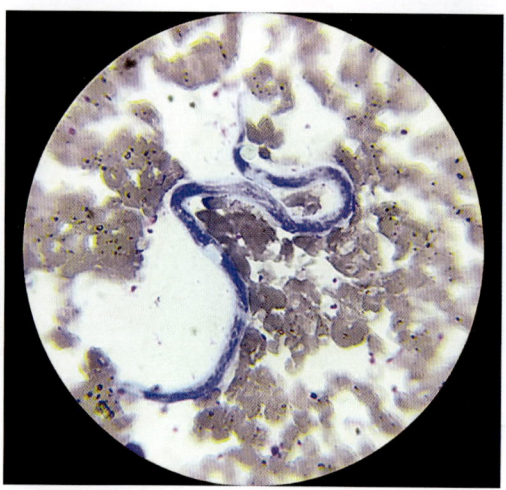

Fig. 35.9: Microfilaria in peripheral blood smear.

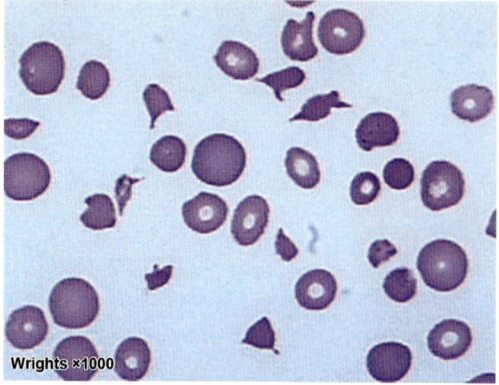

Fig. 33.1: RBCs in normochromic microcytic anemia.

TABLE 44.1: Reaction of antisera with respective blood group.

Reaction: Anti-A	Reaction: Anti-B	Blood group	Agglutination pattern
+	−	A	
−	+	B	
+	+	AB	
−	−	O	

+, Agglutination present; −, No agglutination

Section 1

Pathology

CHAPTER 1

Introduction to Clinical Pathology

Learning Objectives
- Every subject has its own terminology. Knowing basic terms of the subject is essential to understand the subject and hence, develop a keen interest in it. This chapter deals with basic terminology of pathology
- Pathology is a wide subject with many branches or subdivision into it. This chapter also gives introduction of various branches of pathology

Keywords
Histopathology, Cytopathology, Biochemistry, Genetics, Hematology, Immunology, Microbiology, Toxicopathology, Oncology

Pathology is the study of disease process with the aim of understanding their nature and causes. This is achieved by observing blood, urine, feces, and diseased tissue obtained from the living patient or at autopsy by the use of X-rays, and many other techniques. These techniques are studied under clinical pathology. Clinical pathology is thus the application of knowledge gained to the treatment of patients. The great human pathologist Rudolf Virchow is the father of pathology.

Clinical pathology is the key subject in the studies of paramedical sciences. It forms bridge between the preclinical sciences of anatomy, physiology and biochemistry on one hand and clinical branches of medical and surgical disciplines on the other.

Study of pathology is divided into two parts:
1. *General pathology:* It deals with the general principles of disease. It is related to whole body.
2. *Systemic pathology:* It is the study of disease related to the specific organs of the body system.

■ TERMINOLOGY IN PATHOLOGY

- *Health:* Health is a condition when individual is in complete accordance with the surroundings. It is a state of complete physical, mental and social well-being.
- *Disease* (Dis-ease—feeling of uneasiness): State of discomfort to the body is disease.
- *Patient:* Patient is the person affected by disease.
- *Pathology* (Pathos—disease, logos—study): Pathology is the scientific study of diseases.
- *Symptoms:* Symptoms are those, which are narrated by patients and his relatives.
- *Signs:* Signs are those which are observed by clinician or physician.
- *Etiology:* It is a causal factor responsible for the formation of disease.
- *Pathogenesis:* The mechanism by which the disease is produced is termed pathogenesis.
- *Fate:* Outcome of disease.

- *Morphology:* The structural features of the disease
- *Clinical significance:* The functional features of the disease
- *Syndrome:* A syndrome is an aggregate of signs and symptoms or a combination of lesions without which the disease cannot be recognized or diagnosed.
  Examples: Cushing's syndrome: hyperactivity of the adrenal cortex resulting in obesity, hypertension, etc.
- *Primary disease:* Primary disease is the disease without evident cause. Example, primary hypertension is defined as abnormally high BP without apparent cause.
- *Secondary disease:* Secondary disease is the disease which represents a complication of some underlying lesion. For example, secondary hypertension is defined as abnormally high BP as a consequence of some other lesion (e.g. renal artery stenosis).

Introduction to Pathology

Pathology is the study (*logos*) of suffering (*pathos*). Pathology is scientific study of disease.

More specifically, pathology may be defined as the "scientific study of the molecular, cellular, tissue, or organ system in response to injurious agents or adverse influences."

It involves the investigation of the causes (etiology of disease as well as the underlying mechanisms (pathogenesis) that result in the presenting signs and symptoms of the patient.

The purpose of study of pathology is to diagnose, treat, control and prevent the diseases from the knowledge gained through the cause, pathogenesis and effects. These are achieved through examination of tissues from living animals (biopsy) and dead animals/carcass (necropsy) or by experimentation. Thus, pathology deals with disease processes involving etiology, pathogenesis and clinical effects of diseases in animals and tries to explain what went wrong. It is linking the basic knowledge gained in anatomy, histology, physiology and biochemistry and clinical subjects in making diagnosis of diseases and helps in treatment, prevention and control of diseases.

■ BRANCHES OF PATHOLOGY

At the present time, pathology has 14 major areas of activity. These relate either to the methods used or the types of disease which they investigate. The disciplines are:

1. *Anatomical pathology:* It deals with the tissue diagnosis of disease, usually from biopsy materials taken from a patient in the operating theater or on a ward, or from an autopsy (post- mortem). Subspecialties include:
   - *Histopathology (histos—tissue):* Hence, histopathology is the study of microscopic changes or abnormalities in tissues that are caused as a result of diseases.
     A sample of tissue called as biopsy is taken from the body in order to examine it more closely. Biopsies are most often done to look for cancer. But biopsies can help identify many other conditions. Like if a person has chronic hepatitis, it becomes important to know if cirrhosis is present. This is done by histopathological test.
   - *Cytopathology (cyto—cell):* It is a diagnostic technique that examines cells from various body sites to determine the cause or the nature of disease.
     The first cytopathology test developed was the Pap test which has been widely utilized in the last 50 years for screening and diagnosing of cervical cancer and its precursors.
2. *Chemical pathology or biochemistry:* It deals with the entire spectrum of illness, often involving detecting changes in a wide range of substances in blood and body fluids (electrolytes, enzymes and proteins) that change in many diseases.

In addition, it involves detecting and measuring tumor (cancer) markers, hormones, vitamins, poisons and both therapeutic and illicit drugs. Example test: cholesterol and triglycerides to diagnose risk factors for heart disease.

3. *Clinical pathology:* The branch of pathology dealing with the study of disease and disease processes by means of chemical, microscopic, and serologic examinations. Sample test includes complete urine analysis, stool and other body fluid analysis.

4. *Forensic pathology:* It is the subspecialty of Pathology that focuses on medicolegal investigations of sudden or unexpected death. A forensic pathologist is primarily involved identifying the cause of death and reconstructing the circumstances by which the death occurred. This is performed in a meticulous, painstaking manner. A major component of the role involves the performance of autopsy examinations to both the external and internal body organs to discover cause of death. They also look at tissue sample from bodies under the microscope to assist in establishing the underlying pathological basis for the cause of death. Forensic pathologists are occasionally required to visit crime scenes or accidents or to testify in court.

5. *Genetics:* It includes three main branches—cytogenetics (microscopic analysis of chromosomal abnormalities), molecular genetics (uses DNA technology to analyse mutations in genes) and biochemical genetics (specialized biochemical testing to identify specific markers). It involves tests on chromosomes, DNA and specific biochemical markers from body fluids, cells in body fluids and tissues to diagnose genetic diseases.
Example tests: Cystic fibrosis (gene test), Down syndrome (chromosomal test), maple syrup urine disease (biochemical genetic test).

6. *Hematology:* It deals with many aspects of diseases which affect the blood, such as anemia, leukemia, lymphoma and clotting or bleeding disorders. It also encompasses the subspecialty of transfusion medicine, which includes blood typing and compatibility testing and the management and supply of a large range of blood products.
Example test: INR (clotting test) to check warfarin dosage is correct.

7. *Immunology:* Immune function tests can determine whether an individual is allergic, and if so, what to do. Many diseases result from the immune system, defense systems inappropriately targeting normal organs systems resulting in "autoimmune diseases". For this reason, many other immunological tests constitute diagnostic markers for disorders, such as lupus, rheumatoid arthritis, diabetes and thyroid conditions. Other immunological tests monitor tissue injury due to inflammation.
Example test: SLE (lupus).

8. *Microbiology:* It deals with diseases caused by infectious agents, such as bacteria, viruses, fungi and parasites through tests on blood, body fluids and tissue samples. Additional areas involve control of outbreaks of infectious disease and dealing with the problems of infections caused by antibiotic-resistant bacteria. *Example test:* Urine sample to detect urinary tract infection.

9. *General pathology:* It covers all areas of pathology at less specialized levels. *Example test:* Pathology laboratories have general pathologists managing tests from more than one discipline, including chemical and anatomical pathology, hematology and microbiology.

10. *Nutritional pathology:* It is the study of disease processes resulting from

deficiency or excess of essential foods. *Example:* Scurvy—caused by vitamin C deficiency.
11. *Toxicopathology:* It means the study of diseases caused by toxic substances. Toxin may be chemical, biological or physical agent. Example test includes testing of blood for presence of alcohol, presence of drug in athletes.
12. *Oncopathology (onco—tumor):* Branch of science which deals with the study of unusual, developing and multiplying portion of the body that are termed to be tumors is Oncopathology. It studies various tumor marker tests. Basically, it is the branch of science dealing with Cancer.
13. *Molecular pathology:* This branch of pathology studies and diagnoses the molecules that make up the organs and tissues of the body. It includes the study of disease and chromosomal abnormalities at the molecular level to aid in diagnosis and therapeutic intervention of disease processes. There are three areas of testing that includes genetics, hematopathology, and infectious disease. Genetically inherited disease can be prevented by early diagnosis using molecular level.
14. *Oral and maxillofacial pathology:* It is considered as one of the nine specialties of dental medicine, oral pathology studies diseases that affect the oral cavity and its surrounding structure.

CHAPTER 2

Cellular Pathology

Learning Objectives
- Cells are the basic structural and functional unit of the body. This chapter describes detailed structure of cells and its components
- Most of the diseases of mankind could be understood in terms of cellular injury. This chapter overviews cellular injury, cellular adaptation to injury, causes of cell injury, morphology and types of cell injury
- It also discusses types of cell death

Keywords
Cell organelles, Atrophy, Hypertrophy, Hyperplasia, Metaplasia, Hypoxia, Steatosis, Cholesterolosis, Lipofuscin, Melanin, Hemosiderin, Bilirubin, Hyalinosis, Amyloidosis, Apoptosis, Necrosis

INTRODUCTION

Animal cells are eukaryotic. Animal cells have outer boundary known as the plasma membrane. The nucleus and the organelles of the cell are bound by a membrane. The genetic material (DNA) in animal cells is within the nucleus that is bound by a double membrane. The cell organelles have a vast range of functions to perform like hormone and enzyme production for providing energy for the cells.

CELL ORGANELLES

Animal cell contains membrane-bound nucleus, it also contains other membrane-bound cellular organelles. These cellular organelles carry out specific functions that are necessary for the normal functioning of the cell. Animal cells lack cell wall, a large vacuole and plastids. Due to the lack of the cell wall, the shape and size of the animal cells are mostly irregular.

The cell organelles are centrioles, endoplasmic reticulum, golgi apparatus, lysosomes, microfilaments, microtubules, mitochondria, nucleus, peroxisomes, plasma membrane and ribosomes **(Fig. 2.1)**.

Cell Membrane

- A typical cell membrane is 75 Å in thickness.
- It is a semipermeable barrier, allowing only a few molecules to move across it.
- An electron microscopic study of cell membrane shows the lipid bilayer model of the plasma membrane; it also known as the fluid mosaic model.
- The cell membrane is made up of phospholipids which has polar (hydrophilic) heads and nonpolar (hydrophobic) tails
- It encloses cytoplasm in which various cell organelles are present.

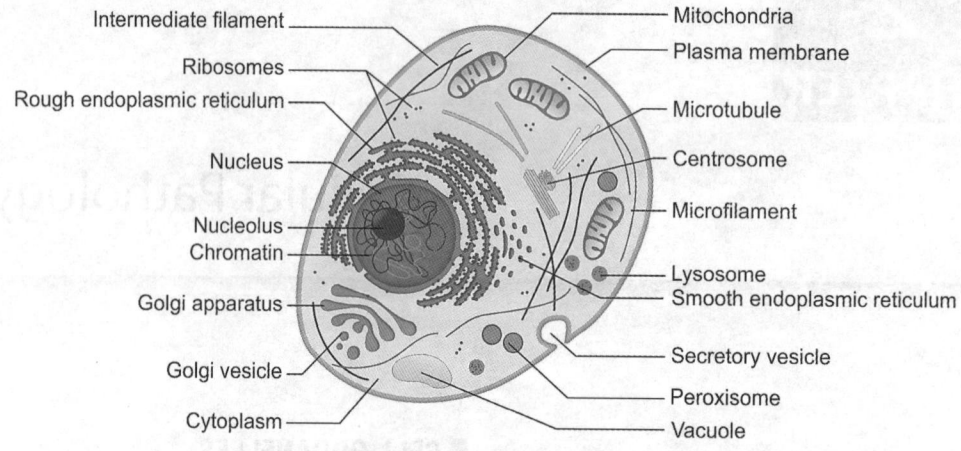

Fig. 2.1: Typical human cell.
(For color version See Color Plate 1)

Cytoplasm

- The fluid matrix that fills the cell is the cytoplasm.
- The cellular organelles are suspended in this matrix of the cytoplasm
- This matrix maintains the pressure of the cell, ensures the cell does not shrink or burst.

Nucleus

- It is a dense spherical structure present in the center of the cell. It is covered with a double-layered membrane called nuclear envelope
- A fluid present within nuclear envelope is called nucleoplasm
- Nucleus is the house for most of the cells genetic material—the DNA and RNA
- The RNA moves in/out of the nucleus through these pores
- Proteins needed by the nucleus enter through the nuclear pores
- The RNA helps in protein synthesis through transcription process
- The nucleus controls the activity of the cell and is known as the control center
- The nucleolus is the dark spot in the nucleus, and it is the location for ribosome formation.

Ribosomes

- Ribosome is the site for protein synthesis where the translation of the RNA takes place
- As protein synthesis is very important to the cell, ribosomes are found in large number in all cells
- Ribosomes are found freely suspended in the cytoplasm and also are attached to the endoplasmic reticulum.

Endoplasmic Reticulum

- Within cytoplasm of the cell is an extensive network of membrane arranged in plates and tubules, collectively called as endoplasmic reticulum (ER)
- ER is the transport system of the cell. It transports molecules that need certain changes and also molecules to their destination
- ER is of two types, rough and smooth
- ER bound to the ribosomes appears rough and is the rough endoplasmic reticulum, while the smooth ER does not have the ribosomes.

Lysosomes

- It is the digestive system of the cell
- They have digestive enzymes helps in break down the waste molecules and also help in detoxification of the cell

- If the lysosomes were not membrane bound the cell could not have used the destructive enzymes
- They are referred to as the suicide bags of the cell. They have digestive enzymes and are involved in clearing the unwanted waste materials from the cell. They also engulf damaged materials like the damaged cells, and invading microorganisms and digest food particles.

Centrosomes

- It is located near the nucleus of the cell and is known as the 'microtubule organizing center' of the cell
- Microtubules are made in the centrosome
- During mitosis the centrosome aids in dividing of the cell and moving of the chromosome to the opposite sides of the cell.

Vacuoles

- They are bound by single membrane and small organelles
- In many organisms vacuoles are storage organelles. They store excess food or water
- Vesicles are smaller vacuoles which function for transport in/out of the cell.

Golgi Bodies

- Golgi bodies are compact and consist of parallel membrane plates and tubule
- It is the site for enzyme secretion. It participates in formation of lysosomes
- The Golgi bodies modify the molecules from the rough ER by dividing them into smaller units with membrane known as vesicles
- It is involved with processing and packaging of the molecules that are synthesized by the cells. The crude proteins that are passed on by the ER to the apparatus are developed by the Golgi apparatus into primary, secondary, and tertiary proteins.

Mitochondria

- Mitochondrion is the main energy source of the cell
- They are called the power house of the cell because energy (ATP) is created here
- All enzymes which are present in Krebs' cycle are present in mitochondria
- Mitochondria consist of inner and outer membrane. It is composed of largely proteins and lipids
- Each mitochondrian is composed of tubular or paired lamellae called cristae
- Its main function is to produce energy for cell by the process of cellular respiration
- It is spherical or rod-shaped organelle.
- It is an organelle which is independent, as it has its own hereditary material.

Peroxisomes

- Peroxisomes are single membrane bound organelle that contain oxidative enzymes that are digestive in function
- They help in digesting long chains of fatty acids and amino acids and help in synthesis of cholesterol.

Cytoskeleton

- It is the network of microtubules and microfilament fibers.
- They give structural support and maintain the shape of the cell.

■ FUNCTIONS OF CELL

The cells perform variety of activities by the aid of the cellular organelles. These cells function as a unit and the cells together form tissues. A group of tissues with similar function form an organ and a group of organs of specific function to perform become an organ system. Thus, the microscopic cells form the basic unit for the activities and coordination and help survival of the organism.

CELL PATHOLOGY

Rudolf Virchow (1821-1902) was a German physician. He is best known as Father of modern Pathology, as he is the founder of cellular pathology.

He pioneered the modern concept of pathological processes by his application of the cell theory to explain the effects of disease in the organs and tissues of the body. He emphasized that diseases arose, not in organs or tissues in general, but primarily in their individual cells. Most of the diseases of mankind could be understood in terms of the dysfunction of cells. Cellular dysfunction leads to organ dysfunction which is further diagnosed by clinical expression.

OVERVIEW OF CELL INJURY

- *Homeostasis:* Cells actively control the composition of their immediate environment and intracellular structure within a narrow range of physiological parameters. This is called as homeostasis
- *Cell adaption:* Under physiological stresses or pathological stimuli ("*injury*"), cells can undergo adaptation to achieve a new steady state that would be compatible to their viability in the new environment
- *Cell death:* If the injury is too severe ("*irreversible injury*"), the affected cells die.

Cellular Adaptation to Injury

Cellular adaptations can be induced and/or regulated at any of the number of regulatory steps, including receptor binding, signal transduction, gene transcription or protein synthesis.

The most common morphologically apparent adaptive changes are:
1. Atrophy (decrease in cell size)
2. Hypertrophy (increase in cell size)
3. Hyperplasia (increase in cell number)
4. Metaplasia (change in cell type).

Atrophy

Atrophy is the shrinkage in cell size by loss of cellular substance. With the involvement of a sufficient number of cells, an entire organ can become atrophic.

Mechanisms of atrophy are not specific, but atrophic cells usually contain increased autophagic vacuoles with persistent residual bodies, such as lipofuscin.

Causes and Examples of Atrophy

Decreased workload (disuse atrophy), loss of innervation (denervation atrophy), diminished blood supply (ischemia), inadequate nutrition (marasmus, cachexia), loss of endocrine stimulation (menopause), aging (senile atrophy), and pressure (enlarging benign tumor).

Hypertrophy

Hypertrophy is an increase in cell size by gain of cellular substance. With the involvement of a sufficient number of cells, an entire organ can become hypertrophic. Not only the size, but also the phenotype of individual cells can be altered in hypertrophy. With increasing demand, hypertrophy can reach a limit beyond which degenerative changes and organ failure can occur.

Causes and Examples of Hypertrophy

Increased workload (skeletal muscle of body builders), cardiac muscle hypertrophy, hormone-induced hypertrophy (in pregnant woman).

Hyperplasia

Hyperplasia constitutes an increase in the number of indigenous cells in an organ or tissue. This results in increase in size of the organ.

Pathological hyperplasia is typically the result of excessive endocrine stimulation.

Hyperplasia is often a predisposing condition to neoplasia.

Causes and Examples of Hyperplasia

Hormonal hyperplasia (female breast at the time of puberty and pregnancy), compensatory hyperplasia (unilateral nephrectomy—at the loss of one kidney, other kidney becomes hyperplasic), erythroid hyperplasia of bone marrow in chronic hypoxia (such as in mountain climbers), excessive hormone stimulation (endometrial hyperplasia is common during menopause), prostatic hyperplasia, viral infections, (such as in papilloma virus—warts).

Metaplasia

Metaplasia is a "reversible" change in which one adult cell type is replaced by another adult cell type.

Metaplasia is a cellular adaptation in which indigenous cells are replaced by cells that are better suited to tolerate a specific abnormal environment.

Because of metaplasia, normal protective mechanisms may be lost. Persistence of signals that result in metaplasia often lead to neoplasia.

Causes and Examples of Metaplasia

It usually occurs in response to stress or chronic irritation. Tobacco smoke (Squamous metaplasia in the respiratory tract is most common), gastric acid reflux (gastric metaplasia of distal esophagus), repeated skeletal muscle injury with hemorrhage—muscle replaced by bone (myositis ossificans).

Cellular Injury

Cell injury is change in morphology and function of cell in response to stress. Cell injury occurs when the limits of cell adaptation have been exceeded or if the cells are not capable to adapt. Cells are complex interconnected systems, and single local injuries can result in multiple secondary and tertiary effects.

Cell function is lost far before biochemical and subsequently morphological manifestations of injury become detectable.

Effect of cell injury depends upon:
A. Type, duration and severity of injury.
B. On the type, status, adaptability and genetic make-up of the injured cell, e. g. brain tissue is very sensitive to hypoxia (2–5 min), skeletal muscles can adapt hypoxia for 2–6 hours.

Causes of Cell Injury

Oxygen Deprivation (Hypoxia or Ischemia)

It occurs usually as a result of ischemia (= loss of blood supply), which occurs; for example, when arterial flow suffers from atherosclerosis or thrombotic occlusion of arteries—most common cause of hypoxia.

Hypoxia is due to inadequate oxygenation, for example, in cardiorespiratory failure. It is caused by loss of oxygen-carrying capacity of the blood, either due to anemia (decreased capacity of the blood for oxygen), or after poisoning with carbon monoxide (CO)= loss of the carrying capacity of the blood depending on the severity of hypoxia—the cell may undergo adaptation, injury or cell death.

Example: If femoral artery is narrowed (due to atherosclerotic or atherothrombotic reduction of the lumen of the affected vessel), skeletal muscles of the leg decrease in size—atrophy. This reduction in size of cell mass may achieve a new balance on the lower level, but severe and prolonged hypoxia will induce severe injury and cell death.

Physical Agents

Many forms of physical energy may give rise to cell and tissue injury, such as mechanical trauma, extremes of temperature, sudden changes in atmosphere pressure, electromagnetic energy, radiation, electric shock and hyperthermia (burns).

Chemical Agents

The list of chemicals that may cause cell and tissue injury includes poisons arsenic, cyanide, mercuric salts, etc. It also includes air pollutants, insecticides and herbicides, alcohol, narcotic drugs, variety of therapeutic drugs and even oxygen in high concentrations.

Chemicals induce cell injury by one of two major mechanisms:
1. Some chemicals act directly by chemical bindings with some critical molecules or cellular organelles; for example, mercuric chloride poisoning (mercury binds directly to sulfhydryl groups of cell membranes)—GIT and kidney or anticancer drugs and some antibiotic drugs also induce cell damage by direct cytotoxic effects.
2. Other chemicals are not biologically active but convert into reactive toxic metabolites (role of free radicals for example).

Infectious Agents

These agents range from the submicroscopic viruses, Rickettsiae to bacteria, fungi and higher forms of parasites.

Viruses induce cellular changes by two general mechanisms:
1. Cytolytic and cytopathic viruses cause various degrees of cellular injury and cell death.
2. Oncogenic viruses stimulate host cell to proliferate and may induce tumors.

Cytopathic effects of viruses cause injury by two major mechanisms:

First is direct cytopathic effect, in which rapidly replicating virus particles interfere with some aspects of cell metabolism and cause cellular damage.

Second mechanism involves the induction of an immunological response-destruction of the cell by either antibody or cell-mediated reactions, for example the damage and death of hepatocytes caused by hepatitis B viruses are mediated by cytolysis induced by T-lymphocytes.

Immunologic Reactions

Immune system works in a defense against biologic agents. Immune reactions may, however, can cause cell injury; for example, anaphylactic reaction—to a foreign protein or drug and reactions to endogenous self-antigens are responsible for a number of autoimmune diseases.

Genetic Derangements

Genetic defects cause a number of diseases. Genetic injury may result in severe defects and congenital malformations (Down syndrome) or in mild derangements and errors of metabolism (lack of a distinctive enzyme), etc.

Nutritional Imbalances

Even now nutritional errors continue to be major cause of cell injury. Protein-calorie deficiencies chiefly among underprivileged population (starvation). Deficiencies of specific vitamins, nutritional excesses have become important in cell injury among overprivileged population (excess in lipids—predisposes to atherosclerosis, causes obesity, influences diabetes mellitus).

Morphology of Cell Injury

Ultrastructural changes include:
- Cellular swelling—it is near-universal manifestation of cell injury
- Formation of cytoplasmic blebs and distortion of microvilli
- Deterioration of cell attachments.

Mitochondrial changes—occur very rapidly in ischemic injury, but are delayed in some types of chemical injury. Early after ischemia—swelling of mitochondria is due to changes in ions. Small to large size amorphous densities in mitochondria—these consist of lipids or lipid-protein complexes—dense granules rich in calcium (appear early after reperfusion).

Endoplasmic reticulum—changes of ER occur early after injury due to changes in ion and water regulation. Detachment of ribosomes and disaggregation of polysomes—result in decrease of proteosynthesis. Progressive fragmentation of ER—results in formation of myelin figures - derived from plasma and organelle membranes (lipoproteins).

Alterations of lysosomes in cell injury—generally appear later. Lysosomes become swollen, and after the onset of lethal injury lysosomes rupture and this event causes leakage of the lysosomal enzymes at this stage it is irreversible cell injury.

General Biochemical Mechanisms of Cell Injury

1. *Loss of energy (ATP depletion, O_2 depletion)*: ATP depletion and decreased ATP synthesis are common with both hypoxic and toxic (or chemical) injury. As a result, Na^+, K^+- ATPase pump activity is reduced. Cellular energy metabolism is changed. There is failure of Ca^{++} pump as result calcium cannot get out of the cell. There is reduced protein synthesis.
2. *Mitochondrial damage:* Mitochondria is concerned with cell respiration and the production of ATP, which is responsible for vital functions of cell, including cellular osmolarity (Na/K), protein synthesis and membrane transport process. Loss of membrane potential results in failed oxidative phosphorylation and loss of ATP. Membrane damage leads to leakage of cytochrome C and other proteins which activate apoptotic pathways.
3. *Loss of calcium homeostasis:* Intracellular Ca^{++} is low and is sequestered in mitochondria and endoplasmic reticulum. Extracellular Ca^{++} is high. These gradients are maintained by Ca^{++} Mg^{++} ATPases. Increased cytosolic Ca^{++} activates enzymes: ATPases, phospholipases, proteases, and endonucleases. This starts breaking apart ATP, lipid membrane, cellular protein and DNA, respectively.
4. *Defects in plasma membrane permeability:* Mitochondrial membrane damage causes increased cytosolic Ca^{++}, oxidative stress, lipid peroxidation, phospholipase activity, loss of membrane potential, leakage of cytochrome C.
   Plasma membrane damage causes loss of osmotic balance, loss of proteins, enzymes and nucleic acids. Injury to lysosome membranes causes leakage of enzymes with destruction of cellular components. This may lead to cell death.
5. Generation of reactive oxygen species (O_2, H_2O_2, OH) and other free radicals. Free radicals are chemical species with a single unpaired electron in an outer orbital. Free radicals are chemically unstable and therefore readily react with other molecules, resulting in chemical damage.
   Free radicals initiate autocatalytic reactions; molecules that react with free radicals are in turn converted to free radicals.
   If not adequately neutralized, free radicals can damage cells by three basic mechanisms:
   1. *Lipid peroxidation of membranes:* Double bonds in polyunsaturated membrane lipids are vulnerable to attack by oxygen free radicals.
   2. *DNA fragmentation:* Free radicals react with thymine in nuclear and mitochondrial DNA to produce single strand breaks.
   3. *Protein cross-linking:* Free radicals promote sulfhydryl-mediated protein cross-linking, resulting in increased degradation or loss of activity.

Types of Cell Injury

Depending on the intensity of the factor causing injury and length of its action, cell injury may be reversible and irreversible, details of which are discussed below and shown in **Flowchart 2.1**.
1. Acute reversible changes
   A. Cellular swelling (hydropic change or vacuolar degeneration)
2. Chronic reversible changes
   A. By intracellular accumulation of lipids:

Flowchart 2.1: Types of cell injury.

```
                        Normal cell
                        (Homeostasis)
        ┌───────────────────┼───────────────────┐
   Adaptation        Reversible cell injury   Irreversible
                                              cell injury
   → Atrophy
   → Hyperplasia    Acute change   Chronic change   Cell death
   → Hypertrophy
   → Metaplasia     Cell swelling                 Apoptosis
                                                  Necrosis

   Intracellular    Pigment         Extracellular       Pathological
   accumulation     accumulation    accumulation        calcification
   of lipids                        of proteins

   → Fatty change   → Lipofuscin    → Hyalinosis
   → Cholesterolosis → Melanin      → Amyloidosis
                    → Hemosiderin
                    → Bilirubin
```

a. Fatty change (steatosis)
b. Cholesterolosis
B. Pigment accumulation:
   a. Lipofuscin
   b. Melanin
   c. Hemosiderin
   d. Bilirubin
C. Extracellular accumulation of proteins:
   a. Hyalinosis
   b. Amyloidosis
D. Pathological calcification (metastatic and dystrophic).
3. Irreversible cell changes (cell death)
   a. Apoptosis
   b. Necrosis

Cellular Swelling

Cellular swelling (synonyms: hydropic change, vacuolar degeneration, cellular edema) is an acute reversible change resulting as a response to nonlethal injuries. It is an intracytoplasmic accumulation of water due to incapacity of the cells to maintain the ionic and fluid homeostasis. It is easy to be observed in parenchymal organs: liver (hepatitis, hypoxia), kidney (shock), myocardium (hypoxia, phosphates intoxication). It may be local or diffuse, affecting the whole organ.

In cellular swelling, at gross examination, the affected organ is enlarged, pale and soft. Microscopically, the cells are enlarged, with a clear cytoplasm (due to the presence of small clear or pale vacuoles, with indistinct shape and limits) and a normal nucleus in central position; blood capillaries are compressed, explaining the organ's pallor.

Fatty Change (Steatosis)

Fatty change or steatosis represents the intracytoplasmic accumulation of triglyceride (neutral fats) of parenchymal organs, such as: liver, myocardium and kidney.

Mechanism: Increase of free fatty acids (starvation, diabetes and chronic ethylism/alcoholism), reduction of free fatty acids oxidation (hypoxia, toxins, chronic ethylism/alcoholism), increase of esterification of free fatty acids into triglycerides (due to increased free fatty acids or reduction of their oxidation, chronic ethylism/alcoholism) and reduced export of triglycerides due to deficiency of lipid binding apoprotein (starvation/malnutrition, toxins). Initially, fatty change does not impair the cells function, being reversible.

At the beginning, the hepatocytes present small fat vacuoles in the vicinity of the endoplasmic reticulum (liposomes). In the late stages, the size of the vacuoles increases pushing the nucleus to the periphery of the cell—macrovesicular fatty change. These vesicles are well delineated and optically "empty" because fat solves during tissue processing (paraffin embedding). Large vacuoles may coalesce, producing fatty cysts, which are irreversible lesions.

Cholesterolosis

Cholesterolosis is an intracellular accumulation of lipids (cholesterol). When cholesterol is in excess in the bile, it passes into the lamina propria where is phagocytized by macrophages. These macrophages become larger and polygonal, with foamy cytoplasm and small, hyperchromatic, central nucleus (xantic cells). Aggregation of xantic cells may enlarge the mucosal folds, producing a polypoid appearance of the mucosal surface. The gallbladder may be affected in a patchy localized form or in a diffuse form. The diffuse form macroscopically appears as a bright red mucosa with yellow mottling (due to lipid), hence the term strawberry gallbladder.

Sometimes, cholesterolosis is associated with inflammation of the gallbladder (cholecystitis) or with gallstones (cholelithiasis).

Lipofuscin

It is insoluble pigment—fine intracytoplasmic granules, yellow-brown called aging pigment, because it is seen mainly in the cells that are undergoing slow regressive changes. Lipofuscin is composed of complex lipids; it is derived of peroxidation of lipids, mostly from cellular membranes in cell injury. Lipofuscin is often associated with atrophy—brown atrophy. There is prominent accumulation of lipofuscin in liver and heart of aging patients, or in patients with severe malnutrition; for example, in cancer cachexia (usually accompanied by shrinkage of the entire organ). Lipofuscin represents indigestible residues of autophagic vacuoles. Lipofuscin itself is not injurious to the cell.

Melanin

It is brown-black in colored pigment, produced in melanocytes. Melanin is derived from tyrosine; the pigment is formed when enzyme tyrosinase catalyzes the oxidation of tyrosine to dihydroxyphenylalanine. The function of melanin is to block harmful UV rays from the epidermal nuclei.

Melanin may accumulate in excessive quantities in non-malignant and malignant melanocytic lesions. In inflammatory skin lesions, melanin may be released from injured basal cells and taken up by dermal macrophages. This give rise to post-inflammatory pigmentation of the skin.

Hemosiderin

It is a golden-yellow to brown granular pigment found in lysosomes within the cell cytoplasm.

Hemosiderin is hemoglobin-derived pigment. It is composed of aggregates of partially degraded ferritin.

Iron metabolism is normally regulated so that the total amount of iron in the body is maintained within relatively narrow range. The body has no effective mechanism for elimination of excess iron. Excess of iron then accumulates in macrophages and parenchymal cell in the form of hemosiderin.

Deposition of hemosiderin in tissue macrophages is termed hemosiderosis.

Localized Hemosiderosis

It is common and results from gross hemorrhages, ruptures of small vessels or from severe vascular congestion, etc.; in this case, hemoglobin is broken down and its iron is deposited locally as hemosiderin. There is no clinical significance; its presence only indicates a site of hemorrhage. A change in color is due to subcutaneous hemorrhage. The tissue affected by hemorrhage is first red-blue (due to lysis of erythrocytes), then becomes green-blue (due to formation of biliverdin and bilirubin). Finally, it appears golden-yellow (due to transformation to hemosiderin). Hemosiderin is picked up by macrophages and deposited in the tissue.

Generalized Hemosiderosis

It is less common, occurs in those conditions when there is an excess iron in the body like following multiple tranfusions, following excessive dietary iron and in some hemolytic anemias. Hemosiderin is deposited in many organs (liver, bone marrow, spleen, lymph nodes) first in macrophages, later also in parenchymal cells. It has usually no clinical significance, except of being an indication of iron overload.

Hemochromatosis

It is uncommon inherited or idiopathic disease characterized by deposits of hemosiderin throughout the body. The mostly affected organs are the liver (cirrhosis), pancreas (diabetes mellitus), and the skin (brown color). Primary defect lies in mucosal cells of the small intestine. These cells usually absorb only limited amount of iron from the food. In hemochromatosis, this control is lost and large amounts of iron are absorbed. Iron is toxic to the tissues and leads to fibrosis and cirrhosis of the liver and fibrosis of pancreas with destruction of Langerhans islands, leading to diabetes mellitus.

Bilirubin

Accumulation of bilirubin is called jaundice (icterus)—yellowish discoloration of skin and sclera—occurs when bilirubin is elevated in the blood and deposited in tissues.

Bilirubin is a bile pigment that represents an end product of hemoglobin molecule destruction; it does not contain iron. Normally majority of bilirubin is formed in the cells of RES, where erythrocytes are destroyed (spleen), minor part of bilirubin is formed in bone marrow and liver then bilirubin is transported into the liver in an unconjugated form (as an indirect bilirubin)—bound to albumin.

In the liver, bilirubin is conjugated with glucuronide to form soluble (direct) bilirubin, which is excreted by liver cells to the bile and then to intestine, where it is changed to urobilinogen (then absorbed by portal blood and returned to the liver or excreted in urine). *Jaundice*—common clinical disorder due to excess of bilirubin within cells and tissues.

Causes of jaundice—may result from three distinct mechanisms:
- Increased production of bilirubin
- Decreased excretion by the liver
- Bile duct obstruction.

Hemolytic Jaundice (Increased Production)

Increased destruction of erythrocytes (for example due to hemolytic anemia) overhelms the capacity of the liver to conjugate bilirubin. This leads to an accumulation of unconjugated (indirect) bilirubin in serum-complexed to albumin, cannot be excreted in the urine—this BR is toxic to brain—soluble in lipids.

Hepatocellular jaundice (decreased uptake, conjugation and excretion): Usually both conjugated and unconjugated bilirubin levels are elevated. Urine levels of bilirubin and urobilinogen are elevated.

Obstructive Jaundice

Biliary tract obstruction results in accumulation of bilirubin in the liver—cholestasis. Bilirubin cannot reach the intestine—this result in a failure of lipid substances to be absorbed. Deposition in connective tissue (skin, sclera, internal organs) result in yellow color typical of jaundice. Deposition in parenchymal cells most important in basal ganglia (so called kernicterus).

Hyalinosis

Hyalin refers to any alteration within the cell or extracellular space which gives a homogenous glassy eosinophilic appearance-hyaline change does not represent specific alteration.
- Intracellular hyaline are hyaline droplets in proximal tubular epithelial cells of kidney that represent reabsorption of proteins which passed through damaged glomerular membrane into primitive urine.
  Alcoholic hyaline are aggregates of cytokeratin intermediate filaments in cytoplasm of hepatocytes in alcoholic liver disease.
- Extracellular hyaline are hyaline of extracellular spaces. Like hyalinization of collagenous fibrous tissue means regressive change that is represented by a decrease of a vascularity and an increase of thickness of collagen fibers occurs for example, in old scars.

Amyloidosis

Amyloidosis is a group of rare but serious conditions caused by deposits of abnormal protein, called amyloid, in tissues and organs throughout the body.

Proteins begin as a string of amino acids that fold themselves into a three-dimensional shape. This 'protein folding' allows them to perform useful functions within our cells.

Amyloid is a description of proteins which have folded abnormally and then collected together. In this form they do not break down as easily as normal proteins and can build up in tissues and organs.

If this build-up causes the tissues or organs to stop working properly, the resulting conditions are called amyloidosis.

The amyloid deposits occasionally only affect one part of the body (localized amyloidosis), but more often several different part of the body are affected (systemic amyloidosis), such as the heart, kidneys, liver, or nerves. Without treatment to address the underlying cause, the amyloid deposits can eventually lead to organ failure and death, sometimes within only a year or two.

There are around 30 different proteins that can misfold and form amyloid, which is why there are many different types of amyloidosis.

■ TYPES OF CELL DEATH

There are two types of cell death—necrosis and apoptosis.

Apoptosis

Apoptosis is a word from Greek language, which originally refers to falling of leaves from trees in the autumn. It is programmed cell death, (cell suicide), since it is active process, it requires energy and protein synthesis. It is an important mechanism for removal of cells.

Apoptosis is dependent on gene activation and new protein synthesis. It is thought that the process is regulated by a number of apoptosis-associated genes. These include bcl-2 protein, which inhibits apoptosis and therefore extends cell survival, p-53 protein which stimulates apoptosis.

Sequence of Events in Apoptosis

1. Elevation of cellular calcium and rapid reduction of volume of the cell (cell shrinkage).
2. Activation of calcium-dependent enzyme endonuclease which cleaves DNA.
3. Fragmentation of DNA is regular with fix intervals (180bp).
4. There is marked condensation of both nucleus and cytoplasm, followed by Membrane bleeping.
5. Formation of apoptotic bodies—small apoptotic bodies are composed of fragments of nuclei with condensed chromatin, larger apoptotic bodies are composed

of both fragments of nuclei and condensed cytoplasm with preserved organelles.
6. Apoptotic bodies are rapidly phagocytosed by epithelial cells in Neighborhood or by macrophages—cell dying by apoptosis are recognized and phagocytosed soon after initiation of apoptosis.

Morphologic Changes in Apoptosis

- Rapid volume reduction and formation of cytoplasmic blebs
- Loss of cell–cell contacts
- Formation of apoptotic bodies
- Phagocytosis of apoptotic bodies by macrophages, within which they undergo hydrolytic phagocytic degradation.

This type of cell death occurs in physiological, embryological and also in pathological processes.

- *Physiological apoptosis:* It occurs in a number of situations
  - Is involved in normal tissue turnover
  - In hormone-induced atrophy (endometrium in menstrual cycle, mammary gland in menopause)
  - In developing tissues.
- *Embryological apoptosis:*
  - Formation of digits (by apoptosis of interdigital tissue).
- *Pathological apoptosis:* It is involved in response to pathologic stimuli, like inflammation and cancer, in an attempt by the body to arrest cell proliferation and tissue damage.
  - Such as viral infection (for example, Councilman bodies in liver cells in viral hepatitis)
  - Tumor regression induced by chemotherapy
  - At times there is involvement of apoptosis in tumor growth.

Necrosis

Necrosis is a word from Greek language, which originally refers to death, the stage of dying, or dead. It is a form of cell injury which results in unprogrammed (premature) death of cells in living tissue.

In contrast with apoptosis, cleanup of cell debris by phagocytes of the immune system is generally more difficult, as the disorderly death generally does not send cell signals which tell nearby phagocytes to engulf the dying cell. This lack of signaling makes it harder for the immune system to locate and recycle dead cells which have died through necrosis. Rather various receptors are activated, and result in the loss of cell membrane integrity and an uncontrolled release of products of cell death into the extracellular space. This initiates in the surrounding tissue an inflammatory response which spread the necrosis and also prevents nearby phagocytes from locating and eliminating the dead cells by phagocytosis. These enzymes are derived either from dying cells themselves. This is called as autolysis or from lysosomal enzymes of leukocytes, referred to as heterolysis.

For this reason, it is often necessary to remove necrotic tissue surgically, a procedure known as debridement. Untreated necrosis results in a build-up of decomposing dead tissue and cell debris at or near the site of the cell death. A classic example of it is gangrene.

Cellular Changes

Cell membrane disappears. Cytoplasm is swollen, mitochondria is rupture, forms myelin figures and may be calcified.

The nuclear changes in necrosis are characteristics by manner in which its DNA breaks down:
- *Karyolysis:* Chromatin of the nucleus fades due to the loss of the DNA by degradation.
- *Pyknosis:* Nucleus shrinks and the chromatin condenses.
- *Karyorrhexis:* The shrunken nucleus fragments to complete dispersal.

Cause of Necrosis

There may be external or internal factor responsible for necrosis.

External factors may involve mechanical trauma (physical damage to the body which causes cellular breakdown), damage to blood vessels (which may disrupt blood supply to associated tissue), and ischemia. Thermal effects (extremely high or low temperature) can result in necrosis due to the disruption of cells like frostbite.

Internal factors causing necrosis include trophoneurotic disorders; injury and paralysis of nerve cells. Pancreatic enzymes (lipases) are the major cause of fat necrosis.

Morphological Types of Necrosis

Coagulative Necrosis

It is most common pattern of necrosis. It is characteristic of hypoxic cell death.

Macroscopic appearance: Firm consistency, yellowish color, dry appearance of the cut section.

This pattern of necrosis, most commonly results from sudden severe ischemia which is encountered mostly in solid organs, such as kidney, heart, spleen and adrenal gland.

Pathogenesis: Nucleus usually disappears, but the shape of cell is preserved. Presumably, the pattern of coagulative necrosis results from severe intracellular acidosis which denaturates not only of structural proteins, but also enzymes (this block rapid proteolysis of the cell). Finally, the necrotic cell breaks into fragments.

The best example of coagulative necrosis is myocardial infarction. Gross appearance of acute myocardial infarct changes with time.

Early infarct can be visualized by various histochemic reactions that may show depletion of oxidative enzymes from infarcted area.

Microscopic appearance: In early acute infarction, cell swelling, pyknosis, eosinophilia of cytoplasm.

Lesser than 8-10 hours, ischemic area is slightly paler, hardly discernable. By 18-24 hours, the infarct becomes apparent grossly - pale, more sharply circumscribed, hyperemic border.

Microscopically, total necrosis with loss of nuclei, heavy infiltrate of leukocytes, and macrophages. By 3-7 days, more apparent hyperemia at the border of infarct, yellow-brown color, soft consistency. At the end of 1st week, infarct becomes circumscribed by highly vascularized scar tissue. Microscopically, there is a prominent fibrovascular reaction in margins.

6th week by total replacement by scar now termed as myofibrosis.

Liquefactive Necrosis

Liquefactive necrosis (or colliquative necrosis) is characterized by the digestion of dead cells to form a viscous liquid by autolysis and heterolysis. This is typical of bacterial, or sometimes fungal, infections because of their ability to stimulate an inflammatory response. The necrotic liquid mass is frequently creamy yellow due to the presence of dead leukocytes and is commonly known as pus. Typically seen in an abscess where there are large numbers of neutrophils present, which release hydrolytic enzymes that break down the dead cells so rapidly that pus forms. Pus is the liquefied remnants of dead cells, including dead neutrophils.

Hypoxic infarcts in the brain presents as this type of necrosis, because the brain contains little connective tissue but high amounts of digestive enzymes and lipids, and cells therefore can be readily digested by their own enzymes.

Gross morphology: Necrotic area becomes very soft and fluidy. These changes are first detectable at about 12 hours.

Within 2-3 day softening and discoloration become more apparent.

In large infarcts, there is a marked swelling, tissue liquefaction result in subsequent pseudocystic degeneration. No fibrous scar is formed, necrotic area changes into postmalatic pseudocyst (postnecrotic pseudocyst) where cystic space is filled with debris and fluid.

Fat Necrosis

This refers to necrosis in adipose tissue due to action of activated lipases. When lipases are released into adipose tissue, triglycerides are cleaved into fatty acids, which bind and precipitate calcium magnesium or sodium, ions forming insoluble salts. These salts look chalky white on gross examination, basophilic in histological sections stained with H and E and are visible on radiographic examinations.

Most common is acute pancreatic necrosis, in which active pancreatic enzymes cause focal necrosis of the pancreas and the adipose tissue throughout the abdomen. Here, lipases are activated and released and destroy not only pancreatic tissue itself but also fat cells in the pancreas and also fat cells throughout the peritoneal cavity.

Caseous Necrosis

It is another distinctive type of necrosis that is a combination of coagulative and liquefactive necrosis. This pattern of cell injury occurs with granulomatous inflammation in response to certain microorganisms (tuberculosis or fungal). The host response to the organisms is a chronic inflammatory response and in the center of the caseating granuloma there is an area of cellular debris with the appearance grossly as soft, friable, whitish-gray debris resembling cheesy material—hence the term caseous necrosis.

Gross morphology: This appearance has been attributed to the specific lipopolysaccharides of the capsule of the agent, tuberculous bacillus *(Mycobacterium tuberculosis):* The exact interactions with dead cells are not completely understood.

Microscopy: Histologically, caseous necrosis appears as amorphous eosinophilic material with cell debris.

Fibrinoid Necrosis

This is a type of connective tissue necrosis that occurs in the wall of arteries in cases of vasculitis. There is necrosis of smooth muscle cells of the tunica media and endothelial damage which allows plasma proteins, (primarily fibrin) to be deposited in the area of medial necrosis. Fibrinoid necrosis is a special form of necrosis usually caused by immune-mediated vascular damage. It is marked by complexes of antigen and antibodies, sometimes referred to as "immune complexes" deposited within arterial walls together with fibrin. Fibrinoid necrosis is characterized by loss of normal structure of collagen fibers.

Gangrenous Necrosis

It is not a distinctive type of necrosis, it is a necrosis secondary modified usually by the attack of bacterial agents. The term gangrene is commonly used in clinical practice to describe a condition when extensive tissue necrosis is complicated by bacterial infection. The necrotic tissue appears as white and friable, like clumped cheese. Dead cells disintegrate but are not completely digested, leaving granular particles. There are three major types of gangrene that are as follows:

1. *Dry gangrene:* Commonly it occurs in extremities as a result of ischemic coagulative necrosis due to arterial obstruction necrotic tissue. It appears black and dry and is sharply demarcated from viable tissue.
2. *Wet gangrene:* It results from severe bacterial infection of necrotic area. It occurs in the extremities due to arterial obstruction, also in the internal organs, such as intestine—most common example—in acute suppurative appendicitis. Grossly, tissue is swollen, reddish-black with extensive liquefaction, wet gangrene is severe complication associated with high mortality rate.
3. *Gas gangrene:* It is a wound infection caused by *Clostridium perfringens* and other types of clostridia.

TABLE 2.1: Differentiation between necrosis and apoptosis.

Characteristics	Necrosis	Apoptosis
Cause	Not programmed (Damage/trauma)	Programmed
Cell size	Cellular swelling	Cellular shrinkage
Cell numbers	Many cells affected	One cell affected
Cell membrane	Loss of cell membrane integrity (cell lysis)	Membrane blebbing but integrity maintained (Apoptopic bodies are formed)
Requires ATP	No	Yes
Inflammation	Yes	No
Cell contents	Ingested by macrophages	Ingested by neighboring cells
Stimuli	Pathologic (hypoxia, toxins)	Physiologic and pathologic

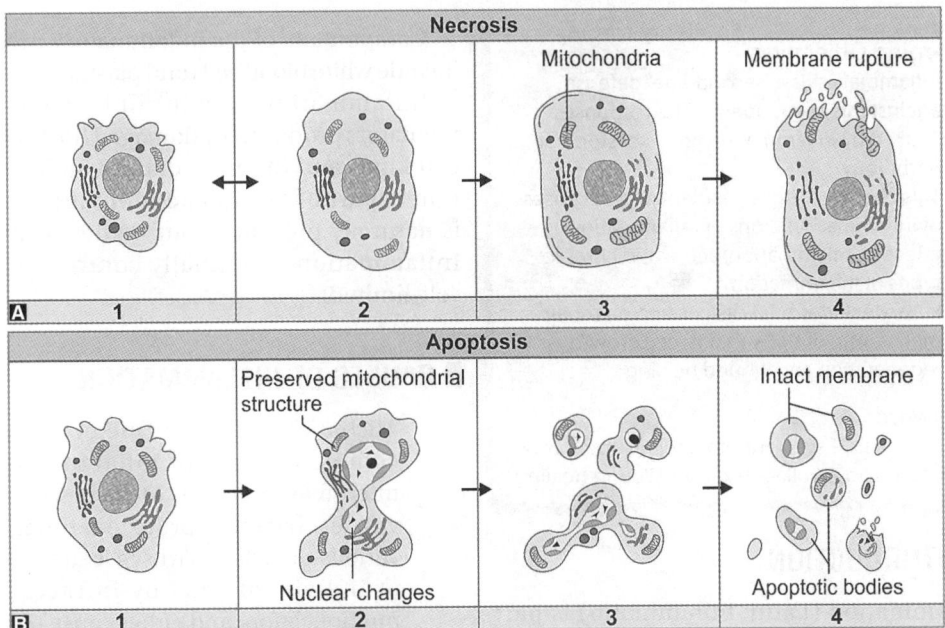

Figs. 2.2A and B: Diagrammatic representation: (A) Necrosis—(1) Normal, (2) Reversible injury, (3) Cell swelling, (4) Lysed necrotic cell; (B) Apoptosis—(1) Normal, (2) Cell condensation (blebbing), (3) Cell fragmentation, (4) Apoptopic bodies.

It is characterized by extensive necrosis and tissue destruction and production of gas by fermentative action of bacteria. Grossly-appearance similar as in wet gangrene with additional presence of gas in tissues.

Table 2.1 and **Figures 2.2A and B** provide differentiating characteristics of necrosis and apoptosis.

CHAPTER 3

Inflammation

Learning Objectives
- Inflammation is a "second-line" defense against infectious agents. The responses evoked by inflammation are a keystone of pathology
- This chapter includes explanation of causes of inflammation, signs of inflammation, effect of inflammation, acute and chronic types of inflammation
- It also includes brief description on repair mechanism of body that is, cell growth, regeneration and wound healing

Keywords
Leukocytosis, Fever, Endotoxemia, Suppuration, Scar formation, Collagenization, Wound healing

▌INTRODUCTION

Inflammation (Latin: inflammatio) is part of the complex biological response of body tissues to injury. It involves host cells, blood vessels and proteins. Inflammation is one of the most common mechanisms of disease. In medical terminology, the suffix "itis" refers to inflammation.

Goals of inflammation are:
- To eliminate the initial cause of cell injury
- To remove necrotic cells and tissue
- To initiate the process of repair

Inflammation is also a potentially harmful process as components of inflammation that are capable of destroying microbes can also injury nearby normal tissue.

Components of the inflammatory process include white blood cells and plasma proteins.

Inflammation is induced by chemical mediators produced by damaged host cells—cytokines and other mediators. Inflammation is part of our innate immunity which is naturally present in our bodies by birth. Inflammation is normally controlled and self-limited.

▌CAUSES OF INFLAMMATION

i. *Microbial infections*: One of the most common causes of inflammation is microbial infection. Microbes include viruses, bacteria, protozoa, fungi and various parasites. Viruses lead to death of individual cells by intracellular multiplication, and either cause the cell to stop functioning and die, or cause explosion of the cell (cytolytic). Bacteria release specific toxins—either exotoxins or endotoxins.

ii. *Hypersensitivity reactions*: A hypersensitivity reaction occurs when an altered state of immunologic responsiveness causes an inappropriate or excessive immune reaction that damages the tissues.

iii. *Physical agents, irritant and corrosive chemicals*: Tissue damage leading to inflammation may occur through physical trauma, ultraviolet or other ionizing radiation, burns or excessive cooling ('frostbite'). Corrosive chemicals (acids, alkalis, oxidizing agents) provoke inflammation through direct tissue damage.

iv. *Tissue necrosis*: Death of tissues from lack of oxygen or nutrients resulting from inadequate blood flow (infarction) is a potent inflammatory stimulus.

The Five Classical Signs of Inflammation

PRISH is a more modern acronym which refers to the signs of inflammation.
- *Dolor*: Latin term for "**P**ain". The inflamed area is likely to be painful, especially when touched. Chemicals that stimulate nerve endings are released, making the area much more sensitive.
- *Rubor*: Which in Latin means "**R**edness". Redness is caused by the dilation of small blood vessels in the area of injury as the capillaries are filled up with more blood than usual.
- *Functio laesa*: Which in Latin means "**I**njured function", which can also mean loss of function or "immobility". Loss of function may result from pain that inhibits mobility or from severe swelling that prevents movement in the area. This feature was noted by German pathologist Rudolf Virchow.
- *Tumor*: A Latin term for "**S**welling". Swelling, called edema, is caused primarily by the accumulation of fluid outside the blood vessels.
- *Calor*: Latin term for "**H**eat". Fever is brought about by chemical mediators of inflammation and contributes to the rise in temperature at the injury.

Dolor, Calor, Rubor, and Tumor were first described and documented by Aulus Cornelius Celsus (ca 25 BC-ca 50), a Roman encyclopedist. These five acute inflammation signs are only relevant when the affected area is on or very close to the skin. When inflammation occurs deep inside the body, such as an internal organ, only some of the signs may be detectable. Some internal organs may not have sensory nerve endings nearby, so there is no pain present, as is the case with some types of pneumonia (acute inflammation of the lung). If the inflammation from pneumonia pushes against the parietal pleura (inner lining of the surface of the chest wall), then there is pain.

■ EFFECTS OF INFLAMMATION

The effects of inflammation can be both local and systemic. The systemic effects of acute inflammation include fever, malaise, and leukocytosis. The local effects are usually clearly beneficial, for example, the destruction of invading microorganisms, but at other times they appear to serve no obvious function, or may even be harmful.

Beneficial effects of inflammation	Harmful effects of inflammation
Dilution of toxins	Persistent cytokine release
Entry of antibodies	Destruction of normal tissues
Fibrin formation	Swelling
Delivery of nutrients and oxygen	Inappropriate inflammatory response
Stimulation of immune response	

Systemic Effects of Inflammation

Both acute and chronic inflammation, even if well localized, can have effects on the whole body.

The main ones are:

Leukocytosis

Leukocytosis is a common feature of inflammatory reactions. Leukocytosis means that there is an abnormally high number of circulating white blood cells. Increased neutrophils indicate a bacterial infection whereas increased lymphocytes are most likely to occur in viral infections.

Fever

Fever is a common systemic response to inflammation. Fever is most often associated with inflammation that has an infectious cause, **(Fig. 3.1)** although there are some non-infectious febrile diseases. Fever is co-ordinated by the hypothalamus and involves a wide range of factors. Here are some of the contributors to fever:

The elevation of body temperature is thought to improve the efficiency of leukocyte killing and may also impair the replication of many invading organisms.

Endotoxemia

Sepsis is the term used for disease due to toxic bacterial products circulating in the blood.

Endotoxemia specifically refers to circulating gram-negative bacterial toxic products.

■ TYPES OF INFLAMMATION

There are two types of inflammation:
Acute and chronic (sometimes called systemic) inflammation.
1. *Acute inflammation*: it arises after a cut or scrape in the skin, an infected ingrown nail, a sprained ankle, acute bronchitis, a sore throat, tonsillitis or appendicitis. It is short-term and the effects subside after a few days.
2. *Chronic inflammation*: it is long-term and occurs in "wear and tear" conditions, including osteoarthritis, and autoimmune diseases, such as lupus and rheumatoid arthritis, allergies, asthma, inflammatory bowel disease and Crohn's disease. Habitual or environmental factors, such as excess weight, poor diet, lack of exercise, stress, smoking, pollution, poor oral health and excessive alcohol consumption can also lead to chronic inflammation.

The Acute Inflammatory Response

Response to acute inflammation is divided into two main categories—vascular changes and cellular changes.
- *Vascular changes*: In the early stages of inflammation, the affected tissue becomes reddened, due to increased blood flow, and swollen, due to edema fluid. These changes are the result of vascular response to inflammation. The vascular events of the acute inflammatory response involve three main processes:
    - Changes in vessel caliber and, consequently, blood flow (hemodynamics): When tissue is first injured, the small blood vessels in the damaged area constrict momentarily, a process called vasoconstriction. Following this transient event, which is believed to be of

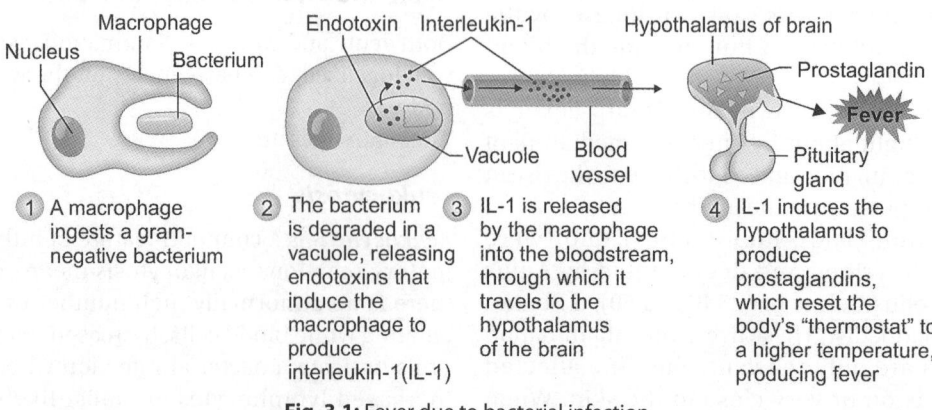

Fig. 3.1: Fever due to bacterial infection.
(For color version See Color Plate 1)

little importance to the inflammatory response, the blood vessels dilate (vasodilation), increasing blood flow into the area. Vasodilation may last from 15 minutes to several hours.

- Increased vascular permeability:
  Next, the walls of the blood vessels, which normally allow only water and salts to pass through easily, become more permeable. Protein-rich fluid, called exudate, is now able to exit into the tissues. Substances in the exudate include clotting factors, which help prevent the spread of infectious agents throughout the body. Other proteins include antibodies that help destroy invading microorganisms.
  There are two mechanisms of increased vascular permeability—
    - Chemical mediators of acute inflammation may cause retraction of endothelial cells, leaving intercellular gaps (chemical mediated vascular leakage).
    - Toxins and physical agents may cause necrosis of vascular endothelium, leading to abnormal leakage (injury-induced vascular leakage).
- Formation of the cellular exudate: As fluid and other substances leak out of the blood vessels, blood flow becomes more sluggish and white blood cells begin to fall out of the axial stream in the center of the vessel to flow nearer the vessel wall. The white blood cells then adhere to the blood vessel wall, the first step in their emigration into the extravascular space of the tissue.
  The movement of leukocytes from the vessel lumen in a directional fashion to the site of tissue damage is called chemotaxis. All granulocytes and monocytes respond to chemotactic factors and move along a concentration gradient (from an area of lesser concentration of the factor to an area of greater concentration of the factor).

- *Cellular changes*: The most important feature of inflammation is the accumulation of white blood cells at the site of injury. Leukocytes become activated during inflammation. Most of these cells are phagocytes, certain "cell-eating" leukocytes that ingest bacteria and other foreign particles and also clean up cellular debris caused by the injury.
  The first step in phagocytosis is adhesion of the particle to be phagocytosed to the cell surface. The phagocyte ingests the attached particle by sending out pseudopodia around it **(Fig. 3.2)**. These meet and fuse so that the particle lies in a phagocytic vacuole (also called a phagosome) bounded by cell membrane. Lysosomes, membrane-bound packets containing the toxic compounds, then fuse with phagosomes to form phagolysosomes. It is within these that intracellular killing of microorganisms occurs.
  The main phagocytes involved in acute inflammation are the neutrophils, a type of white blood cell that contains granules of cell-destroying enzymes and proteins. When tissue damage is slight, an adequate supply of these cells can be obtained from those already circulating in the blood. But, when damage is extensive, stores of neutrophils—some in immature form—are released from the bone marrow, where they are generated.

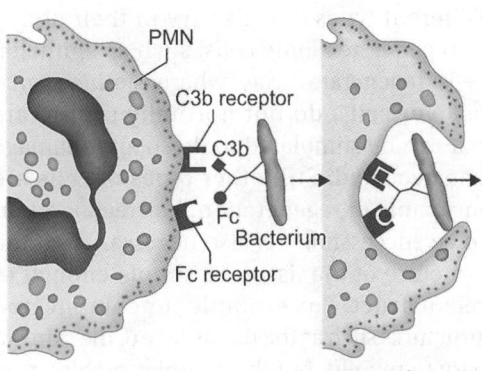

Fig. 3.2: Process of phagocytosis.

Intracellular killing of microorganisms by leukocytes.

Neutrophils and macrophages are specialized cells, containing noxious antimicrobial agents.

Neutrophils produce hydrogen peroxide (bactericidal by itself) which reacts with myeloperoxidase in the cytoplasmic granules to create oxygen radicals which are wickedly damaging. Antibacterial cationic proteins, lysozyme, and defensins all affect bacterial permeability, so the bacteria leak to death.

Release of lysosomal products from the cell damages local tissues and can kill microorganisms outside of the cell. Enzymes such as elastase and collagenase will chew through tissue. Some of the compounds are pyrogens, producing fever by acting on the hypothalamus. Acid hydrolases degrade tissue matrixes.

Events Following Acute Inflammation

Once acute inflammation has begun, a number of outcomes may follow. These include healing and repair, suppuration, and chronic inflammation. The outcome depends on the type of tissue involved and the amount of tissue destruction that has occurred, which are in turn related to the cause of the injury.

Healing and Repair

During the healing process, damaged cells, which are capable of proliferation regenerate. Different types of cells vary in their ability to regenerate. Some cells, such as epithelial cells, regenerate easily, whereas others, such as liver cells, do not normally proliferate but can be stimulated to do so after damage has occurred. Still other types of cells are incapable of regeneration. For regeneration to be successful, it is also necessary that the structure of the tissue be simple enough to reconstruct. For example, uncomplicated structures such as the flat surface of the skin are easy to rebuild, but the complex architecture of a gland is not. In some cases, the failure to replicate the original framework of an organ can lead to disease. This is the case in cirrhosis of the liver, in which regeneration of damaged tissue results in the construction of abnormal structures that can lead to hemorrhaging and death.

Repair, which occurs when tissue damage is substantial or the normal tissue architecture cannot be regenerated successfully, results in the formation of a fibrous scar. Through the repair process, endothelial cells give rise to new blood vessels, and cells called fibroblasts grow to form a loose framework of connective tissue. As repair progresses, new blood vessels establish blood circulation in the healing area, and fibroblasts produce collagen that imparts mechanical strength to the growing tissue. Eventually, a scar consisting almost completely of densely packed collagen is formed. The volume of scar tissue is usually less than that of the tissue it replaces, which can cause an organ to contract and become distorted. For example, scarring of the intestines can cause the tubular structure to become obstructed through narrowing. The most dramatic cases of scarring occur in response to severe burns or trauma.

Suppuration

The process of pus formation, called suppuration, occurs when the agent that provoked the inflammation is difficult to eliminate. Pus is a viscous liquid that consists mostly of dead and dying neutrophils and bacteria, cellular debris, and fluid leaked from blood vessels. The most common cause of suppuration is infection with the pyogenic (pus-producing) bacteria, such as *Staphylococcus* and *Streptococcus*.

Once pus begins to collect in a tissue, it becomes surrounded by a membrane, giving rise to a structure called an abscess. Because an abscess is virtually inaccessible to antibodies and antibiotics, it is very difficult to treat. Sometimes, a surgical incision is necessary to drain and eliminate it. Some abscesses, such as boils, can burst of their own accord. The abscess cavity then collapses, and the tissue is replaced through the process of repair.

The Chronic Inflammatory Response

Chronic inflammatory response is a long time inflammation that follows an acute inflammation that failed to destroy injurious agent or may be chronic in type from the onset (it may occur without a clinically apparent acute phase). It is often an asymptomatic and subclinical response. The duration varies from several months to years **(Table 3.1)**.

Causes of Chronic Inflammation

Acute and Chronic inflammation are compared.
1. Persistent infection—caused by distinctive infectious agents, For example—Mycobacteria, *Treponema pallidum*, some fungi, organisms of low toxicity—intracellular organisms.
2. *Prolonged exposure to undegradable material*: For example, silica particles which, after being inhaled, set up a chronic inflammatory response in lungs called silicosis.
3. *Autoimmune diseases*: immune reaction set up against own tissues or cells—reveal a chronic inflammatory pattern—for example, rheumatoid arthritis.

Morphologic Features and Clinical Signs

Chronic inflammation is an inflammatory response characterized by the presence of lymphocytes, plasma cells and macrophages. It is distinguished from acute inflammation by the absence of cardinal signs such as rubor, calor, dolor, and tumor. Active hyperemia, fluid exudation and neutrophilic emigration are absent. As compared to acute inflammation it is of long duration.

Chronic Inflammatory Cells

1. Macrophages—play central role in chronic inflammatory infiltrate. These include:
   Macrophage activation—this is a multiple-step process governed by mediators of inflammation, such as lymphokines produced by activated T-lymphocytes, bacterial toxins, by various chemicals, fibronectin, etc.
   Morphologic changes in activated macrophages: process of activation results in—increase in the size, increased level of lysosomal enzymes, more active metabolism, greater activity in phagocytosis, more ability in killing microbes.
   Following activation, macrophages produce biologically active products, such as:
   - Enzymes—neutral and acid proteases—some of them may also play a role in immediate inflammatory response—collagenases, elastase which degrade connective tissue components.
   - Chemotactic factors for leukocytes—due to which neutrophilic granulocytes (PMN) are attracted to the site of infection.
   - Growth factors and promoting factors for fibroblasts and blood vessels—thus

TABLE 3.1: Comparison between acute and chronic inflammation.

Features	Acute	Chronic
Causative agents	Physical and chemical damage Pathogenic invasion Tissue necrosis	Persistent infection Presence of foreign bodies Autoimmune diseases
Cardinal signs	Present	Absent
Onset	Rapid	Delayed
Duration	Short (days)	Long (weeks/months)
Fundamental cells	Neutrophil Mast cells Basophil Platelets	B and Lymphocytes Macrophages Plasma cells Antibodies

macrophages may modulate a formation of nonspecific granulation tissue.
- Cytokines such as interleukin I and TNF (tumor necrosis factor), etc.
- Macrophages are the most effective phagocytic cells in acute and chronic inflammatory response.
- Major functions of macrophages—enzymatic degradation and phagocytic activity.
2. Plasma cells—produce antibodies directed against persistent antigens or against altered tissue components.
3. Lymphocytes—when activated by the contact with antigen, lymphocytes release lymphokines—many of them stimulate macrophages. On the other hand, lymphocytes may be stimulated by cytokines released by activated macrophages.
4. Eosinophils—are characteristic of immunologic reaction mediated by IgE and of parasitic infections. The granules of eosinophils contain major basic protein (MBP) which is highly toxic for parasites but may also cause lysis of host epithelial cells, thus eosinophils may contribute to tissue damage particularly in hypersensitivity states.
5. Neutrophils—in chronic inflammation of bone marrow (osteomyelitis)—large numbers of neutrophils may persists for months also chronic inflammation of fallopian tube may have the pattern of chronic suppuration with large numbers of neutrophils.
6. Fibroblasts—fibroblast is fibroproduction and accumulation of extracellular proteins—It is a characteristic feature of chronic inflammatory response.

Morphologic Types

Morphological type of chronic inflammatory response depends on type of injurious agent. In vast majority of cases of chronic inflammations occur in response to an injurious agent that is antigenic, less commonly—inflammatory response due to non-antigenic stimuli.

Immune response is started when antigen enters the body and is reinforced by a subsequent accumulation of antigen. Local persistence of antigen leads to accumulation of activated T-lymphocytes, plasma cells and macrophages. (these cells are also called chronic inflammatory cells). The immune response takes several days to develop because nonsensitized lymphocytes must pass through several cell division cycles before increased number of effector lymphocytes becomes apparent in the tissue.

There are two different types of chronic inflammation in response to antigenic stimuli:
1. Granulomatous inflammatory response, and
2. Nongranulomatous inflammatory response

Granulomatous Chronic Inflammation

It is characterized by formation of epithelioid granulomas. Granuloma—is defined as an aggregate of macrophages. There are two types of granulomas are recognized generally.
i. Epithelioid granuloma—which represents an immune response in which macrophages are activated by T-lymphocytes. Epithelioid cell are activated macrophages. These are large cells with abundant pale foamy cytoplasm, superficial resemblance to epithelial cells. Macrophages aggregation is a function of lymphokines produced by T-lymphocytes. Typical feature of epithelioid granulomas is formation of Langhans-type giant cells which are derived from macrophages. Gamma interferon plays a key role in transformation macrophages into epithelioid cells and giant cells.

Epithelioid granulomas occur in several different diseases.

Infection due to Intracellular Organisms

- Tuberculosis (*Mycobacterium tuberculosis*)—typical granulomatous inflammation.

- Leprosy (*Mycobacterium leprae*)—tissue granulomas composed of epithelioid macrophages with phagocytosed bacilli.
- Syphilis (*Treponema pallidum*)—gumma-foci of necrosis surrounded by histiocytes and plasma cell infiltrate.
- Cat-scratch disease (Gram negative bacillus)—rounded or stellate granulomas usually within lymph nodes containing the central granular debris and leukocytes.
- Several parasitic and fungal infections (schistosomiasis, *Cryptococcus*).

ii. Foreign body giant cell granuloma—which represents non-immune phagocytosis of foreign bodies and particles by non-activated macrophages. When foreign material enters tissue, it can either be phagocytosed by single macrophage or induces formation of foreign body granuloma. Macrophages aggregate around these inert foreign particles. Foreign body granuloma indicates the presence of non-digestible foreign material (talc particles, sutures, etc.).

iii. Disorders due to chemical agents, such as beryllium (berylliosis), silical particles (silicosis).

iv. Disease of uncertain nature, such as Crohn disease.

Nongranulomatous Chronic Inflammation

It is characterized by the accumulation of sensitized lymphocytes (activated specifically by the antigen), plasma cells and macrophages in the affected area. These cells are scattered diffusely and do not form granulomas.

Nongranulomatous chronic inflammation occurs for example:

i. *In chronic viral infections*: Persistent infection of parenchymal cells by viruses evokes an immune response. The affected tissue shows presence of lymphocytes and plasmacytes, cytotoxic effect is mediated either by killer- T-lymphocytes or by cytotoxic antibodies.

ii. *In chronic autoimmune diseases*: Immune response is also mediated by killer- T-lymphocytes or by cytotoxic antibodies. The antigen is a host cell molecule which is recognized as foreign by immune system. Pathologic result is cell necrosis, resulting in fibrosis and lymphocytic and plasmacytic infiltration.

iii. *In chronic inflammation due to chemical toxic substances*: Alcohol may produce chronic inflammation notably of the liver and pancreas. Toxic substance can cause cell necrosis that may result in alteration in host molecule which thus can become antigenic and evoke immune response. Lymphocyte and plasma cell infiltration is slight, dominating feature is fibrosis.

iv. *Chronic nonviral bacterial infections*: In which the causative agents accumulate in cells. For types of inflammation **(Flowchart 3.1)**.

Function of Chronic Inflammation

- Chronic inflammatory response serves to remove injurious agent which is not easily eradicated by the body.
- Destruction of agent is dependent on immune response which is activated—either by direct killing by activated T- lymphocytes or by interaction with antibodies produced by plasma cells.
- Chronic inflammation is characterized by tissue fibrosis which may represent a serious side effect of chronic inflammation (for example, pulmonary fibrosis due to chronic interstitial inflammation may cause respiratory failure).

REPAIR—CELL GROWTH AND REGENERATION

Tissue injuries associated with inflammation are followed by healing. Proper healing

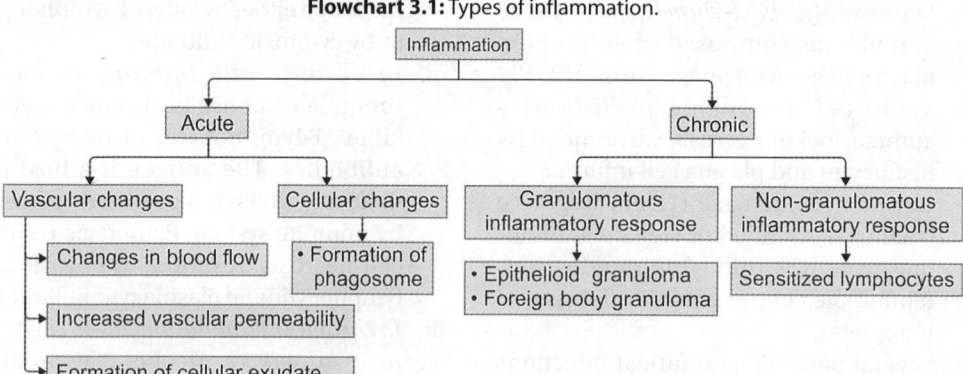

Flowchart 3.1: Types of inflammation.

needs previous removal of inflammatory and necrotic cell debris. If injurious agent was rapidly inactivated (transitory injury)—rapid healing follows—

- *Resolution*: Resolution is removal of debris associated with a complete restoration of the tissue to preinjury state. Inflammatory exudate and necrotic debris are digested by lysosomal enzymes (mostly from leukocytes), then removed by lymphatics. Remaining particles are phagocytosed by macrophages.
- *Regeneration*: It is complete replacement necrotic parenchymal cell by new parenchymal cells after removal of debris. Replacement of lost parenchymal cells is dependent on—
  - Regenerative capacity of the cells
  - Number of surviving cells
  - Maintenance of basement membranes or presence of stem cell layer.

The cell cycle: Proliferating cells occupy several functional states between two mitoses. The cell cycle consists of G1 gap (presynthetic), S (DNA synthesis), G2 gap (premitotic) and M (mitotic) phases.

The cells may leave cell cycle during G1 and then they either cease proliferation, differentiate or eventually die or they enter G0 phase, resting phase from which they can be eventually recruited back to the cycle.

Types of cells: The cells of the body can be divided into three groups on the basis of their regenerative capacity and their relation to the cell cycle.

i. Labile cells (intermitotic)—these are continuously dividing cells—they continue to proliferate, remain all the time in cell cycle. Tissues that contain labile cells are:
   - Stratified squamous epithelium of the skin, oral cavity, vagina cervix, esophagus,
   - Lining epithelial cell of the gland such as salivary glands, pancreas biliary tract,
   - Columnar epithelium of uterus, fallopian tube,
   - Urinary epithelium, lymphoid tissue, hematopoietic tissue.

   Healing in tissues with many labile cells Injury is followed by rapid and complete regeneration.

   For example—surgical removal of endometrium by curettage is followed by complete regeneration from the basal germinative layer within short time or destruction of erythrocytes stimulates rapid erythroid hyperplasia in bone marrow which results in complete regeneration of erythropoiesis.

ii. Stable cells (reversible postmitotic)—they are considered to be in G0 phase, may undergo rapid proliferation after appropriate stimuli, they may be recruited back to the cell cycle.
   - Tissues that contain stable cells are
   - Parenchymal cell of virtually all glandular organs, such as liver, kidney, pancreas,

breast, lung—Mesenchymal cells, such as fibroblasts and
- Smooth muscle cells and vascular endothelial cells

Healing in tissues with prevailing stable cells:

Regeneration in tissues with most stable cell is possible, but there are following conditions:

Sufficient amount of viable tissue must remain. Intact fibrous interstitial network and original basement membranes preserved. If complete necrosis involves both parenchyma and interstitium— no regeneration is possible and necrosis heals by scar formation.

iii. Permanent cells (irreversible postmitotic): These are non-dividing. These cells have left cell cycle and cannot undergo mitotic division. These cells have no regenerative capacity.

This group includes—nerve cells (mature neurons) and skeletal and heart muscle cells.

Healing in tissues with permanent cells:

Injury to tissue with permanent cells is always followed by scar formation, no regeneration is possible.

III. Resolution and regeneration—it is an ideal outcome of healing. It is possible only in the tissues with prevailing labile cells (cells capable of mitotic division—complete regeneration).

If complete resolution and regeneration is not possible, necrotic foci may be replaced by collagen, this process is termed organization (repair by scar formation).

Mechanism of healing depends on the type of inflammation, the extent of necrosis, regenerative capacity of damaged cells, rate of lymphatic flow, amount of fibrin in the inflammatory exudate, etc.

Repair by Scar Formation

Scar is a mass of collagen that is the final result of the process of organization. Repair by scar occurs—if resolution fails, if the injurious agent continuously causes injury in chronic inflammation or if parenchymal necrosis cannot be repaired by regeneration because of prevalence of permanent cells.

Process of repair by scar formation has several steps

i. Preparation—the tissue is prepared by removal of the inflammatory exudate. Debris is liquefied by lysosomal enzymes derived of neutrophil leukocytes, liquefied material is removed by lymphatics, residual particle are phagocytosed by macrophages.

ii. Ingrowth of granulation tissue—granulation tissue is highly vascularized connective tissue composed of newly formed capillaries, proliferating fibroblasts and myofibroblasts, cell debris and residual inflammatory cells. Major role of the granulation tissue is to occupy the tissue defects lost by injury. Granulation tissue is deeply red (because of numerous capillaries) soft, and is composed of thin-wall proliferating capillaries lined by hyperplastic endothelial cells, of fibroblasts, myofibroblasts and fibronectin . It is chemotactic for fibroblasts and promotes formation of capillaries.

iii. Collagenization—collagens are the major fibrillary extracellular proteins. Collagen is synthesized by fibroblasts. There are different types of collagens. The most important in scar formation are interstitial collagens type III and I. Type III composed of thin fibers.

iv. Maturation of the scar—collagen content of granulation tissue progressively increases with the time, particularly the amount of type I collagen steadily increases. The scar becomes less cellular and less vascular. The mature scar is composed of hypovascular poorly cellular collagenous mass-composed mostly of collagen type I.

v. Contraction and strengthening—contraction decreases the size of scar—allows optimal function of the remaining tissue. Strength of scar depends on the amount of collagen type I.

Healing of Skin Wounds

Wound healing is complex phenomena involving number of different processes, including parenchymal cell regeneration, synthesis of extracellular matrix proteins, remodeling of connective tissue, etc.

1. Healing by first intention (primary union)—healing of clean uninfected surgical incision joined by surgical sutures. The incisional space immediately fills with clotted blood containing fibrin
   - Within 24 hours—neutrophils appear, there is an increased proliferation in basal layer of epidermis at the margins of the wound. Epithelial cells migrate and synthesize basement membrane.
   - Day 3—leukocytes disappear and are replaced by macrophages. Granulation tissue progressively invades the incision space, collagen fibers are already present, but do not cross completely the incision space, and the epithelial cells continue to proliferate.
   - Day 5—the incision space is filled with granulation tissue, collagen fibers are abundant and begin to bridge the incision, epidermis recovers to normal thickness.
   - 2nd week—accumulation of collagen continues, but proliferation of fibroblasts and leukocytes slow down. Edema, fluid, and necrotic cells mostly have disappeared, and there is a regression of vascular channels.
   - End of the 1st month—scar covered by intact epidermis is finished. The scar is composed of mature collagenous connective tissue devoid of inflammatory infiltrate.
2. Healing by second intention (secondary union)—healing by second intention differs from primary healing in several aspects:
   - Large tissue defects, such as large infarctions, ulcerations, abscesses, large wounds—have always more fibrin in exudate, thus more intense inflammatory reaction.
   - Much greater amount of granulation tissue is formed.
   - Final scar is much smaller than original wound due to wound contraction (mostly results of activities of myofibroblasts)—tissue retraction.

CHAPTER 4

Pathology Laboratory

Learning Objectives
- Pathology laboratory plays a role of backbone in medical science as it ensures accurate and timely diagnosis of disease by examination of body fluids and tissues
- This chapter provides detailed information on different levels of laboratories, infrastructure of laboratories and safety measures to be followed in laboratories
- Waste generated from pathology laboratory is highly dangerous. This chapter gives brief knowledge about biomedical waste segregation and various methods of disposal of pathology laboratory waste

Keywords
Primary health centers (PHC), Urban health centers (UHC), Biosafety laboratories (BSL), Biomedical waste, Incineration, Autoclaving, Standards for treatment and disposal of biomedical waste

INTRODUCTION

Laboratory services are an integral part of disease diagnosis, treatment, monitoring response to treatment, disease surveillance programs and clinical research. Use of diagnostic techniques aid early diagnosis which enables appropriate and prompt intervention thereby reduces overall disease burden and promotes good health.

Clinical laboratory practices should be categorized in further sections where tests are done on biological specimens for diagnosis, patient care, disease control and research, such as:
- Microbiology and serology
- Hematology and blood banking
- Molecular biology and molecular pathology
- Clinical pathology
- Clinical biochemistry
- Immunology (immunohematology and immunobiochemistry)
- Histopathology/pathology and cytology.

LEVELS OF LABORATORIES

In India, the laboratory services are integrated with the 3-tier public health system at the primary, secondary and tertiary levels. Besides these, there are reference laboratories, research laboratories and specific disease reference laboratories to provide services for complex and special tests. The private sector provides laboratory support at all levels of health care both in rural and urban areas. Each laboratory should identify the scope, functions and the capacity of the services offered by it, and appropriate infrastructure with requisite biosafety measures should be planned. Qualified and trained staff should be employed with periodic upgradation of their skills.

Primary Level

Simple laboratory tests, such as hemoglobin estimation and urine examination for albumin and sugar and some biochemical tests are carried out at primary health centers (PHCs) and urban health centers (UHCs) by laboratory technicians.

Secondary Level

The district hospitals have facilities and manpower for carrying out pathology, clinical pathology, biochemistry, serology, and microbiological investigations. The laboratory staff includes pathologists, microbiologists, cytotechnicians, laboratory technicians, blood bank technicians and laboratory attendants.

Tertiary level

The medical college hospitals and non-teaching large hospitals are equipped with sophisticated diagnostic and investigative facilities to provide tertiary level health care. These hospitals receive referrals from the primary as well as the secondary levels.

Reference Laboratories, Research Laboratories and Specific Disease Reference Laboratories

The reference laboratories, research laboratories and specific disease reference laboratories provide services in a specialized field or area of importance. These may be located in a medical college, research institution or a private institution. They set and should maintain high standards of quality in one or more particular area and therefore receive referrals specific to that field. They also offer consultancy, standardize diagnostic tests and carry out training pertaining to that specific area.

▌INFRASTRUCTURE

Infrastructure of laboratories should be planned according to the services provided by the laboratory. The basic infrastructure facilities include:
- Reception room/area where requisition forms are received and reports disbursed
- Specimen collection room/area, toilets, privacy for special purposes, e.g. semen collection, facilities for disabled persons, toilet for staff
- Quality water supply for analytical purpose
- Uninterrupted power supply
- Analytical work area
- Specimen/sample/slide storage facility, including cold storage where applicable
- Record room/area
- Facility for cleaning of glassware, sterilization/disinfection
- Waste disposal facility, including biomedical wastes
- Fire-safety equipment
- Ventilation, climate control and lighting arrangements
- Separate room/area for meetings/administrative work
- Separate facilities/area for staff for hand washing, eating and storing food, drinks etc.
- Communication facility with referral centers
- Transport of specimen/samples to referral centers
- Additional infrastructure facilities may be added for special tasks as and when needed.

Equipment and Reagents

- Laboratory equipment should be of adequate capacity to meet work load requirement. All analytical equipment should be calibrated
- Standard reagents of certified quality must be used for the purpose of analysis. The batch number of reagents must be recorded.

Specimen Collection

- Specimen collection is the first phase of interaction between the patient and the laboratory. Appropriate counseling should be done before specimen collection and consent taken whenever needed. Specimen collection can be done at the patient's bedside, in the laboratory or in the field.

- Trained manpower/phlebotomist should be employed for specimen collection.

Data Management

Laboratory data management includes recording details of the patient, findings of analysis, reporting of results and archiving the data for future reference. Recording data allows smooth functioning of the internal quality control measures, internal audit and external quality assessment. From the point of view of management, absence of record implies that the work was never done.

■ SAFETY IN LABORATORIES

Personnel working in laboratories may be exposed to risks from various chemicals, infectious materials, fire hazard, gas leak, etc. The environment is also at risk of being contaminated by hazardous materials used and wastes generated in the laboratory. Safety in laboratories therefore includes protection of both the staff and the environment from hazardous materials.

General Safety Measures

- Documentation of laboratory safety policies and procedures
- All laboratory personnel should be aware about the laboratory safety policies and procedures and follow these at all times
- List of hazardous materials used in the laboratory should be prepared. All hazardous materials should be accounted for on a continuous basis
- Laboratory personnel should follow safe hygienic practices which include hand washing, wearing protective clothing, gloves, eye protection, etc.
- Eye wash facility should be available as "stand-alone" facility or attached to sink. Portable, sealed, refillable bottles should also be available
- Biohazard symbol should be used on all container/equipment containing biohazardous material
- Laboratories should ensure proper preservation and security of specimens
- Destruction/disposal of hazardous material should be authorized, supervised and handled according to standard procedures
- Laboratory personnel should be thoroughly trained in managing fire, and nonfire emergencies, such as large spillage, gas leakage, etc.
- Adequate fire extinguishers should be readily available in the laboratory
- Periodic checking of all safety equipment and accessories should be ensured.

Levels of Biosafety Laboratories (BSL)

- **BSL-1** can handle biological materials with minimum biohazard to the laboratory personnel and environment, e.g. laboratories at primary health center (PHC) level, side laboratories in labor rooms or wards. It is considered a cold zone. Access to the laboratory should be limited to laboratory personnel and the staff should use personal protection, such as gowns, gloves, eye protection, e.g. glasses, footwear, use a separate area for hand washing, storing food, drinks, etc. The laboratory work can be carried out on open bench tops and the surface should be decontaminated as per the safety requirements, arthropod and rodent control measures should be followed, mouth pipetting should be replaced with mechanical procedure and techniques which minimize splashes and aerosol formation.
- **BSL-2** laboratories are equipped with facilities to handle biomaterial which pose moderate hazard in the event of injury to skin or exposure to mucous membrane or ingestion. It is also considered a cold zone. All diagnostic and healthcare laboratories in public or private sector should have BSL-2 facilities. In addition to BSL-1

precautions, a biohazard warning sign should be displayed at the entrance. Special care should be exercised while handling sharps and an autoclave should be available for decontamination. Biohazardous material should be handled in class I or II biological safety cabinets (BSC) within the laboratory. Mechanical circulation of air with inward flow is preferred. Chemical, fire, electrical safety measures should be followed. Eyewash station should be conveniently located. All laboratory personnel should undergo pre-employment health check-up and a record of their illnesses and immunization received should be available to the laboratory managers.

- **BSL-3** laboratories are located in teaching and/or research institutions, production and clinical testing facilities. They can handle pathogenic agents which can cause potentially lethal disease when inhaled. They are containment laboratories and are considered a warm or neutral zone. Access to the laboratory should be determined by the laboratory in-charge. Higher degrees of personal protection of the laboratory staff is needed, including respiratory protection in certain instances. The staff should undergo baseline and periodic serum testing for the agent being handled in the laboratory. Laboratory design in addition to BSL-2 facilities should have a ducted exhaust air ventilation system instaled with negative airflow into the laboratory. Heating, ventilation, air-conditioning (HVAC) control systems may be installed to avoid positive pressure in the laboratory. High-efficiency particulate air (HEPA) filtration should be used to re-circulate air into the laboratory. Handling of biohazardous material should be done in BSC class I, II or III. Laboratory staff should be trained to work in BSL-3 laboratories.
- **BSL-4** laboratories or maximum containment laboratories are suitable for handling dangerous and exotic agents with high risk of life-threatening disease associated with aerosol transmission. These laboratories should be located in isolated areas. All biosafety precautions for BSL-3 laboratories should be followed with additional safety practices, including complete change of clothing and shoes prior to entering and exiting from the laboratory. No individual should work alone: Two-person rule should be followed. Staff should be trained to handle personnel injury or illness. All work should be conducted in class III BSC or class II BSC with personal one-piece positive pressure suits fitted with ventilatory support. Ventilation system should be non re-circulating with unidirectional airflow from the area of least hazard to area(s) of greatest potential hazard. HVAC control systems should be installed to monitor airflow in the supply and exhaust systems. The facilities should be negatively pressurized to prevent contamination if airflow system fails.
- High Security Animal Disease Laboratory (HSADL) is India's first BSL-4 laboratory at Bhopal. It conducts research on all kinds of zoonotic diseases and emerging infectious disease threats.
- The Indian Council of Medical Research (ICMR) has established first Bio-Safety Level-4 (BSL-4) laboratory in the premise of Microbial Containment Complex (MCC), National Institute of Virology, Pune with support of Department of Science and Technology (DST), New Delhi.

HANDLING BIOMEDICAL WASTE

All human activities produce waste. We all know that such waste may be dangerous and needs safe disposal. Industrial waste, sewage and agricultural waste pollute water, soil and air. It can also be dangerous to human beings and environment. Similarly, hospitals and other healthcare facilities generate lots of waste which can transmit infections, particularly HIV, hepatitis B and C and tetanus to the people who handle it or come in contact with it.

Most countries of the world, especially the developing nations are facing the grim situation arising out of environmental pollution due to pathological waste arising from increasing populations and the consequent rapid growth in the number of healthcare centers. India is no exception to this. India generates around three million tonnes of medical wastes every year and the amount is expected to grow at eight percent annually.

Biomedical waste means "any solid and/or liquid waste, including its container and any intermediate product, which is generated during the diagnosis, treatment or immunization of human beings or animals".

Biomedical waste poses hazard due to two principal reasons—the first is infectivity and other toxicity.

Biomedical waste consists of the following:
- Human anatomical waste like tissues, organs and body parts
- Animal wastes generated during research from veterinary hospitals
- Microbiology and biotechnology wastes
- Waste sharps like hypodermic needles, syringes, scalpels and broken glass
- Discarded medicines and cytotoxic drugs
- Soiled waste, such as dressing, bandages, plaster casts, material contaminated with blood, tubes and catheters
- Liquid waste from any of the infected areas
- Incineration ash and other chemical wastes.

Segregation

Segregation refers to the basic separation of different categories of waste generated at source and thereby reducing the risks as well as cost of handling and disposal. Segregation is the most crucial step in biomedical waste management. Effective segregation alone can ensure effective biomedical waste management.

- Segregation reduces the amount of waste needs special handling and treatment
- Effective segregation process prevents the mixture of medical waste like sharps with the general municipal waste
- Prevents illegally reuse of certain components of medical waste like used syringes, needles and other plastics
- Provides an opportunity for recycling certain components of medical waste like plastics after proper and thorough disinfection.
- Recycled plastic material can be used for non-food grade applications.
- Of the general waste, the biodegradable waste can be composted within the hospital premises and can be used for gardening purposes.
- Reduces the cost of treatment and disposal (80% of a hospital's waste is general waste, which does not require special treatment, provided it is not contaminated with other infectious waste).

The biomedical waste (BMW) management requires its categorization. The BMW Rules classify the BMW into 10 categories as depicted in **Tables 4.1** and **4.2**.

Collection

The collection of biomedical waste involves use of different types of container from various sources of biomedical wastes like operation theater, laboratory, wards, kitchen, corridor, etc. The containers/ bins should be placed in such a way that 100 % collection is achieved. Sharps must always be kept in puncture-proof containers to avoid injuries and infection to the workers handling them.

Storage

Once collection occurs then biomedical waste is stored in a proper place. Segregated wastes of different categories need to be collected in identifiable containers. The duration of storage should not exceed for 8–10 hours in

TABLE 4.1: Categories of biomedical wastes.

Waste category	Type of waste	Treatment and disposal option
Category 1	Human anatomical waste (Human tissues, organs, body parts)	Incineration @/deep burial*
Category 2	Animal waste (Animal tissues, organs, body parts, carcasses, bleeding parts, fluid, blood and experimental animals used in research, waste generated by veterinary hospitals and colleges, discharge from hospitals, animal houses)	Incineration @/deep burial*
Category 3	Microbiology and biotechnology waste (Wastes from laboratory cultures, stocks or specimen of live microorganisms or attenuated vaccines, human and animal cell cultures used in research and infectious agents from research and industrial laboratories, wastes from production of biologicals, toxins and devices used for transfer of cultures)	Local autoclaving/microwaving/incineration@
Category 4	Waste sharps (Needles, syringes, scalpels, blades, glass, etc. that may cause puncture and cuts. This includes both used and unused sharps)	Disinfecting (chemical treatment@@/autoclaving/microwaving and mutilation/shredding)**
Category 5	Discarded medicine and cytotoxic drugs (Wastes comprising of outdated, contaminated and discarded medicines)	Incineration@/destruction and drugs disposal in secured landfills
Category 6	Soiled waste (Items contaminated with body fluids including cotton, dressings, soiled plaster casts, lines, bedding and other materials contaminated with blood)	Incineration@/autoclaving/microwaving
Category 7	Solid waste (Waste generated from disposable items other than the waste sharps such as tubing, catheters, intravenous sets, etc.)	Disinfecting by chemical treatment@@/autoclaving/microwaving and mutilation/shredding**
Category 8	Liquid Waste (Waste generated from the laboratory and washing, cleaning, house keeping and disinfecting activities)	Disinfecting by chemical treatment@@ and discharge into drains
Category 9	Incineration ash (Ash from incineration of any biomedical waste)	Disposal in municipal landfill
Category 10	Chemical waste (Chemicals used in production of biologicals, chemicals used in disinfecting, as insecticides, etc.)	Chemical treatment @@ and discharge into drains for liquids and secured landfill for solids.

@@ Chemical treatment using at least 1% hypochlorite solution or any other equivalent chemical reagent. It must be ensured that chemical treatment ensures disinfection.
** Mutilations/Shredding must be such as to prevent unauthorized reuse.
@ There will be no chemical pre-treatment before incineration. Chlorinated plastics shall not be incinerated.
* Deep burial shall be an option available only in towns with population less than five lakh and in rural areas.

big hospitals (more than 250 bedded) and 24 hours in nursing homes. Each container may be clearly labeled to show the ward or room where it is kept. The reason for this labeling is that it may be necessary to trace the waste back to its source. Besides, storage area should be marked with a caution sign **(Fig. 4.1)**.

TABLE 4.2: Color coding and type of container.

Color Coding	Type of container	Waste category	Treatment options
Yellow	Plastic bag	Cat. 1, Cat. 2, Cat. 3 and Cat. 6	Incineration/deep burial
Red	Disinfected container/ plastic bag	Cat. 3, Cat. 6, and Cat. 7	Autoclaving/microwaving/chemical treatment
Blue/white translucent	Plastic Bag/puncture proof container	Cat. 4 and Cat. 7	Autoclaving/microwaving/chemical treatment and destruction/ shredding
Black	Plastic bag	Cat. 5, Cat. 9, and Cat. 10 (solid)	Disposal in secured landfill

Note
Label shall be non-washable and prominently visible
Waste collection bags for waste types needing incineration shall not be made of chlorinated plastics
Categories 8 and 10 (liquid) do not require containers/bags
Category 3 if disinfected locally need not be put in containers/bags.

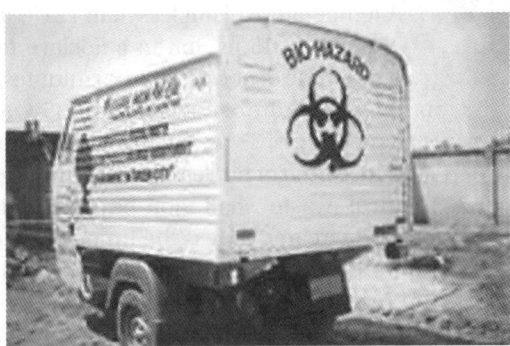
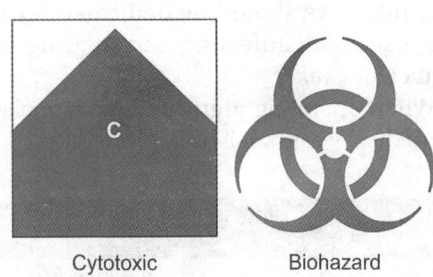

Cytotoxic   Biohazard

Fig. 4.1: Caution signs for biowastes.

Transportation

The waste should be transported for treatment either in trolleys or in covered wheel barrow. Manual loading should be avoided as far as for as possible. The bags/container containing BMWs should be tied/ lidded before transportation. Before transporting the bag containing BMWs, it should be accompanied with a signed document by nurse/doctor mentioning date, shift, quantity and destination.

Special vehicles must be used so as to prevent access to, and direct contact with, the waste by the transportation operators, the scavengers and the public.

Standards for Treatment and Disposal of Biomedical Wastes

Incineration is one of the most widely used techniques for disposal of biomedical wastes. The process involves burning of the waste at very high elevated temperatures (1500°C) under controlled operating conditions in a chamber known as incinerator. The end products generated are carbon dioxide and water with ash as residual material.

All incinerators shall meet the following operating and emission standards:
- **Operating standards**
  - Combustion efficiency (CE) shall be at least 99.00%

- The combustion efficiency is computed as follow:

$$CE = \frac{\%CO_2}{\%CO_2 + \%CO} \times 100$$

- The temperature of the primary chamber shall be 800 ± 50°C.
- The secondary chamber gas residence time shall be at least (one) second at 1050 ± 05°C, with minimum 3% oxygen in the stack gas.
- **Emission standards:** Emission standards for biomedical wastes are depicted in **Table 4.3**.

Standards for Waste Autoclaving

The autoclave should be dedicated for the purposes of disinfecting and treating biomedical waste.

1. When operating a gravity flow autoclave, medical waste shall be subjected to:
   a. A temperature of not less than 121°C and pressure of 15 pounds per square inch (psi) for an autoclave residence time of not less than 60 minutes, or
   b. A temperature of not less than 135°C and a pressure of 31 psi for an autoclave residence time of not less than 45 minutes, or
   c. A temperature of not less than 149°C and a pressure of 52 psi for an autoclave residence time of not less than 30 minutes.
2. When operating a vacuum autoclave, medical waste shall be subjected to a minimum of one prevacuum pulse to purge the Autoclave of all air. The waste shall be subjected to the following:
   a. A temperature of not less than 121°C and pressure of 15 psi for an autoclave residence time of not less than 45 minutes, or
   b. A temperature of not less than 135°C and a pressure of 31 psi for an autoclave residence time of not less than 30 minutes.
3. Medical waste shall not be considered properly treated unless the time, temperature and pressure indicators indicate that the required time, temperature and pressure were reached during the autoclave process. If for any reasons time temperature or pressure indicators indicates that the required temperature, pressure or residence time was not reached, the entire load of medical waste must be autoclaved again until the proper temperature, pressure and residence time were achieved.
4. Spore testing: The autoclave should completely and consistently kill the approved biological indicator at the maximum design capacity of each autoclave unit. Biological indicator for autoclave shall be Bacillus stearothermophilus spores using vials or spore strips, with at least 1×10^4 spores per milliliter.

TABLE 4.3: Emission standards for biomedical wastes.

S. No.	Parameters	Concentration mg/Nm³ at (12% CO_2 correction)
1.	Particulate matter	150
2.	Nitrogen oxides	450
3.	HCl	50
4.	Minimum stack height shall be 30 meters above ground	
5.	Volatile organic compounds in ash not be more than 0.01%	

Note
Suitably designed pollution control devices should be installed with the incinerator to achieve above emission limits, if necessary.
Wastes to be incinerated shall not be chemically treated with any chlorinated disinfectants.
Chlorinated plastics shall not be incinerated.
Toxic metals in incineration ash shall be limited within the regulatory quantities as defined under the Hazardous Waste (Management & Handling Rules), 1989.
Only low sulphur fuel like LDO/LS. HS/Diesel shall be used as fuel in the incinerator.

Routine Test

A chemical indicator strip/tape that changes when a certain temperature is reached can be used to verify that a specific temperature

TABLE 4.4: Standards to dispose of liquid wastes.

Parameters	Permissible limits
pH	6.5–9.0
Suspended solids	100 mg/L
Oil and grease	10 mg/L
Biochemical oxygen demand (BOD)	30 mg/L
Chemical Oxygen Demand (COD)	250 mg/L

has been achieved. It may be necessary to use more than one strip over the waste package at different location to ensure that the inner content of the package has been adequately autoclaved.

Standards for Liquid Waste

The effluent generated from the hospital should conform to the limits enlisted in **Table 4.4**.

Bioassay test 90% survival of fish after 96 hours in 100% effluent these limits are applicable to those hospitals which are either connected with sewers without terminal sewage treatment plant or not connected to public sewers. For discharge into public sewers with terminal facilities, the general standards as notified under the Environment Protection Act, 1986 should be applicable.

Standards of Microwaving

- Microwave treatment shall not be used for cytotoxic, hazardous or radioactive wastes, contaminated animal carcasses, body parts and large metal items
- The microwave system shall comply with the efficacy test/ routine tests and a performance guarantee may be provided by the supplier before operation of the unit
- The microwave should completely and consistently kill the bacteria and other pathogenic organisms that is ensured by approved biological indicator at the maximum design capacity of each microwave unit. Biological indicators for microwave shall be *Bacillus subtilis* spores strips with at least 1×10^4 spores per milliliter.

Standards for Deep Burial

- A pit or trench should be dug about 2 meters deep. It should be half filled with waste, and then covered with lime within 50 cm of the surface, before filing the rest of the pit with soil
- It must be ensured that animals do not have any access to burial sites. Covers of galvanized iron/wire meshes may be used
- On each occasion, when wastes are added to the pit, a layer of 10 cm of soil shall be added to cover the wastes
- Burial must be performed under close and dedicated supervision
- The deep burial site should be relatively impermeable and no shallow well should be close to the site
- The pits should be distant from habitation, and sited so as to ensure that no contamination occurs of any surface water or ground water. The area should not be prone to flooding or erosion
- The location of the deep burial site will be authorized by the prescribed authority
- The institution shall maintain a record of all pits for deep burial.

CHAPTER 5

Tumor Markers

Learning Objectives
- Tumor marker tests can help doctors diagnose cancer and recommend a treatment plan for an individual
- This chapter points out 35 tumor markers which are common in use
- It has information on types of tumor markers, its uses and technique to diagnose along with the limitations

Keywords
Anaplastic lymphoma kinase (ALK), Alpha-fetoprotein (AFP), Beta-2-microglobulin (B2M), Beta-human chorionic gonadotropin (Beta-hCG), *BRCA1* and *BRCA2* gene, Philadelphia chromosome, B-RAF protein, Stem cell factor (SCF), Cancer antigen 15-3, Cancer antigen 19-9, Cancer antigen 125, Calcitonin carcinoembryonic antigen (CEA), Chromogranin A (CgA), Cytokeratin epidermal growth factor, Estrogen receptor (ER), Lactate dehydrogenase, Neuron-specific enolase (NSE), Nuclear matrix protein 22, Programmed death ligand 1 (PD-L1), Prostate-specific antigen (PSA), Chemiluminescent magnetic immunoassay (CMIA)

■ INTRODUCTION

Tumor markers are substances that are produced by cancer or by other cells of the body in response to cancer or certain benign (noncancerous) conditions. Most tumor markers are made by normal cells as well as by cancer cells; however, they are produced at much higher levels in cancerous conditions. These substances can be found in the blood, urine, stool, tumor tissue, or other tissues or bodily fluids of some patients with cancer. Most tumor markers are proteins. However, more recently, patterns of gene expression and in genetic material (DNA, RNA), have also begun to be used as tumor markers.

Many different tumor markers have been characterized and are in clinical use. Some are associated with only one type of cancer, whereas others are associated with two or more cancer types. No "universal" tumor marker that can detect any type of cancer has been found.

■ TYPES OF TUMOR MARKERS

Tumor markers are usually normal cellular constituents that are present at normal or very low levels in the blood of healthy persons. There are five basic types of tumor markers. These are products that are over-expressed (produced in higher than normal amounts) by malignant cells. There are five basic types of tumor markers.

1. **Enzymes:** Many enzymes that occur in certain tissues are found in blood plasma at higher levels when the cancer involves that tissue. Enzymes are usually measured by determining the rate at which they convert a substrate to an end product, while most

tumor markers of other types are measured by a test called an immunoassay. Some examples of enzymes whose levels rise in cases of malignant diseases are acid phosphatase, alkaline phosphatase, amylase, creatine kinase, gamma-glutamyl transferase, lactate dehydrogenase, and terminal deoxynucleotidyl transferase.
2. **Tissue receptors:** Tissue receptors, which are proteins associated with the cell membrane, are another type of tumor marker. These substances bind to hormones and growth factors, and therefore affect the rate of tumor growth. Some tissue receptors must be measured in tissue samples removed for a biopsy, while others are secreted into the extracellular fluid (fluid outside the cells) and may be measured in the blood. Some important receptor tumor markers are estrogen receptor, progesterone receptor, interleukin-2 receptor, and epidermal growth factor receptor.
3. **Antigens:** Oncofetal antigens are proteins made by genes that are very active during fetal development but function at a very low level after birth. The genes become activated when a malignant tumor arises and produce large amounts of protein. Antigens comprise the largest class of tumor marker and include the tumor-associated glycoprotein antigens. Important tumor markers in this class are alpha-fetoprotein (AFP), carcinoembryonic antigen (CEA), prostate specific antigen (PSA), cathepsin-D, HER-2/neu, CA-125, CA-19-9, CA-15-3, nuclear matrix protein, and bladder tumor-associated antigen.
4. **Oncogenes:** Some tumor markers are the product of oncogenes, which are genes that are active in fetal development and trigger the growth of tumors when they are activated in mature cells. Some important oncogenes are BRAC-1, Myc, p53, RB (retinoblastoma) gene (RB), and Ph 1 (Philadelphia chromosome).
5. **Hormones:** The fifth type of tumor marker consists of hormones. This group includes hormones that are normally secreted by the tissue in which the malignancy arises as well as those produced by tissues that do not normally make the hormone (ectopic production). Some hormones associated with malignancy are adrenal corticotropic hormone (ACTH), calcitonin, catecholamines, gastrin, human chorionic gonadotropin (hCG), and prolactin.

■ USES OF TUMOR MARKERS

High tumor marker levels can be a sign of cancer. Along with other tests, tumor marker tests can help doctors diagnose cancer and plan treatment. Tumor markers are most commonly used to do the following:
- **Screen:** Some of the tumor marker may be used to screen people who are at high risk because they have a strong family history or specific risk factors for a particular cancer.
- **Diagnose:** In a person who has symptoms, tumor markers may be used to help detect the presence of cancer and help differentiate it from other conditions with similar symptoms.
- **Stage:** If a person does have cancer, tumor marker elevations can be used to help determine whether the cancer has spread (metastasized) to other tissues and organs and to what extent.
- **Determine prognosis:** Some tumor markers can be used to help determine how aggressive a cancer is likely to be.
- **Guide choice of treatment:** A few tumor markers provide information about which treatments might be effective against a person's cancer. A decrease in the level of a tumor marker or a return to the marker's normal level may indicate that the cancer is responding to treatment, whereas no change or an increase may indicate that the cancer is not responding.
- **Monitor success of treatment and detect recurrence:** Tumor markers can be used to monitor the effectiveness of treatment, especially in advanced cancers. If the

marker level drops, the treatment is working; if it stays elevated, adjustments are needed. (The information must be used with care; however, since other conditions can sometimes cause tumor markers to rise or fall). One of the most important uses for tumor markers, along with guiding treatment, is to monitor for cancer recurrence. If a tumor marker is elevated before treatment, low after treatment, and then begins to rise over time, then it is likely that the cancer is returning. (If it remains elevated after surgery, then chances are that not all of the cancer was removed).

■ LIMITATIONS OF TUMOR MARKERS

Ideally, markers could be used as a screening tool for the general public. The goal of a screening test is to diagnose cancer early, when it is the most treatable and before it has had a chance to grow and spread. For a screening test to be useful, it should have very high sensitivity (ability to correctly identify people who have the disease) and specificity (ability to correctly identify people who do not have the disease). But no tumor marker identified to date is sufficiently sensitive or specific to be used on its own to screen for cancer. Other tests are usually needed to learn more about a possible cancer or recurrence. Some of the limitations of tumor markers are listed below.

- A condition or disease other than cancer can elevate tumor marker levels
- Some tumor marker levels may be high in people without cancer (benign conditions)
- Tumor marker levels may vary over time, making it hard to get consistent results
- The level of a tumor marker may not rise until a person's cancer worsens. This is not helpful for early detection, screening, or watching for recurrence.
- Some cancers do not make tumor markers that are found in the blood. This includes cancers with no known tumor markers. Also, some patients do not have higher tumor marker levels even if the type of cancer they have usually makes tumor markers.

Thus, we can conclude that tumor markers can be very helpful in following response to treatment and recurrence, but they cannot replace physical examination, evaluation of symptoms, and radiologic studies (CT scan, MRI, PET, etc.).

■ LIST OF TUMOR MARKERS

Tumor markers that are currently in common use are listed below:

1. *ALK gene rearrangements and over-expression:* It is a gene that makes a protein called anaplastic lymphoma kinase (ALK), which may be involved in cell growth. Mutated (changed) forms of the ALK gene and protein have been found in some types of cancer, including neuroblastoma, non-small cell lung cancer, and anaplastic large cell lymphoma. These changes may increase the growth of cancer cells. Checking for changes in the ALK gene in tumor tissue may help to plan cancer treatment. Also called anaplastic lymphoma kinase gene.
   - Cancer types: Non-small cell lung cancer and anaplastic large cell lymphoma
   - Tissue analyzed: Tumor
   - How used: To help determine treatment and prognosis.
2. *Alpha-fetoprotein (AFP):* It is a protein normally produced by a fetus. Alpha-fetoprotein levels are usually undetectable in the blood of healthy adult men or women (who are not pregnant). False elevated levels may be seen in pregnancy and liver disease (hepatitis, cirrhosis, toxic liver injury).
   - Cancer types: Liver cancer and germ cell tumors
   - Tissue analyzed: Blood
   - How used: To help diagnose liver cancer and follow response to treatment; to assess stage, prognosis, and response to treatment of germ cell tumors

- Low levels present in both men and non-pregnant women (0-15 IU/ml); generally results >400 are caused by cancer (half-life 4–6 days).
3. *Beta-2-microglobulin (B2M):* It is a small protein normally found on the surface of many cells, including lymphocytes, <2.5 mg/L and in small amounts in the blood and urine. An increased amount in the blood or urine may be a sign of certain diseases, including some types of cancer. False elevated level may be seen in kidney disease and hepatitis.
   - Cancer types: Multiple myeloma, chronic lymphocytic leukemia, and some lymphomas
   - Tissue analyzed: Blood, urine, or cerebrospinal fluid
   - How used: To determine prognosis and follow response to treatment
   - Normal value : < 2.5 mg/L.
4. *Beta-human chorionic gonadotropin (β-hCG):* It is a hormone found in the blood and urine during pregnancy. It may also be found in higher than normal amounts in patients with some types of cancer, including testicular, ovarian, liver, stomach, and lung cancers, and in other disorders. Measuring the amount of beta-human chorionic gonadotropin in the blood or urine of cancer patients may help to diagnose cancer and find out how well cancer treatment is working. Beta-human chorionic gonadotropin is a type of tumor marker. Also called beta-hCG. Flase elevated levels are seen in pregnancy, hypogonadism (testicular failure) and cirrhosis.
   - Cancer types: Choriocarcinoma and germ cell tumors
   - Tissue analyzed: Urine or blood
   - How used: To assess stage, prognosis, and response to treatment
   - Normal value: In men: <2.5 U/mL, In non-pregnant women: < 5.0 U/mL.
5. *BRCA1 and BRCA2 gene mutations:* BRCA1 is a gene on chromosome 17 and BRCA2 is a gene on chromosome 13 that normally helps to suppress cell growth. A person who inherits certain mutations (changes) in these genes has a higher risk of getting breast, ovarian, prostate, and other types of cancer.
   - Cancer type: Ovarian cancer
   - Tissue analyzed: Blood
   - How used: To determine whether treatment with a particular type of targeted therapy is appropriate.
6. *BCR-ABL fusion gene (Philadelphia chromosome):* It is a gene formed when pieces of chromosomes 9 and 22 break off and trade places. The ABL gene from chromosome 9 joins to the BCR gene on chromosome 22, to form the BCR-ABL fusion gene. The changed chromosome 22 with the fusion gene on it is called the Philadelphia chromosome. The BCR-ABL fusion gene is found in most patients with cancer.
   - Cancer type: Chronic myeloid leukemia, acute lymphoblastic leukemia, and acute myelogenous leukemia
   - Tissue analyzed: Blood and/or bone marrow
   - How used: To confirm diagnosis, predict response to targeted therapy, and monitor disease status.
7. *BRAF V600 mutations:* It is a gene that makes a protein called BRAF, which is involved in sending signals in cells and in cell growth. This gene may be mutated (changed) in many types of cancer, which causes a change in the B-RAF protein. This can increase the growth and spread of cancer cells.
   - Cancer types: Cutaneous melanoma and colorectal cancer
   - Tissue analyzed: Tumor
   - How used: To select patients who are most likely to benefit from treatment with certain targeted therapies.
8. *C-kit/CD117:* It is a protein found on the surface of many different types of cells. It binds to a substance called stem cell factor

(SCF), which causes certain types of blood cells to grow. C-kit may also be found in higher than normal amounts, or in a changed form, on some types of cancer cells, including gastrointestinal stromal tumors and melanoma. Measuring the amount of c-kit in tumor tissue may help diagnose cancer and plan treatment. C-kit is a type of receptor tyrosine kinase and a type of tumor marker. Also called CD117 and stem cell factor receptor.
- Cancer types: Gastrointestinal stromal tumor and mucosal melanoma
- Tissue analyzed: Tumor
- How used: To help in diagnosing and determining treatment.

9. *CA 15-3/CA 27.29:* Cancer antigen 15-3 (CA 15-3) is a protein that is produced by normal breast cells. In many people with cancerous breast tumors, there is an increased production of CA 15-3 and the related cancer antigen 27.29. CA 15-3 is shed by the tumor cells and enters the bloodstream, making it useful as a tumor marker to follow the course of the cancer. False elevated values are seen in healthy people with certain conditions like cirrhosis, hepatitis, and benign breast disease.
- Cancer type: Breast cancer
- Tissue analyzed: Blood
- How used: To assess whether treatment is working or disease has recurred
- Normal value: CA 15-3 = <31 units/mL or <31 k units/L, CA 27-29 = <38 units/mL or <38 k units/L.

10. *CA 19-9:* Cancer antigen 19-9 (CA 19-9) is a protein that exists on the surface of certain cancer cells. It is shed by the tumor cells. Small amounts of CA 19-9 are present in the blood of healthy people. False elevated levels are seen in pancreatitis, ulcerative colitis and inflammatory bowel disease.
- Cancer types: Pancreatic cancer, gallbladder cancer, bile duct cancer, and gastric cancer
- Tissue analyzed: Blood
- How used: To assess whether treatment is working
- Normal value: < 37 U/mL is normal and > 120 U/mL is generally caused by tumor.

11. *Cancer antigen-125 (CA-125):* It is a substance that may be found in high amounts in the blood of patients with certain types of cancer, including ovarian cancer. False elevation is seen in pregnancy, menstruation, endometriosis, ovarian cysts and fibroids.
- Cancer type: Ovarian cancer
- Tissue analyzed: Blood
- How used: To help in diagnosis, assessment of response to treatment, and evaluation of recurrence
- Normal value: 0–35 U/mL.

12. *Calcitonin:* It is a hormone formed by the C cells of the thyroid gland. It helps maintain a healthy level of calcium in the blood. When the calcium level is too high, calcitonin lowers it. False elevation is found in chronic renal insufficiency.
- Cancer type: Medullary thyroid cancer
- Tissue analyzed: Blood
- How used: To aid in diagnosis, check whether treatment is working, and assess recurrence
- Normal value: <8.5 pg/mL for men and <5.0 pg/mL for women.

13. *Carcinoembryonic antigen (CEA):* It is a substance that may be found in the blood of people who have colon cancer, other types of cancer or diseases, or who smoke tobacco. Carcinoembryonic antigen levels may help keep track of how well cancer treatments are working or if cancer has come back. It is a type of tumor marker. False elevation is found in cigarette smoking, pancreatitis, hepatitis and inflammatory bowel disease.
- Cancer types: Colorectal cancer and some other cancers
- Tissue analyzed: Blood
- How used: To keep track of how well cancer treatments are working or check if cancer has come back

- Normal value: <2.5 ng/mL in non-smokers, <5 ng/mL in smokers. A CEA over 20.0 ng/mL often means cancer that has metastasized very high levels (sometimes well over 100 ng/mL) are frequently seen with metastases to the pleural cavity, peritoneal cavity, and central nervous system
14. *CD20:* It is a protein found on B cells (a type of white blood cell). It may be found in higher than normal amounts in patients with certain types of B-cell lymphomas and leukemias. Measuring the amount of CD20 on blood cells may help to diagnose cancer or plan cancer treatment.
    - Cancer type: Non-Hodgkin lymphoma
    - Tissue analyzed: Blood
    - How used: To determine whether treatment with a targeted therapy is appropriate.
15. *Chromogranin A (CgA):* It is a protein found inside neuroendocrine cells, which release chromogranin A and certain hormones into the blood. Chromogranin A may be found in higher than normal amounts in patients with certain tumor. False elevation is found in proton-pump inhibitors (medications given to reduce stomach acid)
    - Cancer type: Neuroendocrine tumors, small cell lung cancer, prostate cancer
    - Tissue analyzed: Blood
    - How used: To help in diagnosis, assessment of treatment response, and evaluation of recurrence
    - Normal varies on how tested, but typically <39 ng/L is normal
16. *Chromosomes 3, 7, 17, and 9p21:*
    - Cancer type: Bladder cancer
    - Tissue analyzed: Urine
    - How used: To help in monitoring for tumor recurrence
17. *Circulating tumor cells of epithelial origin:*
    - Cancer types: Metastatic breast, prostate, and colorectal cancers
    - Tissue analyzed: Blood
    - How used: To inform clinical decision making, and to assess prognosis
18. *Cytokeratin fragment 21-1:* It is a type of protein found on epithelial cells, which line the inside and outside surfaces of the body. Cytokeratins help form the tissues of the hair, nails, and the outer layer of the skin. They are also found on cells in the lining of organs, glands, and other parts of the body. Certain cytokeratins may be found in higher than normal amounts in patients with different types of epithelial cell cancers. False elevation is found in other lung disease.
    - Cancer type: Lung cancer, breast, colorectal, bladder, and head and neck cancers
    - Tissue analyzed: Blood
    - How used: To help in monitoring for recurrence
    - Normal value: 0.05–2.90 ng/mL.
19. *EGFR gene mutation analysis:* It is the protein found on the surface of some cells and to which epidermal growth factor binds, causing the cells to divide. It is found at abnormally high levels on the surface of many types of cancer cells, so these cells may divide excessively in the presence of epidermal growth factor. Also called epidermal growth factor receptor, ErbB1, and HER1.
    - Cancer type: Non-small cell lung cancer
    - Tissue analyzed: Tumor
    - How used: To help determine treatment and prognosis.
20. *Estrogen receptor (ER)/progesterone receptor (PR):* These are hormones found inside the cells of the female reproductive tissue, some other types of tissue, and some cancer cells. The hormone estrogen will bind to the receptors inside the cells and may cause the cells to grow.
    - Cancer type: Breast cancer
    - Tissue analyzed: Tumor
    - How used: To determine whether treatment with hormone therapy and some targeted therapies is appropriate.
21. *Fibrin/fibrinogen:* These are proteins found in blood.
    - Cancer type: Bladder cancer
    - Tissue analyzed: Urine

- How used: To monitor progression and response to treatment.
22. *HE4:* It is a protein found on cells that line the lungs and reproductive organs, such as the ovaries. HE4 may be found in higher than normal amounts in patients with some types of cancer, including ovarian epithelial cancer.
    - Cancer type: Ovarian cancer
    - Tissue analyzed: Blood
    - How used: To plan cancer treatment, assess disease progression, and monitor for recurrence.
23. *HER2/neu gene amplification or protein overexpression:* It is a protein involved in normal cell growth. It is found on some types of cancer cells, including breast and ovarian. Cancer cells removed from the body may be tested for the presence of HER2/neu to help decide the best type of treatment. HER2/neu is a type of receptor tyrosine kinase. Also called c-erbB-2, human EGF receptor 2, and human epidermal growth factor receptor 2.
    - Cancer types: Breast cancer, gastric cancer, and gastroesophageal junction adenocarcinoma
    - Tissue analyzed: Tumor
    - How used: To determine whether treatment with certain targeted therapies is appropriate.
24. *Immunoglobulins*
    - Cancer types: Multiple myeloma and Waldenström macroglobulinemia (lymphoplasmacytic lymphoma.)
    - Tissue analyzed: Blood and urine
    - How used: To help diagnose disease, assess response to treatment, and look for recurrence.
25. *KRAS gene mutation analysis:*
    - Cancer types: Colorectal cancer and non-small cell lung cancer
    - Tissue analyzed: Tumor
    - How used: To determine whether treatment with a particular type of targeted therapy is appropriate
26. *Lactate dehydrogenase:* This is one of a groups of enzymes found in the blood and other body tissues and involved in energy production in cells. An increased amount of lactate dehydrogenase in the blood may be a sign of tissue damage and some types of cancer or other diseases. False elevated levels are seen in hepatitis, MI (heart attack), stroke and anemia (pernicious and thalassemia)
    - Cancer types: Germ cell tumors, lymphoma, leukemia, melanoma, and neuroblastoma
    - Tissue analyzed: Blood
    - How used: To assess stage, prognosis, and response to treatment
    - Normal values are 100–333 U/L.
27. *Neuron-specific enolase (NSE):* False elevated levels are seen in proton pump inhibitor treatment, hemolytic anemia and hepatic failure.
    - Cancer types: Small cell lung cancer and neuroblastoma
    - Tissue analyzed: Blood
    - How used: To help in diagnosis and to assess response to treatment
    - Normal <9 µg/L.
28. *Nuclear matrix protein 22:* False elevated levels are seen in BPH (benign prostatic hypertrophy) and prostatitis.
    - Cancer type: Bladder cancer
    - Tissue analyzed: Urine
    - How used: To monitor response to treatment
    - Normal <10 U/mL
29. *Programmed death ligand 1 (PD-L1):*
    - Cancer type: Non-small cell lung cancer
    - Tissue analyzed: Tumor
    - How used: To determine whether treatment with a particular type of targeted therapy is appropriate
30. *Prostate-specific antigen (PSA):* This is a protein made by the prostate gland and found in the blood. Prostate-specific antigen blood levels may be higher than normal in men who have prostate cancer,

benign prostatic hyperplasia (BPH), or infection or inflammation of the prostate gland. False elevated levels are seen in benign prostatic hypertrophy (BPH), nodular prostatic hyperplasia and prostatitis.
- Cancer type: Prostate cancer
- Tissue analyzed: Blood
- How used: To help in diagnosis, assess response to treatment, and look for recurrence
- Normal <4 ng/mL (half life 2–3 days).

31. *Thyroglobulin:* The form that thyroid hormone takes when stored in the cells of the thyroid. If the thyroid has been removed, thyroglobulin should not show up on a blood test. Doctors measure thyroglobulin level in blood to detect thyroid cancer cells that remain in the body after treatment.
    - Cancer type: Thyroid cancer
    - Tissue analyzed: Blood
    - How used: To evaluate response to treatment and look for recurrence.

32. *Urokinase plasminogen activator (uPA) and plasminogen activator inhibitor (PAI-1):* This is an enzyme that is made in the kidney and found in the urine. A form of this enzyme is made in the laboratory and used to dissolve blood clots or to prevent them from forming.
    - Cancer type: Breast cancer
    - Tissue analyzed: Tumor
    - How used: To determine aggressiveness of cancer and guide treatment.

33. *5-Protein signature (OVA1)*
    - Cancer type: Ovarian cancer
    - Tissue analyzed: Blood
    - How used: To pre-operatively assess pelvic mass for suspected ovarian cancer.

34. *21-Gene signature (Oncotype DX)*
    - Cancer type: Breast cancer
    - Tissue analyzed: Tumor
    - How used: To evaluate risk of recurrence.

35. *70-Gene signature (MammaPrint)*
    - Cancer type: Breast cancer
    - Tissue analyzed: Tumor.

■ TESTING OF TUMOR MARKERS

Tumor marker tests are done by analyzers using chemiluminescent Magnetic Immunoassay—CMIA technology.

Chemiluminescent Magnetic Immunoassay (CMIA)

It is an immunoassay technique in which the antigen or antibody is labeled with a molecule capable of emitting light during a chemical reaction; this light is used to measure the formation of the antigen-antibody complex.

Chemiluminescent compounds can also be used to label analytes. Chemiluminescent compounds are distinct from radioactive, fluorescent, and enzymatic labels. A chemiluminescent label produces light when combined with a trigger reagent. Although many instruments in the clinical laboratory are based on chemiluminescent technology, the specific type of label varies and is often patented, and thus performance can vary. In the case of the Abbott ARCHITECT® (from Abbott Laboratories, Chicago, Illinois, USA), for example, the label is a patented acridinium derivative. This label produces high light emission, and thus high sensitivity (it is easier to measure a large amount of light).

The ARCHITECT CEA (carcinoembryonic antigen) assay is a two-step immunoassay to determine the presence of CEA in human serum and plasma, using Chemiluminescent Microparticle Immunoassay (CMIA) technology with flexible assay protocols, referred to as Chemiflex. In the first step, sample and anti-CEA coated paramagnetic microparticles are combined. CEA present in the sample binds to the anti-CEA coated microparticles. After washing, anti-CEA acridinium-labeled conjugate is added in the second step. Pre-Trigger and Trigger Solutions are then added to the reaction mixture; the resulting chemiluminescent reaction is measured as relative light units (RLUs). A direct relationship exists between the amount of CEA in the sample and the RLUs detected by the ARCHITECT.

6 CHAPTER

Electrolytes

Learning Objectives
- Electrolytes are minerals that carry an electric charge when they are dissolved in a liquid such as blood. These electrolytes help to regulate nerve and muscle function and maintain acid-base balance and water balance
- This chapter elucidates principle, procedure and clinical significance of blood and urine sodium, potassium, chloride, phosphorous and calcium ions
- It also has brief information on working of flame photometer, which is used to analyze electrolytes

Keywords
Maruna and Trinder's method, Turbidometric method, Cushing's syndrome, Schoenfeld and Lewellen's method, Gomori's method, Fanconi's syndrome, O-cresolphthalein complexone (OCPC) method, Hypercalcemia, Hypokalemia

INTRODUCTION AND CLASSIFICATION

Electrolytes are positively and negatively charged molecules, called ions. These are found within cells, between cells, in the bloodstream, and in other fluids throughout the body in the form of dissolved salts. Electrolytes help to move nutrients into and wastes out of the body's cells, maintain a healthy water balance and help stabilize the body's pH level.

Electrolyte panel consists of electrolytes with a positive charge—sodium (Na^+), potassium (K^+) calcium (Ca^{++}), and magnesium (Mg^{++}); the negative ions are chloride (Cl^-), bicarbonate (HCO_3^-; sometimes reported as total CO_2) and phosphate (PO_4^{3-}).

Classification of Electrolytes

Electrolyte tests are typically conducted on blood plasma or serum, urine, and diarrheal fluids. Electrolytes can be classified in four different ways.

1. Some electrolytes are intracellular, i.e. tend to exist mostly inside cells, while others are extracellular, i.e. tend to be outside cells. Potassium, phosphate, and magnesium are intracellular, while sodium and chloride are extracellular.
2. A second classification distinguishes those electrolytes that participate directly in the transmission of nerve impulses and those that do not. Sodium, potassium, and calcium are the important electrolytes involved in nerve impulses, and disorders affecting them are most closely associated with neurological disorders.
3. A third classification focuses on electrolytes that are able to form a tight union, or complex, with one another. Calcium and phosphate have the greatest tendency to form complexes with each other. Disorders that cause an increase in either plasma calcium or phosphate can result in the deposit of calcium-phosphate crystals in the soft tissues of the body.

4. A fourth classification concerns those electrolytes that influence the acidity or alkalinity of the bloodstream, also known as the pH. The pH of the bloodstream is normally in the range of 7.35–7.45. A decrease below this range is called acidosis, while a pH above this range is called alkalosis. The electrolytes most closely associated with the pH of the bloodstream are bicarbonate, chloride, and phosphate.

Diagnostic Importance

Electrolyte levels are affected by how much is taken in through the diet, the amount of water in a person's body, and the amount of electrolytes excreted by their kidneys. Balance of the electrolytes in our bodies is essential for normal function of our cells and our organs.

These ions are measured to evaluate symptoms of heart disease and monitor the effectiveness of treatments for high blood pressure, liver disease to assess renal (kidney), endocrine (glandular), and acid-base function, and are components of both renal function and comprehensive metabolic biochemistry profiles.

Knowing which electrolytes are out of balance can help a doctor to determine the cause and treatment to restore proper balance. If left untreated, electrolyte imbalance can lead to dizziness, cramps, irregular heartbeat, and possibly death.

■ SERUM SODIUM AND POTASSIUM

Serum Sodium

Sodium is a major extracellular cation (Na^+) of the body. Sodium salts are necessary to preserve a balance between Ca^{++} and K^+ to maintain normal heart action and equilibrium of the body. Sodium salts regulate the osmotic pressure in the cells and fluids and guard against the excessive loss of water from the tissues. Almost all blood sodium is found in the plasma. There is very little in the red cells.

Method
Modified Maruna and Trinder's method.

Specimen
Serum.

Principle
Sodium from the specimen is quantitatively precipitated as the triple salt uranyl magnesium sodium acetate and the excess of uranyl salt reacts with potassium ferrocyanide to produce brown color. The intensity of brown color produced is inversely proportional to the sodium conc. of the specimen.

Reagent
- Standard sodium chloride solution (equivalent to 300 mg of Na)
- Uranyl magnesium acetate solution
- Acetic acid 1% aqueous solution
- Potassium ferrocyanide 20% solution.

Procedure

Part I: Precipitation step

Take three test tubes and mark them as T, S and B. Add 5 mL of uranyl magnesium acetate solution in each tube. Add 0.1 mL of serum, 0.1 mL of sodium standard and 0.1 mL of distilled water in test, standard and blank, respectively. Mix well and allow it to stand for 5 minutes. Centrifuge for one minute at 3,000 rpm to get clear supernatant.

Reagent	T	S	B
Uranyl magnesium acetate solution	5 mL	5 mL	5 mL
Serum	0.1 mL	—	—
Sodium standard	—	0.1 mL	—
Distilled water	—	—	0.1 mL

Part II: Color formation

Take three test tubes and mark them as T, S, and B. Add 0.2 mL of supernatant from Part 1 in respective tubes. Add 8 mL of acetic acid in each tube. Now add 0.2 mL of potassium ferrocyanide in each tube. Now make up the volume to 10 mL by acetic acid. Read the absorbance of test and standard against blank at 480 nm. Be sure that the readings are taken within 10 minutes of last step.

Reagent	T	S	B
Supernatant from Part I (T)	0.2 mL	—	—
Supernatant from Part I (S)	—	0.2 mL	—
Supernatant from Part I (B)	—	—	0.2 mL
Acetic acid	8 mL	8 mL	8 mL
Potassium ferrocyanide	0.2 mL	0.2 mL	0.2 mL
Acetic acid	1.6 mL	1.6 mL	1.6 mL

Calculation

$$\text{Serum sodium (mg/dL)} = \frac{\text{OD of T}}{\text{OD of S}} \times 300$$

Serum Potassium

Unlike sodium, potassium is the major intracellular cation of the body. Within the cells, it plays an important role in maintenance of acid-base balance, osmotic pressure and water retention. Intracellular potassium is essential for several important metabolic reactions catalyzed by enzymes. It is also very important constituent of the extracellular fluid because it influences muscle activity notably the cardiac muscle.

Method

Turbidometric method.

Specimen

Serum.

Principle

Potassium ions from specimen react with sodium tetraphenyl boron resulting in a turbid suspension. The extent of turbidity is measured photometrically at 620 nm is proportional to the potassium concentration.

Reagent

- Potassium reagent
- Potassium standard (5 mol/L).

Procedure

Take two test tubes and mark them as T and S. Add 3 mL of potassium reagent in each tube. Add 0.1 mL of serum and 0.1 mL of potassium standard in test and standard, respectively. Mix well and allow it to stand for 5 minutes at room temperature. Read the absorbance of T and S against reagent at 620 nm.

Reagent	T	S
Potassium reagent	3 mL	3 mL
Serum	0.1 mL	—
Sodium standard	—	0.1 mL

Another popular method for determination of sodium and potassium is flame photometry.

Reagent

- Stock standard for sodium (1000 mEq/L)
- Stock standard for potassium (100 mEq/L).

Mixed working standards are prepared as follows:
- *Sodium/potassium (120/2.0 mEq/L)*: It contains 120 mEq/L of sodium and 2.0 mEq of potassium in 1 liter distilled water. It is prepared by mixing 12 mL stock standard for sodium and 2 mL stock standard for potassium in 86 mL of distilled water.
- *Sodium/potassium (140/4.0 mEq/L)*: It contains 140 mEq/L of sodium and 4.0 mEq of potassium in 1 liter distilled water. It is prepared by mixing 14 mL stock standard for sodium and 4 mL stock standard for potassium in 82 mL of distilled water.
- *Sodium/potassium (160/6.0 mEq/L)*: It contains 160 mEq/L of sodium and 6.0 mEq of potassium in 1 liter distilled water. It is prepared by mixing 16 mL stock standard

for sodium and 6 mL stock standard for potassium in 78 mL of distilled water.
Note: mEq/day = milliequivalents per day.

Specimen

Serum or heparinized plasma.

Flame Photometer

It is a spectrophotometer in which a spray of metallic salts in solution is vaporized in a very hot flame and subjected to quantitative analysis by measuring the intensities of the spectral lines of the metals present.
- Main unit, and
- Compressor unit are the important components of the equipment.

Main Unit

It consists of—An atomizer, mixing chamber, burner, optical filters, photodetectors, two digital displays, air regulator, gas regulator, gas pressure gauge.

Compressor Unit

It delivers oil free compressed air to the atomizer.

The atomizer and flame are the most important components in the flame photometer. The function of atomizer is to break up the solution into fine droplets so that the atoms will absorb heat energy from the flame and becomes excited.

The gases used for the flame photometer are—a mixture of hydrogen and oxygen, natural gas, acetylene and propane with air or oxygen, liquid petroleum gas (LPG).

Principle

The solution under test is passed carefully, under controlled conditions as a very fine spray in the air supply to nonluminous flame. In the flame, the solution evaporates and the salt dissociates to give natural ions, which emit light of the characteristic wavelength. The flame is simultaneously monitored by both the channel consists of a detector which views the flame through a narrow band optical filter. The photodetector outputs are connected to two independent digital displays, which are calibrated for direct concentration readouts. Initial calibration is done by using at least three standards of different concentrations.

Procedure

Take four test tubes. Mark them as test, standard 1, standard 2 and standard 3. To each tube add 10 mL of distilled water. Add 0.1 mL of serum to test. Add 0.1 mL of standard (120/2.0 mEq/L), 0.1 mL of standard (140/4.0 mEq/L), 0.1 mL of standard (160/6.0 mEq/L) to standard 1, standard 2 and standard 3, respectively.

Put on the main switch and switch on air compressor and adjust the required air pressure, by adjusting the knob meant for air. Introduce the distilled water through atomizer. Put on gas and control the flame by adjusting the knob meant for gas till the flame is divided into five sharp cones. Adjust the proper filters for the simultaneous determination of sodium and potassium. Make zero adjustment by using distilled water. Introduce the standard 120/2.0 mEq/L and by using the knob meant for sodium the digits 120.0 and by using the knob meant for

Reagent	Test	Standard 1	Standard 2	Standard 3
Distilled water	10 mL	10 mL	10 mL	10 mL
Serum	0.1 mL	—	—	—
Standard (120/2.0 mEq/L)	—	0.1 mL	—	—
Standard (140/4.0 mEq/L)	—	—	0.1 mL	—
Standard (160/6.0 mEq/L)	—	—	—	0.1 mL

potassium the digits 2.0. are adjusted. Introduce the standard 140/4.0 mEq/L. If the standards are accurately prepared the digital display will indicate exact concentration for both sodium and potassium. Introduce the standard 160/6.0 mEq/L and confirm the accuracy of the standard. Now introduce the test and record the readings for sodium and potassium.

Normal Value

Sodium (Na): 135–145 mEq/L
Potassium (K): 1–15 years : 3.7–5.0 mEq/L
16–59 years : 3.6–4.8 mEq/L
≥ 60 years : 3.9–5.3 mEq/L

Clinical Significance

Estimation of serum sodium is useful in diagnosis and treatment of dehydration and over hydration. Changes in sodium more often reflect changes in water balance. Increased sodium values (hypernatremia) are observed in conditions, such as:
- Severe dehydration
- Diabetes insipidus
- Salt poisoning
- Cushing's syndrome
- In certain postrenal conditions like enlarged prostate leading to obstruction of urine flow.

Decreased sodium values (hyponatremia) are observed in conditions such as:
- Severe prolonged diarrhea and vomiting
- Salt losing nephritis
- Addison's disease.

Estimation of serum potassium is very useful in paralysis, severe fluid and electrolyte loss, diabetic coma, renal failure, etc. Increased potassium values (hyperkalemia) are observed in conditions, such as:
- Addison's disease
- Renal glomerular disease
- In anuria and oliguria
- Familial hyperkalemic paralysis
- Acute acidosis
- Decreased insulin
- Intravascular hemolysis.

Decreased potassium values (hypokalemia) are observed in conditions, such as:
- Cushing's syndrome
- Renal tubular damage
- Metabolic alkalosis
- Malnutrition.

■ URINE SODIUM AND POTASSIUM

Urine Sodium

To determine urine sodium value, the method used is flame photometry. The procedure is exactly same as that of serum sodium. Use undiluted urine instead of serum.

Calculation

24 hours excretion of urine sodium =

$$\frac{24 \text{ hours urine volume (mL)}}{100}$$

Normal Value

Urine sodium: 40–220 mEq/24 hour

Increased in diuretics, high sodium diet, acute tubular necrosis (ATN), salt-losing nephritis, Addison's disease, hypothyroidism, *syndrome inappropriate ADH secretion* (SIADH), CHF and liver failure.

Decreased in fasting, some fevers and chronic nephritis.

Urine Potassium

To determine urine potassium value, the method used is flame photometry. The procedure is exactly same as that of serum potassium. Use diluted urine (1:10) instead of serum.

Calculation

Urine potassium, mEq/L = reading × 10

24 hours urine excretion =

$$\frac{\text{Urine potassium mEq/L} \times 24 \text{ hours urine volume (mL)}}{1000}$$

Normal Value

Urine potassium: 25–100 mEq/24 hour

Increased in primary or secondary aldosteronism, glucocorticoids, alkalosis, renal tubular acidosis, excess potassium intake.

Decreased in acute renal failure, potassium sparing diuretics, diarrhea, and hypokalemia.

▪ SERUM AND URINE CHLORIDE

Serum Chloride

Chloride is the major extracellular anion of the body. Its primary role in the body is to maintain proper water distribution, osmotic pressure and normal anion-cation balance in the plasma. In gastric juice, chloride also plays important role in the production of HCl. The chloride ions are ingested through the food (regular salt) and filtered or reabsorbed by the kidney as per the body need.

Method

Modified Schoenfeld and Lewellen's method.

Specimen

Serum or heparinized plasma.

Principle

Chloride ions react with mercuric thiocyanate to form mercuric chloride, an undissociated salt to liberate thiocyanate ions. These thiocyanate ions react with the ferric ions to form ferric thiocyanate, which is colored compound. The color formed is proportional to the chloride content of the specimen. The absorbance can be read at 520 nm. The final color is stable for half an hour:

$Hg(SCN)_2 + 2Cl^- \longrightarrow HgCl_2 + 2SCN^-$

$3 SCN + Fe^{3+} \longrightarrow Fe(SCN)_3$
(colored compound)

Reagent

- Chloride reagent
- Chloride standard (100 mEq/L).

Procedure

Take three test tubes and mark them as T, S and B. Add 2 mL of chloride reagent in each tube. Add 0.1 mL of serum, 0.1 mL of chloride standard and 0.1 mL of distilled water in test, standard and blank, respectively. Mix well and keep at room temperature for 2 minutes. Read the absorbance of test and standard against blank at 505 nm.

Reagent	T	S	B
Chloride reagent	1 mL	1 mL	1 mL
Serum	0.1 mL	—	—
Chloride standard	—	0.1 mL	—
Distilled water	—	—	0.1 mL

Calculations

$$\text{Serum chloride mEq/dL} = \frac{\text{OD of T}}{\text{OD of S}} \times 100$$

Normal value: 96–109 mEq/dL

Clinical Significance

Serum chloride is very useful to assess electrolyte, acid-base and water balance. Serum chloride is increased in metabolic acidosis associated with prolonged diarrhea, renal tubular diseases, respiratory alkalosis, some cases of hyperparathyroidism, diabetes insipidus, dehydration, and in conditions causing decreased renal blood flow, i.e. congestive heart failure.

Serum chloride levels are decreased in prolonged vomiting (loss of HCl), salt losing renal diseases, chronic respiratory acidosis, burns, and effect of certain drugs like corticosteroids, bicarbonates, etc.

Urine Chloride

To determine urine chloride value, the method used is modified Schoenfeld and Lewellen's method. The procedure is exactly same as that of serum chloride. Use undiluted urine instead of serum.

Calculation

Chloride excretion, mg/24 hours =

$$\frac{\text{Urine chl mEq/L} \times 24 \text{ h urine volume (mL)}}{1000}$$

(chl: chloride, h: hours)

Normal Values

The normal range is 20–250 mEq/day. This range is highly dependent on salt intake and the state of the individual's hydration.

Clinical Significance

Increased urine chloride excretion may be caused by—increased salt intake, postmenstrual diuresis, pharmacologic diuresis, salt-losing nephritis, adrenocortical insufficiency.

Decreased urine chloride excretion may occur with—decreased salt intake, adrenocortical hyperfunction, extrarenal fluid loss (such as diarrhea, vomiting, sweating, and gastric suction), salt retention.

■ SERUM AND URINE PHOSPHORUS

Serum Phosphorus

Most of the phosphorus in the blood exists as inorganic phosphate. About 80% of the total phosphorus is combined with calcium in bones and teeth. It is found in every cell of the body. About 10% is combined with proteins, lipids and carbohydrate and other compounds in blood and muscle. The remaining 10% is widely distributed in various chemical compounds.

Method

Gomori's method.

Principle

Protein in serum is first removed by treating with TCA. Protein free filtrate is then treated with an acid molybdate, which reacts with inorganic phosphate to form phosphomolybdic acid. The color reagent, metol reduces phosphomolybdic acid to give a blue colored compound. The intensity of the color is measured at 660 nm.

Reagents

- Trichloroacetic acid (10 g/dL)
- Molybdate reagent
- Color reagent, metol
- Phosphorus standard (5 mg/dL).

Procedure

Take two centrifuge tubes. Mark them as test and diluted standard. Add 4.5 mL TCA reagent in each tube. Add 0.5 mL of serum in test and 0.5 mL of standard in diluted standard tubes. Mix and centrifuge to get clear filtrate. Pipette in the tubes as follows:

Test	Standard	Blank
Filtrate 2.5 mL	—	—
Diluted standard —	2.5 mL	—
Distilled water —	—	2.5 mL
Molybdate reagent 0.5 mL	0.5 mL	0.5 mL
Color reagent 0.5 mL	0.5 mL	0.5 mL

Mix thoroughly and keep in the dark for 10 minutes. Read the intensities at 660 nm.

Calculation

Serum inorganic phosphorus

$$(\text{mg/dL}) = \frac{\text{OD of T}}{\text{OD of S}} \times 5$$

Normal Value

Neonates   : 045–100 mg%
1–19 years   : 120–240 mg%
20–29 years : 144–275 mg%
30–39 years : 165–295 mg%
40–49 years : 177–350 mg%
50–59 years : 160–330 mg%
> 69 years   : 170–300 mg%

Clinical Significance

Decreased serum phosphorus values are observed in preliminary hyperparathyroidism, rickets (vitamin D deficiency) and in Fanconi's syndrome (defect in reabsorption of phosphorus). Increased serum phosphorus levels are found in hypervitaminosis-D, hypoparathyroidism and in renal failure.

Urine Inorganic Phosphorus

The daily excretion of inorganic phosphorus on an average diet is about 1 g. There is increased excretion of phosphorus in urine in hyperparathyroidism, and it is reduced in hypoparathyroidism. Phosphate excretion is also reduced in rickets, due to impaired absorption of phosphorus.

Method

Gomori's method.
Reagents and principle are same as that of serum inorganic phosphate.

Specimen

A 24-hour urine sample with thymol crystals added as a preservative.

Procedure

Dilute the urine sample to 1: 100 in TCA reagent. Also dilute the standard 5 mg/dL in TCA reagent. If proteins are present, a preparation of protein free filtrate is must; if proteins are absent, then directly proceed for the part II step of the serum inorganic phosphate procedure.

Calculation

Urine inorganic phosphorus

$$(mg/dL) = \frac{OD\ of\ T}{OD\ of\ S} \times 5$$

Inorganic phosphorus excretion, mg/24 hrs =

$$\frac{\text{Urine calcium mg/dL} \times \text{vol. of 24 hours urine}}{100}$$

Clinical Significance

High urinary phosphorus (i.e. increased renal losses) occurs in primary hyperparathyroidism, vitamin D deficiency, renal tubular acidosis, diuretic use. Phosphates are among the substances, which may be lost in the Fanconi syndrome. Renal loss of phosphate may itself lead to rickets or osteomalacia.

Low in hypoparathyroidism, pseudohypoparathyroidism, vitamin D intoxication.

■ SERUM AND URINE CALCIUM

Serum Calcium

Calcium is the major constituent of bone. Calcium in serum is present in ionized form or as a complex with protein or other inorganic substances like citrate, phosphate and others. Calcium plays many important roles in physiology of the body like it activates many enzymes and plays a key role in blood coagulation.

Method

O-cresolphthalein complexone (OCPC) method.

Specimen

Serum or heparinized plasma. It should be separated as soon as possible.

Principle

Calcium in an alkaline medium reacts with O-cresolphthalein complexone to form an intense chromophore, which is of purple color. Read the absorbance at 575 nm.

Reagents

- O-cresolphthalein complexone reagent
- Buffer solution
- Calcium standard (10 mg/dL).

Procedure

First of all prepare working solution by mixing equal amounts of reagent 1 and reagent 2. This is to be freshly prepared as it is stable only for one day. Take three test tubes and mark them as T, S and B. Add 6 mL of freshly prepared working reagent in each tube. Add 0.05 mL of serum, 0.05 mL of calcium standard and 0.05 mL of distilled water in test, standard. and blank, respectively. Mix well and keep at room temperature for exactly 10 minutes. Read the absorbance of test and standard against blank at 575 nm.

Reagent	T	S	B
Working reagent	6 mL	6 mL	6 mL
Serum	0.05 mL	—	—
Calcium standard	—	0.05 mL	—
Distilled water	—	—	0.05 mL

Calculations

$$\text{Serum calcium (mg/dL)} = \frac{\text{OD of T}}{\text{OD of S}} \times 10$$

Normal Value

1–3 years   : 8.7–9.8 mg/dL
4–11 years : 8.8–10.1 mg/dL
12–13 years : 8.8–10.6 mg/dL
14–15 years : 9.2–10.7 mg/dL
> 16 years : 8.9–10.7 mg/dL

Clinical Significance

Determination of serum calcium level is useful in diagnosis of parathyroid dysfunction, hypercalcemia of malignancy, 90% of cases of hypercalcemia are due to hyperparathyroidism, neoplasms or granulomatous diseases. Hypercalcemia of sarcoidosis adrenal insufficiency and hyperthyroidism tend to be found in clinically evident disease. Blood calcium should be monitored in renal disease, effects of various drugs, acute pancreatitis, postoperative thyroidectomy and parathyroidectomy.

Calcium levels are found to be low in hypoparathyroidism, malabsorption of calcium and vitamin D, chronic renal disease with uremia, bone disease, late pregnancy, asphyxia, infants of diabetic mothers, cerebral injuries, malignant disease, etc.

Urine Calcium

The same method can be used to determine urine calcium.

Specimen

A 24 hour of urine sample preserved with thymol crystals.

Calculations

$$\text{Urine calcium (mg/dL)} = \frac{\text{OD of T}}{\text{OD of S}} \times 10$$

For the determination of 24-hour calcium excretions, measure the urine volume and calculate the result as follows:

Calcium excretion, mg/24 hours =

$$\frac{\text{Urine calcium mg/dL} \times \text{vol. of 24 hour urine}}{100}$$

Normal value: 100–300 mg/dL in 24 hour of urine sample.

Clinical Significance

Determination of urine calcium level is useful in diagnosis of hypercalciuria causing renal calculi. High calcium levels in urine are seen in—hyperparathyroidism, excess milk intake, high calcium diet, rapidly progressive osteoporosis, multiple myeloma, Paget's disease, etc. Hypercalciuria without hypercalcemia are due to medullary sponge kidney, renal tubular acidosis, hyperthyroidism, etc.

Low calcium level in urine is due to renal failure, hypoparathyroidism, rickets, osteomalacia, metastatic carcinoma of prostate, etc.

CHAPTER 7

Body Fluid

Learning Objectives
- The analysis of body fluids plays a critical role in the diagnosis and prognosis of a disease. A change in concentration or composition of a particular constituent in body fluids is used as an indicator of a pathological condition. A particular component in body fluids can thus be considered as a marker for the detection of a disease
- Different types of body fluids- their function, sample collection, detailed analysis, normal and specific constituents are discussed here
- This chapter throws light upon pathologically important body fluids, such as seminal fluid, amniotic fluid, cerebrosipnal fluid (CSF), pericardial fluid, Pleural fluid, peritoneal fluid and synovial fluid.

Keywords
Oligospermia, Necrozoospermia, Azoospermia, Amniocentesis, Serous fluid, Transudates, Exudates, Pericarditis, Chylous effusion, Empyema, Chyliform effusion, Thoracentesis, Markers of Pleural tuberculosis (TB), Systemic lupus erythematosus (SLE), Ascites, Paracentesis, Arthrocentesis

■ INTRODUCTION

Body fluids are defined as the fluids that are present within the human body. There are different types of body fluids that are present in the human body. In healthy adult men, the total body water is about 60% of the total body weight.

The role of different body fluids test is to help detect, isolate, identify any physiological abnormality or other pathogenic microorganisms present in the body. It can also be done on other types of body fluids because they give a better idea of the kind of disease or disorders present in certain parts of the body. Pathologically important body fluids are discussed in this chapter.

■ SEMINAL FLUID

Semen is the bodily fluid in the urethra of the penis which is released during ejaculation. This cloudy, white substance is created by secretions from the male reproductive organs. During ejaculation sperm will move through the ejaculatory ducts to mix with fluid from the prostate, seminal vesicles and bulbourethral glands, forming semen.

The average semen volume in an ejaculation is 2–5 mL. Semen from one ejaculation contain around 40–600 million sperms depending on the length of time the ejaculation lasts and the volume of the ejaculation.

Most of the fluids in semen are made from secretions of male reproductive organs. The contributions and components of semen are:

Gland	Approximate %	Description
Testes	2–5	Around 200–500 million spermatozoa (sperm) are produced in the testes and released during ejaculation
Seminal vesicle	65–75	Citrate, amino acids, flavins, enzymes, fructose (2–5 mg/mL of semen). This is the main energy source for sperm
Prostate	25–30	Citric acid, acid phosphatase, prostate specific antigen, zinc and proteolytic enzymes. Zinc helps to stabilize chromatin that contains DNA in sperm. Zinc deficiencies can lower fertility because sperm will become more fragile
Bulbo-urethral glands	Less than 1	Mucus which increases sperm mobility in the cervix and vagina by making the channel more viscous so that the sperm can swim

Sample Collection

- Masturbation
- Sex with a condom
- Sex with withdrawal before ejaculation
- Ejaculation stimulated by electricity.

Precautions While Collecting Sample

- Ask patient to avoid ejaculation for 24–72 hours before the test
- Also to avoid alcohol, caffeine and drugs such as cocaine and marijuana two to five days before the test
- The semen must be kept at body temperature
- The semen must be delivered to the testing facility within 30–60 minutes of leaving the body.

Analysis

- The appearance should be whitish to gray and opalescent. Semen that has a red-brown tint could indicate the presence of blood while a yellow tint could indicate jaundice or be a medication side effect.
- The typical volume of semen collected is between 1.5 and 5.5 milliliters (mL) of fluid per ejaculation. Decreased volume of semen would indicate fewer sperm, which diminishes opportunities for successful fertilization and subsequent pregnancy. Excessive seminal fluid may dilute the concentration of sperm.
- The semen should initially be thick and then liquefy within 15–30 minutes. If this does not occur, then it may impede sperm movement.
- Sperm concentration (also called sperm count or sperm density) is measured in millions of sperm per milliliter of semen. Normal is at least 20 million or more sperm per mL, with a total ejaculate volume of 80 million or more. Fewer sperm and/or a lower sperm concentration may impair fertility. Following a vasectomy, the goal is to have no sperm detected in the semen sample. Sperm can be counted either manually or by automated methods. Although, automated counting has some advantages for assessment of motility parameters, manual counting is still performed by most clinical laboratories. Hemocytometer (which is used to calculate blood cells) is used to count sperm manually. Calculate the total number of sperm in 5 large squares in both chambers of the hemocytometer. Divide the total number of sperm in the 10 large squares (5 large squares per 2 chambers) by 100 to estimate the number of millions of sperm.
- Motility is the percentage of moving sperm in a sample and graded based on speed and direction travelled. At least 50% should be motile one hour after ejaculation, moving forward in a straight line with good speed. The progression of the sperm, best measured using an automated system, is rated on a basis from zero (no motion) to 4, with 3–4 representing good motility.

Motility can be observed manually by hanging drop technique. Place a drop of semen on a coverslip over cavity slide. Examine with low and high power objective.

Description	Sperm concentration in ejaculate
Mild oligospermia	10 million–20 million sperm/mL
Severe oligospermia	0–5 million sperm/mL
Necrozoospermia	Sperm present but immobile
Azoospermia	0 sperm

- Morphology analysis is the study of the size, shape and appearance of the sperm cells. The analysis evaluates the structure of the sperm, whereby greater than 50% of those cells examined must be normal in size, shape and length. The more abnormal sperm that are present, the lower the likelihood of fertility. Abnormal forms may include defective heads, midsections, tails and immature forms. More than 14% should have normal heads. A microscope slide is prepared with a very thin coating of semen. The slide is stained to make the sperm clearly visible and several hundred sperms are then viewed under high magnification and individually scored normal or abnormal based on their shape. A nigrosin-eosin stain is commonly used because it is effective, simple and, in addition to allowing sperm to be readily visualized. The nigrosin-stain produces a dark background on which the sperm stand out as lightly colored objects. Normal live sperm exclude the eosin stain and appear white in color, whereas "dead" sperm (i.e. those with loss of membrane integrity) take up eosin and appear pinkish in color.

Normal sperm morphology: A normal sperm has following parts **(Fig. 7.1)**:
- *Head:* The head is almost conical in shape and is formed of acrosome and nucleus.
    - Acrosome: This is found at the anterior tip of the sperm. The acrosome forms a cap like structure called the head cap. The acrosome itself is bounded by a unit membrane. It consists of a number of hydrolytic enzymes such as acid phosphatase, hyaluronidase and others. These enzymes help in tissue lysis (dissolving) and this facilitates the penetration of the sperm into the egg membrane. The enzymes are proteolytic and help in dissolving the egg membrane.
    - Sperm nucleus: The nucleus occupies most of the available space of the sperm head.
- *Neck:* The head is followed by a short neck to separate the middle piece of the sperm. The neck consists of just two granules (centrioles).
- *Middle piece:* The middle piece of the sperm consists of the upper portion of the axial filament which contains alpha, beta and gamma fibers. These are the sites of various enzymes.
- *Tail:* The tail usually is the longest part in the sperm.

Morphological defects (Fig. 7.2):
Head defects: Large head, small head, double head, elongated head, vacuolated head, irregular head, amorphous head, small acrosome, no acrosome.

Neck defects: Bent, thin, thick, irregular, cytoplasmic droplet.

Tail defects: Coiled, short, hairpin, broken, duplicated, terminal droplet.
- Semen pH should be between 7.2 and 7.8, fructose at 150–600 mg/dL. A pH of 8.0 or higher may indicate an infection, while a pH less than 7.0 suggests contamination with urine or an obstruction in the ejaculatory ducts. There should be fewer than 2000 white blood cells per mL.
- Agglutination of sperm occurs when sperm stick together in a specific and consistent manner (head to head, tail to tail, etc.) Clumping of sperm in a nonspecific manner may be due to bacterial infection or tissue contamination.

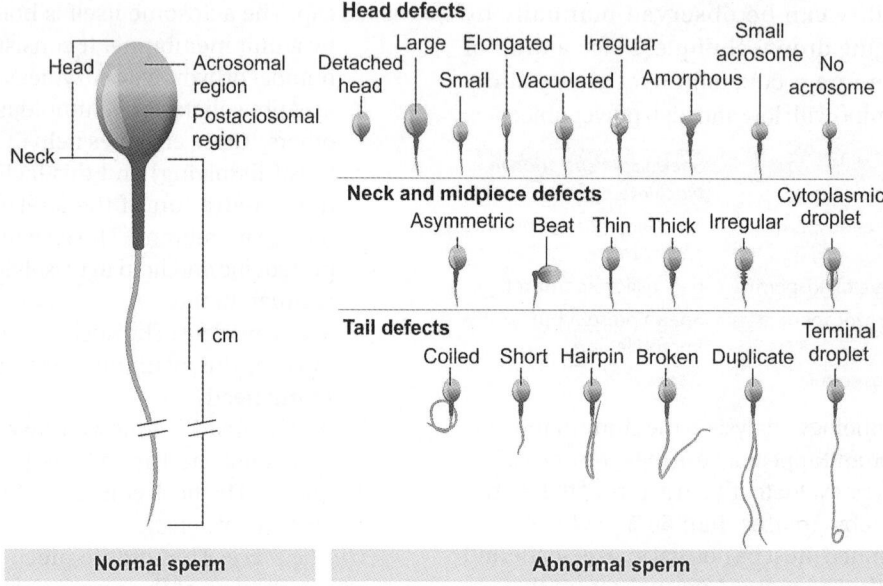

Fig. 7.1: Normal sperm. **Fig. 7.2:** Abnormal sperm.

Clinical Significance

A semen analysis is often recommended when couples are having problems getting pregnant. The test will help a doctor determine if a man is infertile. The analysis will also help determine if low sperm count or sperm dysfunction is the reason behind infertility. Men who have had a vasectomy undergo semen analysis to make sure no sperm are in their semen.

Abnormal sperm will have trouble reaching and penetrating eggs, making conception difficult. Abnormal results could indicate—infertility, infection, hormonal imbalance, disease such as diabetes, gene defects or exposure to radiation.

Computer Assisted Semen Analysis

The use of computer assisted semen analysis has advanced the ability to study and understand sperm function as it relates to human infertility. The major advances have been in the ability to more accurately determine sperm concentration (counts) and motility (movement). Generally, sperms are "looked" at by a computerized digitizing tablet through a microscope. The computer has been "taught" by the laboratory personnel what sperm look like and how they move. When the computer then "sees" a sperm under the microscope, it is able to draw a digitized picture of each individual sperm, including the speed and path this sperm takes while moving under the microscope. A great deal has been learned about the normal and abnormal "micro characteristics" of sperm employing this method. The method is, however, not foolproof. The computer is only as intelligent as its programmer. Small changes in the computer program can alter the sperm calculations significantly. The computers must constantly be monitored and updated.

Additional Testing

Sperm viability, seminal fluid fructose, anti-sperm antibodies, microbial testing, chemical testing, post-vasectomy analysis and sperm function tests.

■ AMNIOTIC FLUID

Amniotic fluid is present in the amnion, a membranous sac that surrounds the fetus. It surrounds, protects, and gives nourishment to the fetus during gestation period. Amniotic fluid keeps are increasing throughout the pregnancy. At 10 weeks of gestation, it is about 30 mL whereas, in full term, volume may exceed 1500 mL.

Sample Collection

Amniotic fluid is collected by amniocentesis. Amniocentesis is done during the 14th, 16th, and 18th weeks of gestation. Amniotic fluid needs to be refrigerated. It is collected in amber colored tube to avoid amniotic fluid from light for the estimation of bilirubin.

The purpose of the test is—to diagnose chromosomal abnormalities, diagnose inherited metabolic disorders like cystic fibrosis. Thus, amniocentesis help for elective abortion in the defective fetus. It also measures bilirubin in Rh sensitization for erythroblastosis fetalis, Analysis of the amniotic fluid for bilirubin level is also useful in the Rh-negative mothers in later weeks of the gestation gives the severity of anemia due to Rh-incompatibility. Genetic abnormalities like sickle cell anemia, thalassemia, and Down's syndrome are diagnosed.

Procedure for Amniotic Fluid Collection

Amniotic fluid is aspirated by the needle into the amniotic sac is called amniocentesis. This is transabdominal amniocentesis. Another route is transvaginal amniocentesis. This method carries a great risk of infection.

30 mL of amniotic fluid is collected in the sterile syringes. The first 2 to 3 mL collected is discarded because this may be contaminated by the maternal blood, tissue fluid, and cells.

Complications of the procedure are there may be a miscarriage, there are chances for injury to the fetus or there may be a leak of amniotic fluid.

Normal Amniotic Fluid Findings

General test	Result
Appearance	Clear, pale to straw yellow
AFP (alpha fetoprotein)	14 to 16 weeks = <5.2 mg/dL, 22 weeks = <3.0 mg/dL
Bilirubin	<0.2 mg/dL
Creatinine	>2.0 mg/dL after 37 weeks
Chromosomal abnormality	Absent
Phosphatidylglycerol	Positive (negative in immature)
Lecithin/Sphingomyelin ratio	Mature >2.0, Immature <2.0, Diabetic mother >3.5
Microscopic examination	There are amniotic epithelial cells from the lining of the sac. Fetal squamous cells originating from fetal skin, oral mucosa, and vagina.

Abnormal Amniotic Fluid Findings

Lab findings	Findings	Clinical significance
Appearance	Yellow	Erythroblastosis (due to the presence of bilirubin)
	Red-brown (dark red-brown)	Indicate fetal death
	Amber color	Indicates bilirubin
	Green color	Due to meconium, fetal hypoxia
	Pink-red (blood-streaked)	Blood contamination, traumatic tap, intra-amniotic hemorrhage
Volume	Increased	Hydramnios due to fetal abnormality

(Contd...)

(Contd...)

Lab findings	Findings	Clinical significance
	Decrease	Oligohydramnios is associated with rupture membranes and fetal abnormality, urinary tract deformities
Presence of cells	Long bipolar cells, multiple filamentous pseudopodia, large vacuolated cells with inclusions	Neural tube defect
Bilirubin	At 28 weeks = >0.075 mg/dL	Erythroblastosis fetalis, hepatitis
	At 40 weeks = <0.025 mg/dL	Maternal infection, sickle cell crises
Saturated phosphatidylcholine	>500 µg/L	Respiratory distress syndrome
AFP	Increased, >2.5 MoM	Open spinal defects (neural tube defect)
Creatinine	>2.0 mg/dL	Indicates fetal maturity and the maternal level is normal

Chromosomal Anomalies Diagnosis

Trisomy 21	Down's syndrome
Trisomy 13	Patau's syndrome
XO 45	Turner's syndrome
XXY 47	Klinefelter's syndrome
Trisomy 18	Edward's syndrome

CEREBROSPINAL FLUID

Cerebrospinal fluid (CSF) is a clear fluid, circulates in the brain and spinal cord. Normal adult has 90–150 mL and newborn 10–60 mL of CSF.

Function

Cerebrospinal fluid acts as buffer, regulates intracranial pressure, carries nutrients to the nervous system and serves as excretory channel for metabolic wastes in the CNS.

Collecting a specimen: Invasive test with potential harm to patient. It is done only for serious reasons like to diagnose meningitis, brain hemorrhage and diagnosis of neurological disease or malignancy. Only a physician collects CSF as it involves risk to patient. Careful handling of specimen is necessary. Three separate tubes of about 5 mL are collected and numbered in sequence.

It acts as blood-brain-barrier. CSF is not an ultrafiltrate of plasma. Many drugs do not enter the CSF from the blood. Some electrolytes are more concentrated, others are less concentrated.

Protein is found only in very small amount. Chemistry tests and microbial examination is done from the first tubes and the last one is for cell counts.

The CSF samples should never be refrigerated. Certain viral studies may require immediate freezing at very low temperatures. Never discard CSF until all tests are done.

Gross appearance: Normal CSF is crystal clear and the consistency of water.

Turbidity: May indicate white cells, bacteria, excess protein or fat. Radiographic dye will give the CSF an oily look. Clotting may be from a traumatic tap.

Color: Bloody fluid—can be from a traumatic tap or may indicate subarachnoid hemorrhage, xanthochromia—may indicate bleeding, lysed RBCs or high protein levels.

CSF cell counts: Normally very few cells are found in CSF—no RBCs, 0–8 WBCs.

PMNs are seen in bacterial infection and lymphocytes are seen in viral infection.

The cells are usually counted manually, with undiluted specimen.

Morphologic Examination

When a cell count is over 30 white cells/microliter a differential count is done smear is made from centrifuged sediment and stained. Cytospin yields better cell count with small amount centrifuged sediment may be used.

Chemistry tests: CSF contains same chemicals that are found as in plasma. Normal values are different because of selective filtration.

Proteins: Protein tests and electrophoresis are common tests of many disease states. Normal range is 12–60 mg/dL (less than 1% of plasma concentration).

Increased protein levels are seen in infections, decreased levels, and leakage of fluid from CNS.

Glucose: Usually about 60–80% of blood glucose should be measured at the same time difference is significant. Bacteria utilize glucose therefore glucose level reduced in bacterial meningitis, but not in viral. Glucose is elevated in diabetic coma.

Other Chemical Tests

Glutamine: Indirect measure of waste products. It is seen in some liver disorders, bilirubin and chloride and lactate dehydrogenase.

Microbiological examination: Gram stains and cultures are useful to diagnose acute bacterial meningitis. Organisms can be seen in the Gram stain, acid fast stains for TB, India ink that stains *Cryptococcus*.

Serous Fluid

It includes pleural, pericardial and peritoneal fluids contained within closed cavities of the body. This fluid fills space between layers of cells to lubricate the surfaces as they move against each other. The fluids are formed and reabsorbed as volume is very small. Increased volume is referred as an effusion.

Transudates: Increase in fluid volume (effusion) occurs in many conditions. Transudate is usually the result of a systemic disease. Transudates result from abnormal movement of fluid across a membrane.

Exudates: The effusions result from an inflammatory response serous effusions are classified as transudate or exudate by protein content. Transudates usually have less than 3 g/dL exudates usually over 8 g/dL.

Collection: Strictly antiseptic conditions are needed. It is collected by aspiration. It may be collected for diagnostic purposes or to relieve excess accumulation. EDTA tube for cell counts, morphology and differential, anticoagulated sample for chemical analysis, sterile tube for Gram stain and culture are needed. Keep extra tubes for cytology tumor studies.

■ PERICARDIAL FLUID

Pericardium is a tough double walled sac surrounding the heart. It protects heart from mechanical injuries and external shocks.

Pericardium consists of two membranes, the outer layer is fibrous parietal pericardium and the inner layer is serous visceral pericardium. A fluid is present in between these two layers. It is called as pericardial fluid and the space where it is present is called as pericardial cavity.

Pericardial fluid is produced by inner serous visceral pericardium. The pericardial fluid reduces friction within the pericardium by lubricating the epicardial surface. This allows the membranes to glide over each other with each heartbeat.

Normal values of pericardial fluid

Pericardial fluid	Normal value
Appearance	Clear
Volume	15–50 mL
Color	Pale yellow
Glucose	Parallel serum values
Red blood cell count	None seen
White blood cell count	Less than 300/mm^3
Culture	No growth
Gram stain	No organisms seen
Cytology	No abnormal cells seen

The fluid is made up of a high concentration of lactate dehydrogenase (LDH), protein and lymphocytes.

Pericardial fluid analysis is needed in two conditions:
- In case of inflammation of the pericardium called as pericarditis and/or
- Excessive accumulation of pericardial fluid called as pericardial effusion.

Pericardial effusion develops either from:
- *Increased accumulation of fluid*: This happens when there is:
  - Increased capillary permeability
  - Increased venous pressure
  - Decreased protein (oncotic pressure).
- Decreased clearance of fluid: This happens when there is:
  - Increased lymphatic obstruction.

There are two main types of pericardial fluid:
1. *Transudate:* The fluid that accumulates when there is an imbalance between the pressure within blood vessels (which drives fluid out of blood vessels) and the amount of protein in blood (which keeps fluid in blood vessels) in such case, the fluid is called as transudate.
2. *Exudate:* The fluid that accumulates when there is an injury or inflammation of the pericardium, in such case the fluid is called as exudate.

Transudate	Exudate
90% of pericardial fluids are transudates	10% of pericardial fluids are exudates
Fluid appears clear	Fluid may appear cloudy
Albumin level—low	Albumin level—higher than in transudates
Cell count—few cells are present	Cell count—increased
Transudates are most often caused by congestive heart failure or cirrhosis	Exudates may be the result of conditions such as infection (bacterial, viral or fungal), malignancies (metastatic cancer, lymphoma, mesothelioma), or autoimmune disease

Differentiation between the types of fluid is important because it helps diagnose the specific disease or condition. Initial set of tests (cell count, protein or albumin level and appearance of the fluid) is used to distinguish between transudates and exudates. Once the fluid is determined to be one or the other, additional tests may be performed to further pinpoint the disease or condition causing pericarditis and/or pericardial effusion.

Causes

The cause of pericarditis is unknown or unproven in many cases. It mostly affects men ages 20–50. Pericarditis is often the result of an infection such as—viral infections that cause a chest cold or pneumonia, such as echovirus or coxsackievirus and influenza, some bacterial or fungal infection. The condition may be seen with diseases such as—cancer (including leukemia), autoimmune diseases, kidney failure, TB, heart attack, heart surgery or trauma to the chest, esophagus, or heart, swelling or inflammation of the heart muscle, etc.

Symptoms

The symptoms produced by a pericardial effusion depend on the speed with which the effusion is formed, as well as the size of the effusion. Many small to moderate effusions formed over a long period of time will be relatively asymptomatic.
- Chest pain is almost always present. The chest pain may be made worse by deep breathing and lessened by leaning forward
- Palpitations (sensation that the heart is pounding or beating fast)
- Light-headedness or passing out
- Fever, chills, or sweating if the condition is caused by an infection
- Fatigue
- Muscle aches
- Shortness of breath
- Nausea, vomiting, and diarrhea (if viral illness is present)

- Anxiety and confusion
- Hiccoughs.

Complications of Pericarditis

Two serious complications of pericarditis are cardiac tamponade and chronic constrictive pericarditis.
1. Cardiac tamponade occurs if too much fluid collects in the pericardium (the sac around the heart). The extra fluid puts pressure on the heart. This prevents the heart from properly filling with blood. As a result, less blood leaves the heart, which causes a sharp drop in blood pressure. If left untreated, cardiac tamponade can be fatal.
2. Chronic constrictive pericarditis is a rare disease that develops over time. It leads to scar-like tissue forming throughout the pericardium. The sac becomes stiff and cannot move properly. In time, the scarred tissue compresses the heart and prevents it from working well.

Diagnosis of Pericardial Effusion

Because pericardial effusions often cause no symptoms, they are frequently discovered after routine tests are abnormal. Various tests can suggest the possibility of a pericardial effusion:
- *Physical examination:* When the pericardium is inflamed, the amount of fluid between its two layers of tissue increases. Its common sign is the pericardial rub. This is the sound of the pericardium rubbing against the outer layer of the heart. By placing a stethoscope on chest sounds that are signs of fluid in the pericardium (pericardial effusion) can be listened.
- *Electrocardiogram:* This simple test detects and records heart's electrical activity. Certain ECG results suggest pericarditis. Electrodes placed over the chest produce a tracing of the heart's electrical activity. Certain patterns on ECG can suggest a pericardial effusion or pericarditis is present. The classic sign of pericarditis—a concave upwards ("saddle") ST-segment elevation throughout the 12 leads or in leads that do not correspond to the territory perfused by a single coronary artery. Low voltages suggest the possibility of effusion. There may also be diminished QRS and T-wave voltages, PR-segment depression.
- *Chest X-ray:* A chest X-ray creates pictures of the structures inside chest, such as heart, lungs, and blood vessels. The pictures can show whether there is an enlarged heart. This is a sign of excess fluid in pericardium. A chest X-ray (CXR) can help to rule out a tuberculous cause of pericarditis and exclude significant effusion.
- *Echocardiography:* An echocardiogram (ultrasound of the heart is painless test which uses sound waves to create pictures of heart). The pictures show the size and shape of heart. This test can show whether fluid has built up in the pericardium.
- *Cardiac CT (computed tomography):* This is a type of X-ray that takes a clear, detailed picture of heart and pericardium. A cardiac CT helps rule out other causes of chest pain.
- *Cardiac MRI (magnetic resonance imaging):* This test uses powerful magnets and radio waves to create detailed pictures of organs and tissues. A cardiac MRI can show changes in the pericardium.
- *Blood tests*: Blood cell count (WBC count is raised), ESR, blood culture, blood tests for immune markers, such as the antinuclear cytoplasmic antibody (ANCA), and C-reactive protein, cardiac enzyme test are commonly asked among blood tests.
- *Pericardial fluid analysis*: Pericardial fluid is analyzed for different parameters.

Pericardiocentesis: It is process of removal of pericardial fluid from the pericardial sac with a needle and syringe. An intravenous (IV) line may be started and the person may be given medications prior to the sample collection. The patient is positioned lying down. A local anesthetic is applied, then the doctor inserts a needle into the space between the ribs (fifth to sixth intercostals space) on the left side of the chest and into the pericardial sac and removes a fluid sample. An ultrasound may be used to help guide the needle.

It can be used to relieve pressure from pericardial effusions or for diagnostic purposes, revealing the cause of abnormalities such as: Cancer, cardiac perforation, cardiac trauma and congestive heart failure.

Pericardial Fluid Tests

Following tables interprets different aspects of pericardial fluid analysis.

Gross Appearance

Clear to pale yellow	Normal
Milk-colored (Chylous)	Lymphatic system involvement
Cloudy/turbid	- Primary bacterial infection - Presence of white blood cells
Bloody tap	- Benign or malignant tumor - Hemorrhagic pericarditis, perforated ulcer - Internal bleeding

In the analysis of pericardial fluid, the first step should be to separate effusions into transudates and exudates by determining the following:

Characteristic	Transudate	Exudate
Appearance	Clear	Cloudy or turbid
Specific gravity	Less than 1.015	Greater than 1.015
Total protein	Less than 2.5 g/dL	Greater than 3.0 g/dL
Fluid-to-serum protein ratio	Less than 0.5	Greater than 0.5
LDH	Parallels serum value	Less than 200 units/L
Fluid-to-serum LDH ratio	Less than 0.6	Greater than 0.6
Fluid cholesterol	Less than 55 mg/dL	Greater than 55 mg/dL
White blood cell count	Less than 100/mm^3	Greater than 1,000/mm^3

Pericardiocentesis Biochemistry

- Pericardial adenosine deaminase activity (ADA) >667 nkat/L (40 U/L) suggests tuberculous pericarditis. As cultures are less sensitive, this indirect test has become the standard test in the diagnosis of pericardial tuberculosis.
- Pericardial interferon-gamma (IFN-gamma) >200 picograms/L suggests tuberculous pericarditis.

	Levels	Interpretation
Triglyceride	Elevated	- Malignant tumor, lymphoma, TB - Parasitic infection, hepatic cirrhosis
Glucose	Parallel to serum level	Lowered in case of infection

Microscopic examination: Normal pericardial fluid has small numbers of white blood cells (WBCs) but no red blood cells (RBCs) or micro-organisms. Results of an evaluation of the different kinds of cells present may include:

- Total cell counts—quantity of WBCs and RBCs in the sample. Increased WBCs may be seen with infections and other causes of pericarditis.
- WBC differential—determination of percentages of different types of WBCs. An increased number of neutrophils may be seen with bacterial infections.
- Cytology—a cytocentrifuged sample is treated with a special stain and examined under a microscope for abnormal cells. This may be done when a mesothelioma or metastatic cancer is suspected. The presence of certain abnormal cells, such as tumor cells or immature blood cells, can indicate what type of cancer is involved.
- Viral PCR is used to identify specific viral elements.
- Gram stain and culture: Culture is more sensitive than Gram stain for bacterial infections, but when either reveals a specific pathogen it is very helpful.
- In fungal infections, a positive fungal pericardial fluid culture confirms the

diagnosis and provides guidance when selecting antifungal medication.
- Pericardial adenosine deaminase activity (ADA) >667 nkat/L (40 U/L) suggests tuberculous pericarditis. The sensitivity is 88% and specificity 83%. As cultures are less sensitive, this indirect test has become the standard test in the diagnosis of pericardial tuberculosis.
- Pericardial interferon-gamma (IFN-gamma) >200 picograms/L suggests tuberculous pericarditis.

PLEURAL FLUID

Lungs have protective covering of visceral and parietal pleural membranes within the thoracic cavity.

Pleural fluid is secreted by parietal layer of pleura. It acts as a lubricant between two membranes and facilitates movement between lungs and chest wall. This is a straw colored fluid. The normal value of pleural fluid is 10–20 mL. It enters in the pleural space from systemic capillaries in the parietal membrane and exits via parietal lymphatics and stomas. Pleural fluid accumulates when too much fluid enters or too little exits the pleural space.

Abnormal accumulation of fluid in pleural space is called pleural effusion. There can be two main reasons for fluid accumulation:
1. An imbalance between the pressure within blood vessels (which drives fluid out of the blood vessel) and the amount of protein in blood (which keeps fluid in the blood vessel) can result in accumulation of fluid called as transudate. Fluid that accumulates as a result of imbalance in these pressures produces transitive effusions. Transudates are most frequently caused by congestive heart failure, hepatic cirrhosis, hypoproteinemia, nephrotic syndrome, acute atelectasis, myxedema, etc.
If the fluid is determined to be a transudate, then usually no more tests on the fluid are necessary.
2. Injury or inflammation of the pleurae may cause abnormal collection of fluid called as an exudate.

Exudative effusions are caused by local processes leading to increased capillary permeability resulting in exudation of fluid, protein, cells and other serum constituents. Causes are numerous; the most common are pneumonia, cancer, pulmonary embolism, viral infection and TB. Yellow nail syndrome is a rare disorder causing chronic exudative pleural effusions, lymphedema and dystrophic yellow nails—all thought to be the result of impaired lymphatic drainage.

An accurate diagnosis of the cause of the effusion, transudate versus exudate, relies on a comparison of the chemistry in the pleural fluid to those in the blood, using Light's criteria. According to Light's criteria (Light, et al. 1972), a pleural effusion is likely exudative if at least one of the following exists:
- The ratio of pleural fluid protein to serum protein is greater than 0.5
- The ratio of pleural fluid LDH and serum LDH is greater than 0.6
- Pleural fluid LDH is greater than 0.6 or 2/3 times the normal upper limit for serum.

The sensitivity and specificity of Light's criteria for detection of exudates have been measured in many studies and are usually reported to be around 98% and 80%, respectively.

According to the types of fluid, following exudate effusions are there:
- **Chylous effusion (chylothorax)** is a milky white effusion high in triglycerides caused by traumatic or neoplastic (most often lymphomatous) damage to the thoracic duct. Chylous effusion also occurs with the superior vena cava syndrome.
- **Chyliform (cholesterol or pseudochylous) effusions** resemble chylous effusions but are low in triglycerides and high in cholesterol. Chyliform effusions are thought to be due to release of cholesterol from lysed RBCs and neutrophils in long-standing

effusions when absorption is blocked by the thickened pleura.
- **Hemothorax** is bloody fluid (pleural fluid Hct > 50% peripheral Hct) in the pleural space due to trauma or, rarely, as a result of coagulopathy or after rupture of a major blood vessel, such as the aorta or pulmonary artery.
- **Pyothorax or empyema** is pus in the pleural space. It can occur as a complication of pneumonia, thoracotomy, abscesses (lung, hepatic, or subdiaphragmatic), or penetrating trauma with secondary infection. Extension of empyema leads to chest wall infection and external drainage.
- **Trapped lung** is a lung encased by a fibrous peel caused by empyema or tumor. Because the lung cannot expand, the pleural pressure becomes more negative than normal, increasing transudation of fluid from parietal pleural capillaries. The fluid characteristically is borderline between a transudate and an exudate; i.e. the biochemical values are within 15% of the cut-off levels for Light's criteria.
- **Iatrogenic effusions** can be caused by migration or misplacement of a feeding tube into the trachea or perforation of the superior vena cava by a central venous catheter, leading to infusion of tube feedings or IV solution into the pleural space.
- **Urinothorax** (*pl.* **urinothoraces**) means urine in the pleural space. It is a rare case of pleural effusion. The urine arrives in the pleural space either retroperitoneally under the posterior diaphragm, or via the retroperitoneal lymphatics.
- **Pneumothorax:** Air in pleural space.
- **Hydrothorax:** Serous fluid in pleural space.

Symptoms

Pleural Effusion

It is excess fluid that accumulates in the pleural cavity, the fluid-filled space that surrounds the lungs. This excess can impair breathing by limiting the expansion of the lungs.

Some pleural effusions are asymptomatic and are discovered incidentally during physical examination or on chest X-ray.

Many cause dyspnea, chest pain, usually a sharp pain that is worse with cough or deep breaths, cough, fever, hiccups, rapid breathing, shortness of breath and fatigue.

Thoracentesis

Once a pleural effusion is diagnosed, the cause must be determined. Pleural fluid is drawn out of the pleural space in a process called thoracentesis, and it should be done in almost all patients who have pleural fluid that is ≥10 mm in thickness on CT, ultrasonography, or lateral decubitus X-ray and that is new or of uncertain etiology. In thoracentesis, a needle is inserted through the back of the chest wall in the sixth, seventh, or eighth intercostal space on the midaxillary line, into the pleural space. The needle used is fine bore (21G) with 50 mL syringe.

The person is positioned sitting upright with arms raised and supported. A local anesthetic is applied and then the doctor inserts the needle into the pleural cavity and the sample is removed.

The fluid may then be evaluated for the following:
- Physical characteristics of the fluid
- Chemical composition including protein, lactate dehydrogenase (LDH), albumin, amylase, pH, and glucose
- Gram stain and culture to identify possible bacterial infections
- Cell count and differential
- Cytopathology to identify cancer cells, but may also identify some infective organisms
- Other tests as suggested by the clinical situation—lipids, fungal culture, viral culture, specific immunoglobulins.

The sample collected should be distributed to different sections of the laboratory as:
- 5 mL for physical inspection in heparinized tube

- 5 mL in sterile container for microbiology
- 5 mL in serum/heparin for biochemistry
- Remaining (20–40 mL) in EDTA for cytology.

If infection is suspected, some of the pleural fluid should be sent in blood a culture bottle which increases diagnostic accuracy, particularly for anaerobic organisms.

Normal Findings

Appearance	Clear
Color	Pale yellow
Amylase	Parallels serum values
Cholesterol	Parallels serum values
CEA	Parallels serum values
Glucose	Parallels serum values
LDH	Less than 200 units/L
Fluid LDH-to-serum LDH ratio	0.6 or less
Protein	3 g/dL
Fluid protein-to-serum protein ratio	0.5 or less
Triglycerides	Parallel serum values
pH	7.37–7.43
RBC count	NIL
WBC count	Less than 1,000/mm^3
Culture	No growth
Gram stain	No organisms seen
Cytology	No abnormal cells seen

(CEA: carcinoembryonic antigen; LDH: lactate dehydrogenase; RBC: red blood cell; WBC: white blood cell)

Pleural Fluid Analysis

Following abnormal findings are associated with different clinical conditions:

Color:
- Milky appearance may point to lymphatic system involvement.
- Reddish pleural fluid may indicate the presence of blood.
- Cloudy, thick pleural fluid may indicate the presence of microorganisms and/or white blood cells.

Amylase: Amylase levels may increase (as compared to upper normal limit for serum) with pancreatitis, esophageal rupture or malignancy.

Cholesterol: Normal cholesterol value runs parallel with serum values. It is above 200 mg/dL in case of pseudochylothorax and usually low in case of chylothorax.

Tumor markers: Normal value of tumor marker runs parallel with serum values.

For a definite diagnosis a panel of pleural fluid tumor markers including CEA, CA-125, CA 15-3 and CYFRA has been shown to reach a combined sensitivity of only 54%. Thus negative results do not help in investigation or monitoring. Mesothelin is a glycoprotein tumor marker that is present at higher mean concentrations in the blood and pleural fluid of patients with malignant mesothelioma than in patients with other causes of pleural effusion. Positive results have also been recognized in bronchogenic adenocarcinoma, metastatic pancreatic carcinoma, lymphoma and ovarian carcinoma. A positive serum or pleural fluid mesothelin level is highly suggestive of pleural malignancy but a negative result cannot be considered reassuring.

Glucose: In the absence of pleural pathology, glucose diffuses freely across the pleural membrane and the pleural fluid glucose concentration is equivalent to blood. A low pleural fluid glucose level (<3.4 mmol/L) may be found in complicated parapneumonic effusions, empyema, rheumatoid pleuritis and pleural effusions associated with TB, malignancy and esophageal rupture. The most common causes of a very low pleural fluid glucose level (<1.6 mmol/L) are rheumatoid arthritis and empyema.

LDH: Lactate levels can increase with infectious pleuritis, either bacterial or tuberculosis.

Triglyceride: Triglyceride levels may be increased with lymphatic system involvement and in case of chylothorax.

pH: Pleural fluid acidosis (pH <7.30) occurs in malignant effusions, complicated pleural infection, connective tissue diseases (particularly rheumatoid arthritis), TB and esophageal rupture. In isolation, it does not distinguish between these causes. Pleural fluid acidosis reflects an increase in lactic acid and carbon dioxide production. Increased consumption of glucose without replacement in the same conditions means that pleural fluid often has both a low pH and low glucose concentration.

Microscopic examination: Normal pleural fluid has small numbers of white blood cells (WBCs) but no red blood cells (RBCs) or microorganisms. Results of an evaluation of the different kinds of cells present may include:

Total cell counts—the WBCs and RBCs in the sample are counted. Increased WBCs may be seen with infections and other causes of pleuritis. If the pleural fluid differential cell count shows a predominant lymphocytosis (>50% cells are lymphocytes), the most likely diagnoses worldwide are malignancy and tuberculosis (TB). Cardiac failure, cirrhosis and other causes of transudates would also have lymphocyte predominance being chronic conditions.

Very high lymphocyte proportions (>80%) occur most frequently in TB, lymphoma, chronic rheumatoid pleurisy, sarcoidosis and late post-coronary artery bypass grafting (CABG) effusions.

- Increased RBCs may suggest trauma, malignancy, or pulmonary infarction.
- WBC differential—determination of percentages of different types of WBCs. An increased number of neutrophils may be seen with bacterial infections like in parapneumonic effusions, pulmonary embolism, acute TB and benign asbestos pleural effusions. An increased number of lymphocytes may be seen with cancers and tuberculosis. Pleural effusions in which >10% of cells are eosinophils are defined as eosinophilic; most common cause of which is air or blood in the pleural space. It can also occur in parapneumonic effusions, drug-induced pleurisy, benign asbestos pleural effusions, Churg-Strauss syndrome, lymphoma, pulmonary infarction and parasitic disease.
- Cytology—a cytocentrifuged sample is treated with a special stain and examined under a microscope for abnormal cells. This is often done when a mesothelioma or metastatic cancer is suspected. The presence of certain abnormal cells, such as tumor cells or immature blood cells, can indicate what type of cancer is involved. Infectious disease tests—these tests may be performed to look for microorganisms if infection is suspected:
    - Gram stain—for direct observation of bacteria or fungi under a microscope. There should be no organisms present in pleural fluid.
    - Bacterial culture and susceptibility testing—if bacteria are present, susceptibility testing can be performed to guide antimicrobial therapy. If there are no microorganisms present, it does not rule out an infection; they may be present in small numbers or their growth may be inhibited because of prior antibiotic therapy.

Specific Conditions and Tests

Tuberculous Pleurisy

When pleural biopsies are taken, they should be sent for both histological examination and culture to improve the diagnostic sensitivity for TB. Tuberculous effusion result from hypersensitivity reaction to mycobacterial protein and the mycobacterial load in the pleural fluid is usually low. Pleural fluid microscopy for acid-fast bacilli therefore has a sensitivity of <5% and pleural fluid culture of 10–20%. Thoracoscopic pleural biopsy has been shown to have a sensitivity of >70% for culture of pleural tissue and overall diagnostic sensitivity approaches 100% when evidence of caseating granulomas on pleural biopsy histology is combined with culture.

Diagnostic Markers of Pleural TB

It is desirable to consider diagnosis of tuberculosis in patients with lymphocytic effusions. In patients who are unsuitable for invasive investigations, pleural fluid or blood biomarkers of infection can be useful.

- **Adenosine deaminase (ADA)** is an enzyme present in lymphocytes, and its level in pleural fluid is significantly raised in most tuberculous pleural effusions. Raised ADA levels can also be seen in empyema, rheumatoid disease and occasionally in malignancy. Measurement of isoenzyme ADA-2 can reduce the false positives significantly. ADA is very cheap and quick to perform and remains stable when stored at 48°C for up to 28 days. It is useful in patients with HIV or those immunosuppressed (e.g. renal transplant). Being a highly sensitive test ADA is a useful 'rule out' test in countries with low prevalence of TB.
- **Interferon gamma release assays (IGRAs)** have been studied with sensitivities as high as 90%, but specificity is limited by an inability of the tests to distinguish latent from active TB. The commercial tests are not yet validated for fluids other than blood. Comparatively ADA is easier to perform and cost effective.

Connective Tissue Diseases

Rheumatoid arthritis and systemic lupus erythematosus (SLE) are the most common connective tissue diseases to involve the pleura. Pleural effusions occur due to primary autoimmune pleuritis or secondary to renal, cardiac, thromboembolic disease or drug therapy.

Rheumatoid Arthritis-associated Pleural Effusions

Pleural involvement occurs in 5% of patients with rheumatoid arthritis rheumatoid factor can be measured on the pleural fluid and often has a titer of >1:320. Most chronic pleural effusions secondary to rheumatoid arthritis have a very low glucose level of <1.6 mmol/L (29 mg/dL).

Rheumatoid arthritis-associated pleural effusions occur more frequently in men, although the disease itself is more common in women. Chronic rheumatoid effusions are the most common cause of pseudochylous (high cholesterol) effusion but they can also be serous or hemorrhagic in appearance. The measurement of triglycerides and cholesterol in milky effusions will confirm the diagnosis of a pseudochylous picture. Eighty percent of rheumatoid pleural effusions have a pleural fluid glucose to serum ratio of <0.5 and a pH <7.30.

Measurement of C4 complement in pleural fluid may be of additional help, with levels <0.04 g/L in all cases of rheumatoid pleural disease.

Systemic Lupus Erythematosus

Pleuritis is the first manifestation of systemic lupus erythematosus (SLE) in 5–10% of patients and an early feature in 25–30%, and is usually accompanied by multisystem involvement. Pleural effusions are frequently small and are bilateral in 50% of patients.

No definitive test distinguishes SLE pleuritis from other causes of exudative effusions. Elevated pleural fluid antinuclear antibodies (ANA) and an increased pleural fluid to serum ANA ratio is suggestive of SLE pleuritis, but elevation is also sometimes seen in malignant effusions.

PERITONEAL FLUID

Peritoneum is a tough semi-permeable membrane lining abdominal and visceral cavities. The organs of abdomen are enclosed in the peritoneum.

The peritoneum is important in osmoregulation.
- It controls passive diffusion of water and solute (up to a certain size).

- It maintains osmotic and chemical equilibrium with blood and lymph.

A fluid is present in between the layers of peritoneum; this is called as peritoneal fluid.

It is produced by mesothelial cells in the abdominal membranes. Peritoneal fluid acts to moisten the outside of the organs and to reduce the friction of organ movement during digestion.

Normal values of peritoneal fluid

Appearance: Light yellow, clear

Volume: Less than 50 mL

RBCs: Negative

WBCs: Less than 300/L

Protein: Less than 4.1 g/dL

Glucose: 70-100 mg/dL

Amylase: 138-404 units/L

Ammonia: Less than 50 mcg/dL

Alkaline phosphatase:

Female less than 45 years old: 76-196 units/L

Female more than 45 years old: 87-250 units/L

Male: 90-240 units/L

Lactate dehydrogenase (LDH): Should equal LDH blood levels

Cytology: Negative for the presence of abnormal cells

Bacteria: Negative

Fungi: Negative

Carcinoembryonic antigen (CEA): Negative for the presence of CEA.

Peritoneal fluid analysis is needed in two conditions:
1. In case of inflammation of the peritoneum called as peritonitis and/or
2. Excessive accumulation of peritoneal fluid called as peritoneal effusion or ascites.

Ascites develops either from:
- *Increased accumulation of fluid*: This happens when there is:
  - Increased capillary permeability
  - Increased venous pressure
  - Decreased protein (oncotic pressure)
- *Decreased clearance of fluid*: This happens when there is:
  - Increased lymphatic obstruction.

There are two main types of peritoneal fluid:
1. *Transudate:* The fluid that accumulates when there is an imbalance between the pressure within blood vessels (which drives fluid out of blood vessels) and the amount of protein in blood (which keeps fluid in blood vessels) in such case, the fluid is called as transudate.
2. *Exudate:* The fluid that accumulates when there is an injury or inflammation of the peritoneum, in such case the fluid is called as exudate.

Transudate	Exudate
90% of ascitic fluids are transudates	10% of ascitic fluids are exudates
Fluid appears clear	Fluid may appear cloudy
Albumin level—low	Albumin level—higher than in transudates
SAAG values above 1.1 g/dL	SAAG values less than 1.1 g/dL
Cell count—few cells are present	Cell count—increased
Transudates are most often caused by congestive heart failure or cirrhosis	Exudates may be the result of conditions such as infection (bacterial, viral or fungal), malignancies (metastatic cancer, lymphoma, mesothelioma), or autoimmune disease

Differentiation between the types of fluid is important because it helps to diagnose the likely cause of fluid accumulation. Initial set of tests (cell count, albumin level, and appearance of the fluid) is used to distinguish between transudates and exudates. Once the fluid is determined to be one or the other, additional tests may be performed to further pinpoint the disease or condition causing ascites.

Symptoms

Following symptoms can indicate peritoneal fluid accumulation:

- Abdominal pain and bloating
- Abdominal tenderness
- Fever
- Low urine output
- Chills
- Joint pain
- Nausea and vomiting

Diagnosis

Along with peritoneal fluid analysis, blood culture and CT scan or ultrasound of abdomen is to be done.

Sample Collection

A sample collection procedure of peritoneal fluid is called as paracentesis.

Paracentesis is the removal of peritoneal fluid from the abdominal cavity with a needle, tubing, and a container that may have a vacuum. The patient is positioned lying down with the head of the bed raised. A local anesthetic is applied and then the doctor inserts the needle into the abdominal cavity and the sample is removed.

Peritoneal Fluid Tests

Following tables interprets different aspects of peritoneal fluid analysis.

Gross Appearance

Clear to pale yellow	Normal
Milk-colored (Chylous)	- Malignant tumor, lymphoma, TB - Parasitic infection, hepatic cirrhosis
Cloudy/turbid	- Peritonitis, primary bacterial infection - Perforated bowel, appendicitis, pancreatitis - Strangulated or infarcted bowel
Bloody tap	- Benign or malignant tumor - Hemorrhagic pancreatitis, perforated ulcer - Internal bleeding

Paracentesis Biochemistry

	Levels	Interpretation
Triglyceride	Elevated	- Malignant tumor, lymphoma, TB - Parasitic infection, hepatic cirrhosis
Protein	- 0.3–4.0 g/dL - >4 g/dL	- Normal - TB, SBP (small bowel perforation)
Glucose	- 7–10 - <6	- Normal - TB and malignancy
Amylase	- 50% of serum level - Increased (up to 5 × serum level)	- Normal - Pancreatitis, pancreatic pseudocyst, pancreatic trauma or Intestinal strangulation
Alkaline phosphatase	Increased	Small bowel perforation and strangulation

Exudate Serum: Ascites Ratios

- *Evidence for these ascites*: Serum ratio is controversial
  - Ascitic fluid protein/serum protein >0.5
  - Ascitic fluid LDH/serum LDH >0.6
  - Ascitic fluid LDH >400.
- Presence of any 2 of these three findings is usually associated with TB, malignancy or pancreatitis.
- Absence of all three usually indicates hepatic cause.

The Serum-Ascites Albumin Gradient

- The serum-ascites albumin gradient (SAAG) is the most useful index for evaluating peritoneal fluid and can help distinguish ascites caused by portal hypertension (cirrhosis, portal vein thrombosis, Budd-Chiari syndrome, etc.) from other causes of ascites. In portal hypertension, the SAAG is >1.1 g/dL while ascites from other causes shows SAAG of less than 1.1 g/dL.
- Simple calculation:
  - Serum albumin—ascites albumin = SAAG.

SAAG > 1.1 mg/dL	SAAG < 1.1 mg/dL
- Cirrhosis - Alcoholic hepatitis - Cardiac ascites - "Mixed ascites" - Massive liver metastasis - Fulminant hepatic failure - Budd-Chiari syndrome - Portal vein thrombosis - Veno-occlusive disease - Myxedema - Fatty liver of pregnancy	- Peritoneal carcinomatosis - Tuberculous peritonitis - Pancreatic ascites - Bowel obstruction - Biliary ascites - Nephrotic syndrome - Postoperative lymphatic leak - Serositis in connective tissue disease

Microscopy and Analysis

Red cell count	Interpretation
- None - >100/µL - >100,000/µL	- Normal - Malignancy, TB - Intra-abdominal trauma (DPL-diagnostic peritoneal lavage)
White Cell Count	**Interpretation**
- <300/µL - >300/µL - >25% neutrophils - >25% lymphocytes - Mesothelial cells - Gram positive cocci - Gram negative	- Normal - Abnormal - SBP (90%), cirrhosis (50%) - TB or chylous ascites - TB peritonitis - Primary peritonitis - Secondary peritonitis

■ SYNOVIAL FLUID

Synovial fluid is formed as an ultrafiltrate of plasma across the synovial membrane. This is often referred to as joint fluid which is the viscous fluid found in the cavities of the moveable joints. This filtration is nonselective except for the exclusion of high molecular weight proteins. The contents of the synovial fluid are similar to the plasma values. This synovial fluid normally does not clot. But in inflammation due to increased fibrinogen may clot. The synovial cells lining the synovium secrete a mucopolysaccharide containing the hyaluronic acid and a small amount of the protein. This hyaluronic acid causes noticeable viscosity of the synovial fluid. The smooth articular cartilage and synovial fluid reduce friction between the bone during joint movements.

Sample Collection

Synovial fluid analysis is done to diagnose the cause of synovial fluid formation. Swelling and pain are the complaints from patients. It helps to differentiate inflammatory to non-inflammatory causes and arthritis due to crystals like gout and pseudogout. It is also done to monitor chronic arthritic diseases and to study malignant tumor involving the joint.

Synovial fluid is the aspirated fluid from the synovial spaces is called Arthrocentesis.

Collect specimen in three tubes:
1. Tube 1 sterile tube for culture.
2. Tube 2 for microscopy, add heparin and not use EDTA.
3. Tube 3 for chemistry, plain tube.

For glucose, the patient should have 6 hours fast.

Synovial fluid can be aspirated from joint of: Knee, Shoulder, Elbow, Wrist, Ankle, and Hip.

Procedure to collect sample:
- Sterile the area with an antiseptic solution, local anesthesia can be given to decrease the pain.
- Lay the patient on his or her back with the joint fully exposed.
- During aspiration, the joint may be wrapped with an elastic bandage to compress free fluid within a certain area to get maximum fluid.
- Insert a sterile needle into the joint space and get the synovial fluid for analysis.

Synovial fluid is present normally in a very small amount. The amount in the large knee joint is less than 3.5 mL. This fluid collection can increase in the inflammation and maybe around 25 mL. Synovial fluid contains mucopolysaccharides called hyaluronic acid which is responsible for the viscosity of the synovial fluid and lubricates the joints. An increase in a synovial fluid enough to aspirates is due to some disease.

Normal Constituents of the Synovial Fluid

Features	
Physical Features	
Volume	<1.5 mL
Color	Pale yellow
Clarity	Clear
Viscosity	• Can form a string 4 to 6 cm long due to high concentration of hyaluronic acid • Good mucin clot
Microscopic	
RBC count	<2000/cmm (0 to 2000/cmm)
White cell count	<200 /cmm (0 to 200/cmm)
Polys	<20% of the differential
Lymphocytes	<15% of the differential
Monocytes	65% of the differential
Macrophages	Variable in number
Crystals	Negative
Chemicals	
Glucose	<10 mg/dL lower than the blood level
Total protein	<3 g/dL (1 to 3 g/dL)
Lactate	<250 mg/dL
Uric acid	This is equal to the blood level (male = 2 to 8 mg/dL and female = 2 to 6 mg/dL)
Culture	Negative

Damage to the articular membrane produces pain and stiffness in the joints, this is referred to as arthritis.

There are following types of arthritis:

Etiological classification	Clinical significance
Non-inflammatory	Degenerative joint disease (Osteoarthritis) seen in old age
Inflammatory	An immunologic disorder like Rheumatoid arthritis, and SLE
Septic	Due to microbial infection like TB/viral/fungal
Hemorrhagic	Coagulation factor deficiency, and traumatic injury
Due to crystals	Increased fluid uric acid in gout, increased monocytes

Laboratory Tests Performed on Synovial Fluid

- Fluid analysis including:
  - WBC count: The differential of the cells.
  - Generally WBCs <200/cmm and RBCs <2000/µL.
  - Rheumatoid arthritis shows more lymphocytes (lymphocytosis).
- A glucose level may be done. Also, take the blood at the same time to estimate the serum glucose level (after the patient has fasted for 6 hours).
  - Glucose level falls in inflammation and lowest in septic arthritis.
  - In septic arthritis, this maybe 50% less than the blood glucose level.
  - Low glucose level is also seen in rheumatoid arthritis.
- Complement level may also be advised. The complement level is decreased in SLE, rheumatoid arthritis, and other immunologic arthritis.
- Estimate on synovial fluid protein, uric acid, and lactate.
  - Increased uric acid level indicates gout.
  - Increased protein and lactate level indicates a bacterial infection. In bacterial arthritis, there is an increased level of protein and lactate.
- Gram stain is done for the diagnosis of gonorrhea.
- AFB stain is done to rule out tubercle bacilli.
- Culture and sensitivity is advised for bacteria and the fungus.
- The calcium pyrophosphate dihydrate crystals are birefringent in pseudogout (blue on red background).
- Complement level is done which is low in—systemic lupus erythematosus and rheumatoid arthritis.

Characteristics of Synovial Fluid in Different Type of Arthritis

Test	Non-inflammatory	Inflammatory	Septic	Hemorrhagic
Color	Yellow, clear	Yellow to white	Yellow to green	Red to brown
Viscosity	High (good)	Low	Low	Low
TLC (cmm)	<5000	10,000 to 100,000	10,000 to 200,000	50 to 10,000
Etiology (causative agent)	Degenerative joint disorder	Immunologic, rheumatoid, lupus	Staph. aureus, H. influenzae, Strep, pneumococci, Neisseria	Trauma, anticoagulant therapy
Polys (%)	<25	>50	>75	>25
Protein (g/dL)	<3.0	>3.0	>3.0	>3.0
Lactate (mg/dL)	Normal	Normal to high	>250 positive	Normal
Glucose serum/fluid (mg/dL)	<10	>25	>25	<10
Glucose	Normal	Decreased	Decreased	Normal

In case of non-inflammatory joint disease as seen in osteoarthritis, traumatic arthritis and in neurogenic joint disease, the fluid is clear and viscous, with low cell count and glucose and protein are normal.

In case of inflammatory joint disease, rheumatoid arthritis and lupus arthritis the fluid is cloudy, yellow with low viscosity, moderately high cell count. Glucose is normal and protein is high. Cholesterol crystals are found in rheumatoid arthritis.

Synovial infections include mostly bacterial infections. The fluid is cloudy, may be yellow or green and milky with low viscosity, very high cell count, low glucose and high protein.

Polarized microscopy is performed for the presence of crystals.

Crystal-induced effusion is seen in gout and pseudogout. Here, the fluid is yellow, cell count may be increased, crystals seen. Monosodium urates seen in gout and calcium pyrophosphate dihydrate in pseudogout.

Hemorrhagic effusion is presence of red blood cells in traumatic injury, coagulation deficiencies and anticoagulation therapy.

CHAPTER 8

Urine Analysis

Learning Objectives
- A urinalysis is an important and cost-effective laboratory test for the assessment of kidney dysfunctions, various types of urinary tract diseases and may provide information about other systemic diseases, such as liver failure and hemolysis. Although it's used most frequently as a screening test, it can also be utilized for monitoring response to treatment or progression of a disease state
- This chapter includes detailed interpretation of Physical, Chemical and Microscopic examination of urine.
- Microscopic examination is illustrated with all possible and simplified diagrams

Keywords
Polyuria, Oliguria, Specific gravity, Albumin, Glucose, Glycosuria, Ketone bodies, Bile salts, Bile pigment, Urobilinogen, Occult blood, Casts, Crystals, Parasites

The normal urine is clear and yellow, amber colored due to the presence of pigment urochrome. An average healthy adult passes 1,000 to 1,600 mL of urine in 24 hours. Normally, the urine is clear when freshly voided but may be cloudy due to phosphates and growth of bacteria. All urine samples become cloudy or turbid upon standing and so freshly passed urine should be examined. First morning specimen after getting up from bed is best for routine examination. Post-prandial specimen is collected one and half to three hours after principal meal.

■ COLLECTION AND PRESERVATION

Containers used for collection of urine should be chemically clear. Urine for bacteriological examination should be collected aseptically, into sterile containers without preservation. Mid-stream of urine is preferred as it contains very few contaminating bacteria.

Urine may be preserved for quantitative examination in a refrigerator or a small piece of camphor or thymol is added. Other preservatives include 2% toluene and formalin. For microscopic examination one to two drops of formalin (for 30 mL of urine) can be used.

■ PHYSICAL EXAMINATION

Physical examination includes: Quantity, color, odor, appearance, reaction and specific gravity.

Quantity

Urinary output of a healthy adult male is 1500 mL/day. However, variations may occur. Women and children excrete less urine. A greater amount of urine is voided during day than at night.

a. **Daily output more than 2000 mL is known as polyuria**
   Causes of polyuria
   1. Excessive fluid intake particularly in cold weather
   2. Nervousness, excitement
   3. Diabetes mellitus and insipidus
   4. Hyperparathyroidism
   5. Renal failure.
b. **Daily output less than 500 mL is known as oliguria**
   Causes of oliguria
   1. Dehydration
   2. Cardiac decompensation
   3. Pyrexia with poor fluid intake
   4. Acute glomerulonephritis.
c. **Complete absence of urine formation is known as anuria**
   The different physiological conditions lead to anuria.

Color

Normal urine is pale yellow colored. Following abnormalities in different conditions are observed.

Color	Causes
Orange	Concentrated urine (restricted fluid intake), urobilin
Dark brown	Altered blood, myoglobin porphyrin
Red	Blood, beet root, aniline dyes
Brownish black	Methemoglobin, melanin
Cream	Carbolic acid, biliverdin, santonin
Milky	Chyle in urine
Cloudy	Phosphates, urates, bacterial contamination

Odor

Normal urine has aromatic odor, and on standing it is ammonical, due to ammonia released by the activity of bacteria.

Pathologically

- *Fruity or sweetish*: Ketone bodies
- *Putrid*: H_2S liberation, pus cells
- *Fecal*: Due to contamination with feces or coliforms
- *Ammonical*: Due to bacterial action.

Appearance

Normal urine is clear. It may develop slight turbidity on standing. These clouds settle at the bottom of the container, which consists of pus cells, RBCs, epithelial cells and mucus. Bacteria in large number cause uniform cloudiness. Turbidity is due to presence of urates, phosphates, hematuria and chemicals.

Reaction or pH

Normal urine is slightly acidic with pH 6 to 6.8. After full meal, the reaction may be alkaline or amphoteric. Reaction is measured by litmus paper or by nitrazine paper. It turns blue in alkaline and red in acidic urine. Nitrazine paper develops certain colors, which are then matched with standard colors.

Specific Gravity

The specific gravity varies inversely with quantity of urine. Normal average is 1.010 to 1.025. It is determined by urinometer or refractometer **(Fig. 8.1)** as:
- Take urine in a cylinder, up to nearly full; remove the froth of bubbles by filter paper. Float the urinometer, so that it does not touch the bottom or sides. Take the reading from lower meniscus.
- If the urine is insufficient, dilute it with an equal volume of distilled water, mix and take the specific gravity. The last two figures of the reading are multiplied by 2.

Example:
If the reading is 1.008, the specific gravity is,
$$08 \times 2 = 16$$
That is, = 1.016.
Albumin increases the specific gravity. In such cases, a correction by deducting 0.001 for every 1% of albumin in urine should be made.

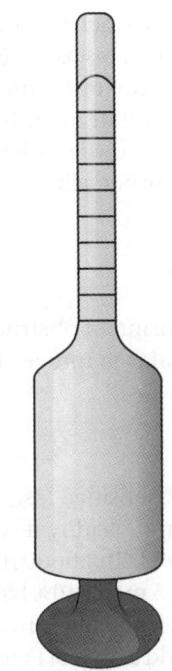

Fig. 8.1: Urinometer.

- High specific gravity is seen in excess sweating, glycosuria, acute nephritis, albuminuria and all causes of oliguria.
- Low specific gravity is seen in (less than 1.001) excessive water intake, chronic nephritis, diabetes insipidus, etc.

CHEMICAL EXAMINATION

It includes test for albumin, glucose, ketone bodies, bile salts, bile pigments, urobilinogen, etc.

Albumin

Normal urine may contain trace, i.e. up to 2 to 3 mg/100 mL of urine.

Albuminuria means presence of albumin and globulin in the urine. Following methods can detect albumin in urine.

a. *Heat and acid test:* Make urine slightly acidic by adding few drops of 10% acetic acid. Fill 3/4th of a test tube with clear and fresh urine, filter, if necessary, and boil the upper part. Turbidity indicates protein as phosphates. Add a few drops of 10% acetic acid, if the turbidity disappears, it was caused by phosphates and persistence or increasing cloudiness indicates albumin in urine.

False negative results may be obtained if the reaction of urine is alkaline or it has a low specific gravity.

If entire specimen of urine coagulates, the albumin usually amount 2 to 3%.

b. *Sulfosalicylic acid test:* The reagent contains sodium sulfate (750 g) and sulfosalicylic acid 50 g in 1000 mL of distilled water. Mix equal quantities of urine and reagent gently by the side of the tube. A white cloud indicates presence of protein. Sulfosalicylic acid precipitates urinary protease, polypeptides and Bence Jones proteins. A heavy precipitate to solid coagulation suggests 0.5% or more protein.

Causes of Albuminuria

Prolonged exposure to cold, pregnancy, severe muscular exertion, drugs and chemical poisoning, nephritis, tuberculosis or carcinoma of kidney, urethritis, prostatitis, etc.

Glucose

Normal urine does not contain glucose. Glucosuria means presence of glucose in urine. Following methods can detect glucose in urine.

Test for Glucose

(For reducing substances like fructose, lactose, galactose and pentose)

Benedict's test (Qualitative): Take 5 mL of Benedicts' qualitative reagent in test tube and add 0.5 mL of urine. Boil the content of tube. Let it stand on the rack for 5 to 10 minutes. The appearance of a yellow or red deposit indicates the presence of reducing substances, i.e. sugar. Cupric sulfate is reduced to cuprous oxide by boiling with reducing agents.

Report: A slight green color, light turbidity or a bluish white ppt or no change is reported as negative. A greenish color with a little yellow deposit is reported as a trace (+), green yellowish (++), orange (+++), and brick red (++++).

Nowadays, paper strips are available commercially, which are dipped in urine as directed and the color produced is matched against the color chart supplied.

Causes of Glycosuria

Diabetes mellitus, non-diabetic glycosuria includes emotional disturbances, hyperthyroidism, pregnancy, after ingestion of considerable carbohydrates, either anesthesia, in some infections, like pneumococcal pneumonia, etc.

Ketone Bodies

Ketone bodies comprise of acetone, acetoacetic acid and β-hydroxy-butyric acid. Ketone bodies are products of incomplete fat metabolism and their presence is indicative of acidosis. Ketonuria is commonly seen in uncontrolled diabetes mellitus, vomiting and diarrhea. It is also present in vomiting of pregnancy and in hunger strikers.

Following methods can detect ketone bodies in urine.

Rothera's Test

Saturate 10 mL urine with Rothera's mixture consisting of 99 parts of ammonium sulfate and 1 part of sodium nitroprusside. Add slowly about 2 mL of strong ammonia. Allow it to stand for 5 minutes. A purple color indicates presence of ketone bodies.

Nowadays acetest tablets are available for the detection of ketone bodies. In positive cases, addition of one drop of urine on this tablet results in the violet color formation within 30 seconds.

Presence of ketone bodies in urine is known as ketonuria. The causes include uncontrolled diabetes mellitus, starvation, dehydration and malnutrition, vomiting and diarrhea, etc.

Bile Salts (Hay's Test)

Bile salts consist of glycocholic acid and taurocholic acid. They lower the surface tension of the fluid and thus cause sulfur particles to sink.

Take about 3 to 5 inch column of urine in a small beaker or in a test tube. Sprinkle finely powered dry sulfur over the surface from a height of about half inch. If bile salts are present, the sulfur powder will sink at bottom.

The presence of bile salts indicates obstructive jaundice.

Bile Pigments

It is present in urine in obstructive jaundice and hepatocellular jaundice. The detection tests include:

Fouchet's Test

This is the most sensitive test. If the urine is alkaline or neutral, acidify it with few drops of (2%) acetic acid. To about 10 mL of acidic urine add about 5 mL or 10% barium chloride solution. Mix well and filter. To the residue on the filter paper add a drop of Fouchet's reagent. A green or blue color indicates presence of bile pigments, i.e. biliverdin and bilirubin respectively.

Urobilinogen

If the urine sample contains bile pigment it should be removed by addition of 1 part of 10% aqueous solution of calcium chloride to 4 parts of urine and filtering it.

To 10 mL of fresh urine add 1 mL of Ehrlich aldehyde reagent. Allow it to stand for 3 minutes. If red/cherry color is obtained, it indicates presence of urobilinogen in urine.

Occult Blood

Centrifuged urine deposit is the best to find the RBCs in the urine. Presence of more than one RBC per high power field (HPF) should be regarded as abnormal.

MICROSCOPIC EXAMINATION (FIG. 8.2)

For microscopical examination a fresh concentrated specimen, preferably overnight sample with restricted fluid intake, should be

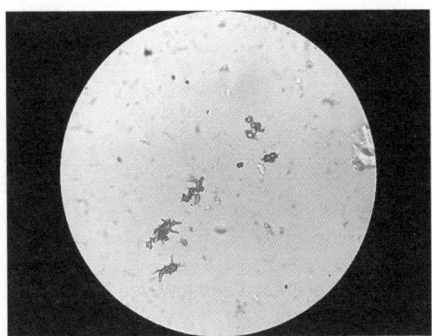

Fig. 8.2: Ammonium biurate crystals in urine.

examined for cells, casts and crystals. If the urine is diluted or contaminated, cells and casts dissolve very quickly.

Cells (Figs. 8.3A and B)

- *RBCs:* More than one per high power field is abnormal.
- *WBCs:* More than one per high power field is abnormal.
- *Epithelial Cells:* Squamous epithelial cells which may be excreted in moderate number are of no pathological importance.
  All other cells should be regarded as pathological.

Casts

Casts have paralleled edges, ends, round or broken. They may be straight or curved, long or short. The finding of cast is very important. Its presence is usually indicated in some form of kidney disorder. Following casts can be seen in different abnormal cases **(Figs. 8.4 and 8.5)**:
- *Hyaline casts:* It is colorless, homogenous, semi-transparent and cylindrical in shape. More than 1 per low power field is abnormal.
- *Granular casts:* These are hyaline casts, filled with granules.
- *Waxy casts:* These are more opaque than hyaline casts. It is usually seen in advanced chronic nephritis and amyloid disease.

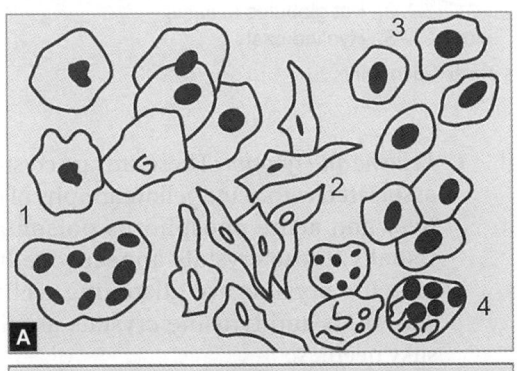

1. Transitional epithelial cells
2. Caudate epithelial cells
3. Renal epithelial cells
4. Renal epithelial cells with fatty degeneration

1. Pus cells in alkaline urine
2. Pus cells in acidic urine
3. Renal epithelial cells in acidic urine
4. Fresh RBCs
5. RBCs in urine with high specific gravity

Figs. 8.3A and B: Cells observed in urine.

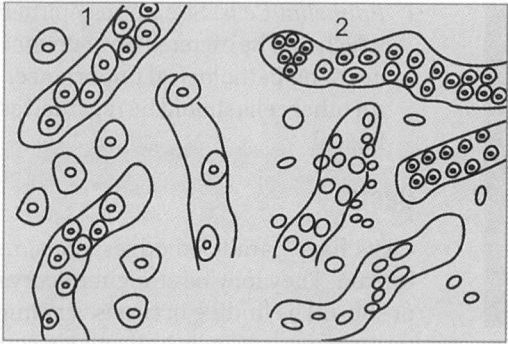

1. Epithelial casts and few free renal casts
2. Blood casts and few free RBCs

Fig. 8.4: Casts observed in urine.

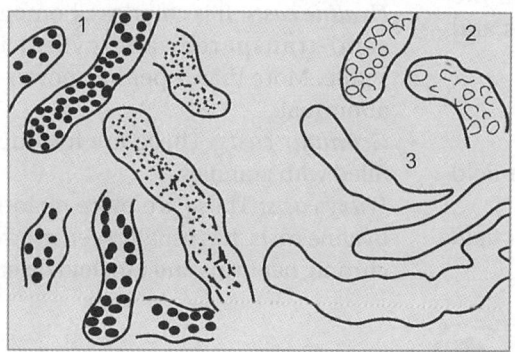

1. Coarse and fine granular casts
2. Fat globules in casts
3. Hyaline casts

Fig. 8.5: Casts observed in urine.

- *Epithelial casts:* These contain epithelial cells in it.
- *Fatty casts:* These contain numerous fat droplets.
- *Pus casts:* These are composed of pus cells.
- *Blood casts:* These contain RBCs in it.

Crystal

In acidic urine, uric acid and urates are found in different forms, usually colored. The crystals include (**Figs. 8.6 to 8.8**):
- *Oxalate:* They are in the form of envelopes and sometimes can be seen as dumb-bells or biscuit shaped, i.e. calcium oxalate.
- *Cystine:* They are colorless and hexagonal. These are soluble in alkalis. Their presence is pathogenic.
- *Leucine and tyrosine:* These are rare crystals, associated with acute yellow atrophy of the liver and acute phosphorus poisoning. Usually, these crystals appear together. Leucine crystals are glistening; yellow spheroids and tyrosine crystals are fine silky needles.

In alkaline urine, following crystals are found.
- *Amorphous calcium and magnesium phosphates:* It is the commonest urinary sediments in the alkaline urine. It has no significance. It looks like small colorless granules.
- *Ammonium, magnesium (Triple) phosphate crystals:* It appears as incomplete, irregular and colorless prisms, which vary in size and shapes.

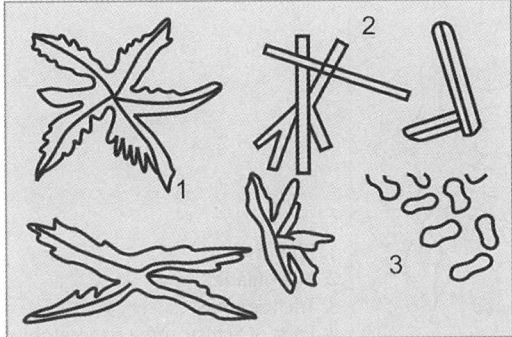

1. Triple phosphate crystals
2. Unusual urinary crystals
3. Calcium carbonate

Fig. 8.6: Crystals observed in urine.

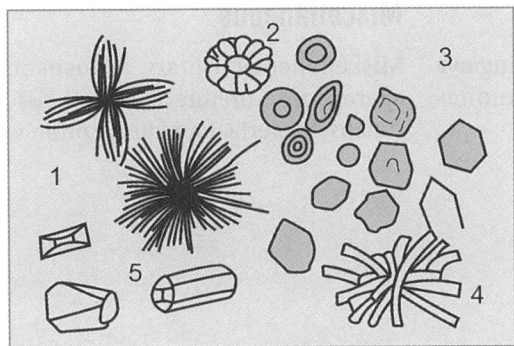

1. Tyrosine crystals
2. Leucine spheres
3. Cystine crystals
4. Calcium phosphate crystals
5. Triple phosphate crystals

Fig. 8.7: Crystals observed in urine.

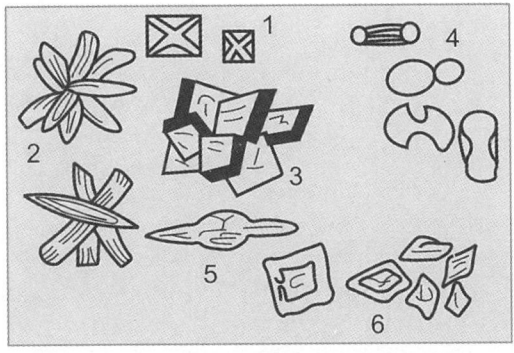

1. Calcium oxalate crystal
2. Rosette form of uric acid crystal
3. Whetstone form of uric acid crystal
4. Envelope shaped calcium oxalate crystal
5 and 6. Rhombic and pointed uric acid crystals

Fig. 8.8: Crystals observed in urine.

- *Magnesium phosphates:* These are elongated rhomboid flakes, large and refractive. Some are with rough edges and surfaces.

- *Calcium carbonate:* Sometimes this is found in alkaline urine. It is a dumb-bell shaped, often found in pairs.

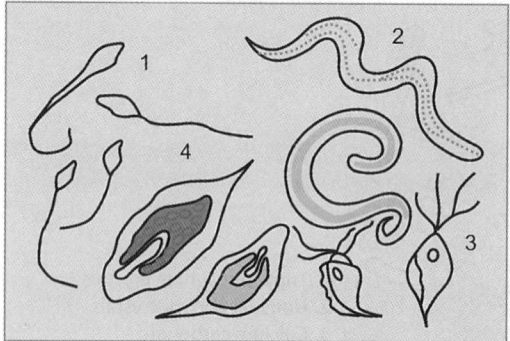

1. Sperms
2. Microfilaria
3. Trichomonas
4. Eggs of Schistosoma haematobium

Fig. 8.9: Miscellaneous things observed in urine.

Parasites

Urinany parasites are very few, including ova of schistosoma, microfilaria, trichomonas vaginalis and *Echinococcus* **(Fig. 8.9)**.

Miscellaneous

Miscellaneous urinary deposits includes—spermatozoa, urethral filaments, tissue debris, mucus, bacteria, hair, dust, cotton wool, etc.

CHAPTER 9

Stool Analysis

Learning Objectives
- A stool analysis is a series of tests done on a stool (feces) sample to help diagnose certain conditions affecting the digestive tract. These conditions can include infection (such as from parasites, viruses, or bacteria), poor nutrient absorption, or cancer.
- This chapter includes detailed interpretation of Macroscopic, Chemical and Microscopic examination of stool

Keywords
Calculus, Parasites, Crystals, Concentration method for ova and cyst, Occult blood

■ INTRODUCTION

The stool of a healthy adult on an ordinary mixed diet is well formed, semisolid in consistency, reaction is alkaline or neutral, and brown in color. The feces are normally, composed of 25% of fecal matter while rest of it is water. In certain diseases, the feces may contain such substances which are not normally present in healthy individual such as blood, mucus, parasites, intestinal calculi, pus, and pathogenic organisms (bacteria, fungi and viruses), etc.

The amount of adult stool is nearly 150 to 250 g/day. Stool should be collected in a clean, dry covered container and should not be mixed with urine.

The stool should be examined for macroscopic examination, chemical examination, and microscopic examination.

■ MACROSOPIC EXAMINATION

Stool should be examined macroscopically for following points:

Color

Normal stool is light, or dark brown in color. Following abnormal colors are found:

Green—in infantile diarrhea.

Clay—in obstructive jaundice, excess of fat, tuberculous peritonitis.

Dark brown or bright red—bleeding from distal colon.

Streaks of bright red blood—piles, fissures, carcinoma of rectum.

Black—gastrointestinal bleeding, tuberculosis.

Odor

Odorless after use of oral antibiotics, foul smelling in acute enteritis, malignant ulcer in rectum and distal colon.

Mucus

Mucus is seen in bacillary dysentery.

Pus

Pus with blood and mucus present in ulcerative colitis, bacillary dysentery, regional enteritis.

Calculus

Gallstones may be seen in feces.

Blood

Impart a dark red to black color and a terry consistency.

It is indicative of ulceration or presence of any other pathology like malignancy.

Parasites

Segments of tapeworm and roundworm may be seen in respective infections.

CHEMICAL EXAMINATION

Normally, pH of stool is 6.8 to 7.3 on mixed diet. Excess of carbohydrate diet produces acidity and excess of proteins produce alkalinity.

Occult Blood Test

Make a suspension of feces and boil for two minutes to destroy, oxidize and inactivate bacteria or enzymes. Cool and add 2 mL of saturated solution of benzidine in glacial acetic acid, mix well and add 1 mL (30%) hydrogen peroxide. Orthotolidine or guaiac solution can be used instead of benzidine solution.

A deep blue color indicates the presence of hemoglobin.

The presence of blood in the stool is of great significance in diagnosing the disease of inflammatory, neoplastic or ulcerative origin of gastrointestinal tract.

Iron may affect the test, so patient should not take meat diet, green vegetable, or iron in any form.

MICROSCOPIC EXAMINATION (FIGS. 9.1 AND 9.2)

Saline or iodine preparation should be made and examined with the low and high power objectives.

Various ova or cysts may be seen (**Fig. 9.3**) as abnormal constituents of stool. This includes ovas of following parasites:

i. Hookworm
ii. Ascaris (Roundworm)
iii. *Trichuris trichiura*
iv. *Taenia*
v. *E. vermicularis*
vi. *H. nana*

Other Abnormalities

- Vegetable cells and fibers—in case of indigestion.
- Starch granules—in carbohydrate dyspepsia.
- Muscle and elastic fiber.
- Fats and fatty acids in fatty dyspepsia.
- Cells—abnormal cells in stool includes— epithelial, pus cells, macrophages, short cells, eosinophils, RBCs.

Crystals

The abnormal crystals includes:
- Calcium oxalate, triple phosphate crystals, fatty acid crystals.
- Needle shaped crystals is seen in ulcerative conditions of intensive dysentery, malignant ulcers, etc.

Besides these, various bacteria, protozoa, metazoa, yeast and fungi may also be seen in stool examination.

Concentration Methods for Ova and Cyst

Take about one gram of feces and thoroughly emulsify with super saturated sodium chloride solution in water in a suitable container. The container should have diameter as well as depth of about one inch. The container is so filled with the emulsion that a slide placed on it just touches the preparation. The slide is

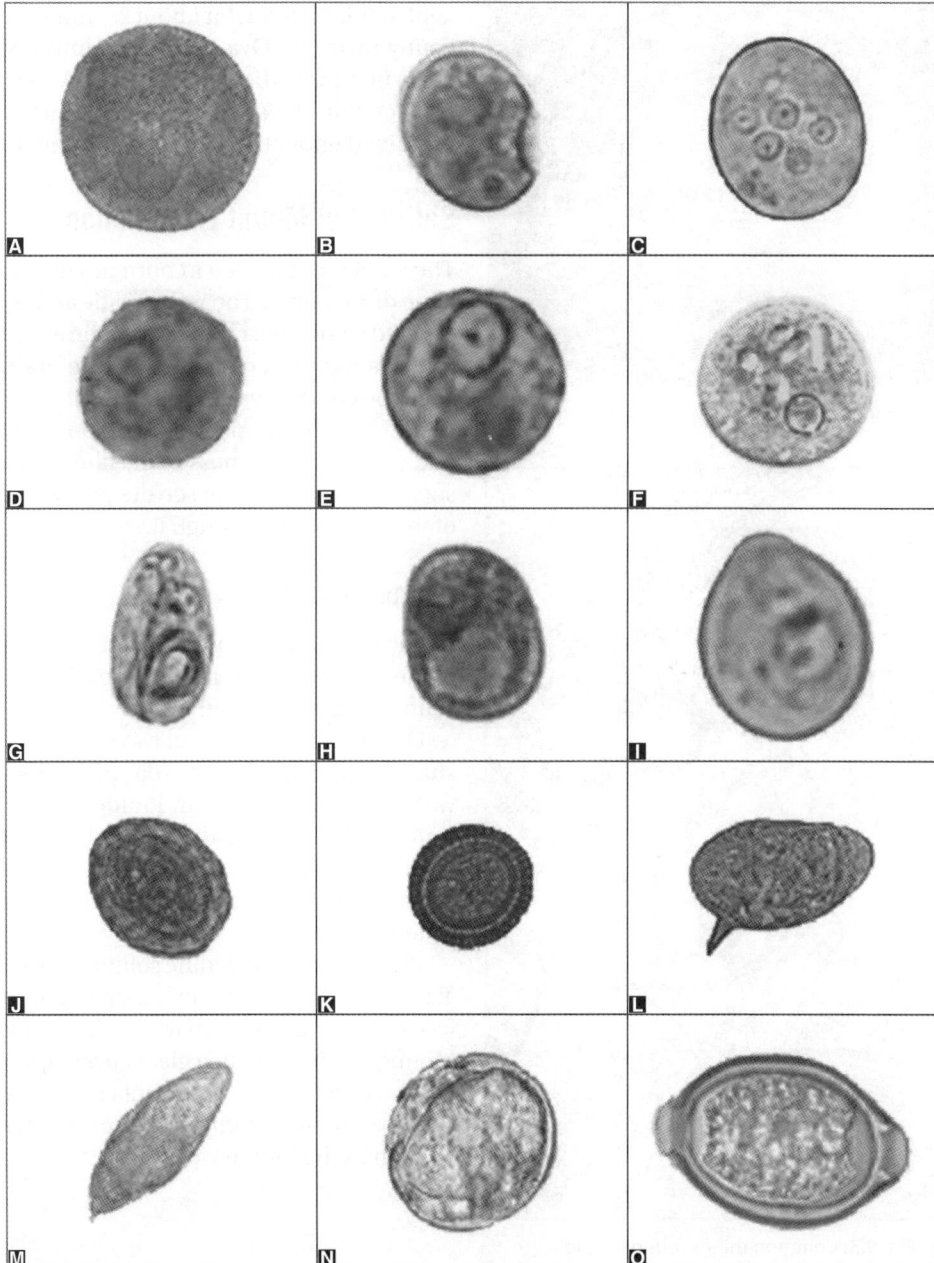

Figs. 9.1A to O: Microscopic images of each of the 15 types of parasites to recognize. (A) *Balantidium coli* cyst; (B) *Endolimax nana* cyst; (C) *Entamoeba coli* cyst; (D) *Entamoeba hartmanni* cyst; (E) *Entamoeba histolytica* cyst; (F) *Entamoeba polecki* cyst; (G) *Giardia lamblia* cyst; (H) *Iodamoeba butschlii* cyst; (I) *Chilomastix mesnili* cyst; (J) *Ascaris* egg; (K) Tapeworm egg; (L) *Schistosoma mansoni* egg; (M) *Schistosoma intercalatum* egg; (N) *Schistosoma japonicum* egg; (O) Whipworm egg.

(For color version See Color Plate 2)

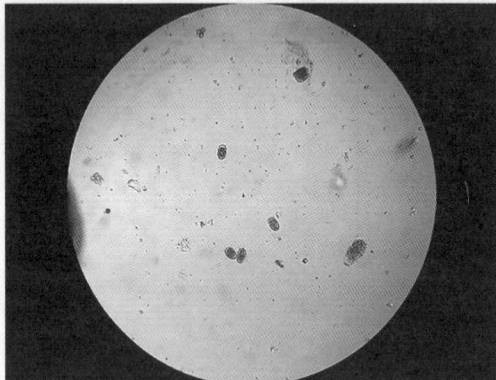

Fig. 9.2: Ova of hook worm in stool.

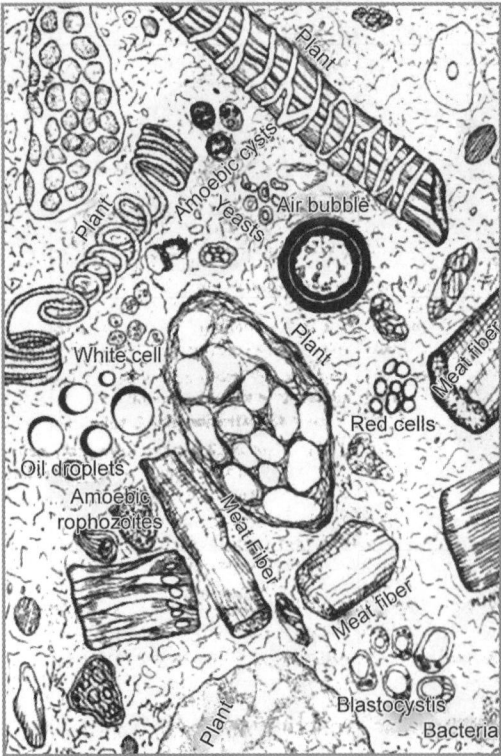

Fig. 9.3: Common things found in stool.

kept in this position for about 25 minutes, and gently inverted. Ova of many helminths will float and stick to the slide **(Fig. 9.1)**. A coverslip is placed on the slide and the preparation is examined under the low power of microscope.

Saline Wet Mount Examination

The stool is emulsified in normal saline and a large drop is placed on a glass slide and is then covered with a cover slip. This is then examined under a light microscope. It is preferable to keep the condenser down and the intensity of the light low for proper visualization of the ova and cysts. The thickness of the film should be such that one is able to see the printed letters of the newspaper through it.

Iodine Preparation

Iodine preparation leads to better visualization of morphological details of ova and cysts as it stains the glycogen in them.

One gram of iodine and two gram of potassium iodide is mixed in 100 mL of distilled water. At first, Potassium iodide is mixed in water and then the iodine crystals are added and it is shaken vigorously. The solution is then filtered into a dark glass bottle and kept away from light.

Place one drop of iodine solution on a clean glass slide. Thoroughly mix a small portion of feces or fecal suspension with iodine solution. Mount specimen with a glass coverslip.

It however has the disadvantage that the live trophozoites of *Entamoeba histolytica* cannot be seen as the iodine kills it.

CHAPTER 10

Sputum Examination

Learning Objectives
- Clinical diagnostic sputum examination aim to detect the causes of lower respiratory tract infections and some other diseases. It also provides an efficacious tool for monitoring the effectiveness of clinical treatment
- This chapter introduces different invasive and noninvasive methods of sputum collection and physical analysis of sputum
- Different staining techniques and microscopic analysis to observe mainly tuberculosis bacteria are also discussed in this chapter

Keywords
Bronchoscopy, Mucopurulent, Ziehl-Neelsen staining, Acid-fast bacilli, Auramine-Rhodamine method, Gram staining, Bronchogenic carcinoma, Sputum culture

▌INTRODUCTION

Respiratory tract consists of trachea and a pair of bronchi. Trachea (windpipe) connects mouth to lungs. It splits into separate channels called bronchi, which funnel air into lungs. Mucus is produced in the respiratory tract by goblet cells and seromucous glands of epithelium.

The presence of infection can increase and change the nature of mucus leading to sputum or phlegm formation. Smoke or air pollution can stimulate its production.

Normal Content and Function

Sputum is made up from mucus, dead cells, foreign matter that is breathed into the lungs, such as tar from cigarettes and air pollutants, white blood cells and other immune cells. Immune cells serve to kill or engulf bacteria so that they are unable cause infections in lung.

The thickness of sputum serves to trap foreign material so that the cilia in the respiratory tract can clear it from the lungs by moving it up through the mouth where it can be swallowed or coughed out. Coughing is body's natural mechanism to get rid of sputum or phlegm.

▌CLINICAL SIGNIFICANCE

Sputum examination is done for identification of causative agent or organism associated with a particular suspected infection of the lower respiratory tract, e.g.
- Suspected tuberculosis
- Pneumonia especially if severe or in an immunocompromised host such as— *Pneumocystis carinii* pneumonia in HIV-positive patients
- Suspected fungal infection
- Infective exacerbation of a chronic disease like bronchiectasis.

Cytological examination is carried out for the investigation of viral infections in cytomegalovirus and herpes simplex infections, fungal infection, asbestosis and malignant cells.

Collection of Sputum Sample

Specimens should be collected in containers of capacity 30 to 50 ml that are sterile, clear, plastic and leak-proof.

Sputum samples can be obtained using a non-invasive or invasive method. Ideally it should be collected before antibiotics are started. During specimen collection, patients produce an aerosol that may be hazardous to healthcare workers or other patients in close proximity. For this reason, precautionary measures for infection control must be followed during sputum collection.

Noninvasive Method

- Patients should be provided with an explanation of the specimen required, pointing out the difference between oral secretions and sputum.
- A leaflet with photographs explaining sputum collection is recommended.
- Sputum sample is ideally collected in the morning (since secretions accumulate overnight), soon after awakening and before taking any mouthwash or food.
- Ask the patient to take several deep breaths—breathing through the nose and exhaling through the mouth, to help loosen secretions.
- Ask the patient to force a deep cough to ensure a sample is obtained from the lower respiratory tract.
- The patient should expectorate into the specimen pot and secure the lid to prevent contamination. Ensure the specimen is sputum rather than saliva, which can be misleading.
- Collect 3 deeply coughed sputum specimens on 3 separate days (in a gap of 8 to 24 hours).
- Label container as surname, first given name, date of birth and the date/time of collection.

Invasive methods of sputum collection include induced sputum and bronchoscopy.

Induced: For patients unable to cough up sputum, deep sputum-producing coughing may be induced. This can be done by inhalation of 10 ml of an aerosol of warm, sterile, hypertonic saline (3–5% NaCl) via an ultrasonic nebulizer. Because induced sputum is very watery and resembles saliva, it should be labeled "induced" to avoid any confusion.

Bronchoscopy: A bronchoscopy (bronchi and scope-to-view) is a medical procedure that allows visualization of the inside of a person's respiratory tract (bronchi). Bronchoscopy might be needed for specimen collection, especially if previous results have been negative and doubt exists as to be positive.

Bronchoscopy is performed as follows:
- A local anesthetic is sprayed into nose and throat to numb them.
- A sedative might be given to help relax to patient. General anesthesia is not usually needed for bronchoscopy.
- The bronchoscope is a soft, small tube with a light and magnifying glass on the end. Doctor inserts it through nose or mouth, into lungs.
- Doctor can look inside the lungs using a magnifying glass, and they can use the scope to remove a sample of sputum.

Sputum thus collected has to be processed within four hours of collection. If any delay, it can be kept in refrigerator for 24 hours. In case transportation is needed, it is suggestible to transport after preparing slide from the sample. Special transportation medium is used if sputum sample has to be transported at greater distance or kept for longer duration. This serves to liquefy and decontaminate sputum. It can preserve sputum for 8 days.

Composition of transport medium	N-cetylpyridinium chloride	0.5 g
	Sodium chloride	1.0 g
	Distilled water	100 mL

Transport medium and sputum sample should be mixed in equal quantities.

Sputum Analysis

Sputum analysis is used to screen for disease and to monitor patient response to drug and nondrug therapy. It consists of macroscopic and microscopic assessments of the sputum.

■ MACROSCOPIC ASSESSMENT

Sputum is described by its color and consistency. Following terminology is used to describe it.

Mucoid	Containing or resembling mucous
Purulent	Containing pus
Mucopurulent	Containing pus and mucous
Frothy	Visible froth
Frothy	Visible froth
Viscous	Thick and sticky

Sputum can be of many colors and consistency. This can help define certain conditions.

Examples are:
- *Clear sputum:* Clear sputum is usually normal, although it may be increased in some lung diseases.
- *Dark yellow/green sputum:* Bacterial infections of the lower respiratory tract, such as pneumonia, may result in the production of green sputum. Yellow-green sputum is common with cystic fibrosis.
- *Brown sputum:* Brown sputum is due to the presence of tar, is sometimes found in people who smoke. Sputum may also appear brown or black due to the presence of old blood. Brown sputum is also common with "black lung disease." These diseases, called pneumoconiosis, occur from inhaling substances like coal into the lungs.
- *Pink sputum:* Pink, especially frothy pink sputum may come from pulmonary edema, a condition in which fluid and small amounts of blood leak from capillaries into the alveoli of the lungs.
- *Bloody sputum:* Coughing up blood (hemoptysis) can be the first sign of lung cancer. Bloody sputum may also occur with a pulmonary tuberculosis and lung abscess.
- *Uniformly rusty:* Appearing purulent sputum is indicative of pneumococcal (*Streptococcus pneumoniae*) pneumonia.

Odor

Normal sputum is odorless. Foul-smelling sputum is indicative of a bacterial infection.

Viscosity

Normal sputum is thin and watery. Patients with asthma have very thick, sticky, tenacious sputum.

Volume

Very little sputum is produced normally. The volume of sputum is increased in a variety of diseases, including bronchitis, pneumonia, and tuberculosis.

■ SPUTUM MICROSCOPY

Sputum microscopy refers to the microscopic investigation of sputum. This is one of the most efficient methods of identifying tuberculosis infection.

Ziehl-Neelsen Technique (Acid-Fast Bacilli Staining)

Ziehl-Neelsen staining method is an acid-fast staining method used to determine the presence of acid fact bacteria such as the *Mycobacterium tuberculosis*, which causes tuberculosis. The bright field microscopy is used for this technique.

Principle

Acid-fast bacteria like *Mycobacterium* have a lipoid capsule that gives its cell wall a waxy appearance. The cell wall also contains large amounts of mycolic acids and fatty acids. Due to these compounds in the cell wall of acid-fast bacteria, it requires a special technique with regards to staining. During staining, the primary stain is able to penetrate and enter the cell wall of acid fast bacteria because the stain is lipid soluble. Heating also enhances this. When a decolorizer is used (sulphuric acid), acid-fast bacteria retain the primary stain because of the characteristic of their cell wall while the non-acid fast microorganism loses the stain. When the counter stain is used, it is readily taken up by the non-acid fast microorganisms, but not the acid-fast bacteria.

Procedure

- Make sure to use a pair of gloves when handling biological fluids like sputum
- Carefully open the container (that contains the sputum sample) and using a laboratory burning stick (dry) obtain and spread a small amount at the central part of a microscope glass slide. Use rotational movement to create a good smear
- Place the slide on a drying rack and allow it to dry for about 30 minutes or use a dryer to dry the smear faster
- Pass the slide over the Bunsen burner flame 3 to 4 times to heat fix it
- Place the slide on the staining rack and pour the carbol fuchsin stain (primary stain) to cover the smear and heat until it starts evaporating—do not overheat
- Allow the slide to stand for between 4 and 7 minutes then wash with water
- Pour 20% sulphuric acid (decolorizer) on the smear and allow it to stand for a minute. Repeat this until the smear appears pink in color
- Wash the slide with water and cover the slide with malachite green stain or methylene blue (counter or secondary stain) and allow the slide to stand for about 2 minutes
- Wash the slide with water and allow the slide to dry on the drying/draining rack—use a tissue paper to clear the slides and back of the slide
- Observe the slide under the microscope using 100x oil immersion objective.

Observation

Reading of smears must be systematic and standardized to ensure that a representative area of the smear is examined. To ensure that an area is covered only once, the smear should be examined in an orderly manner and the following procedure is recommended:

Focus the stained slide under low power objective lens (5x or 10x) and, observe the staining quality and evenness of smear. Select the field where the smear is evenly distributed and WBCs and mucus can be seen. Apply a drop of immersion oil on the stained smear and focus the smear using 100x. Make a series of systematic examination over the length of the smear. After examining a microscopic field, move the slide longitudinally so that the neighboring field to the right can be examined. Search each field thoroughly. Examine a minimum of 100 fields before the smear is reported as negative. If the bacteria is present in the sample, it will appear as pink rods that are either straight or slightly curved while the background will appear bluish in color.

Grading of AFB smears as per WHO recommendation:

- No of acid-fast bacilli (AFB) in 100 immersion fields Negative
- 1-9 AFB in 100 immersion fields Positive scanty record exact figure
- 10 to 99 AFB in 100 immersion fields 1+
- 1 to 10 AFB per field (examine 50 fields) 2+
- More than 10 AFB per field (examine 20 fields) 3+

Fluorescence Microscopy

A fluorescence microscope is a compound microscope that applies the use of fluorescence and phosphorescence to observe the object. With this microscopy technique, the specimen under investigation is the source of light. This technique is also important for sputum microscopy.

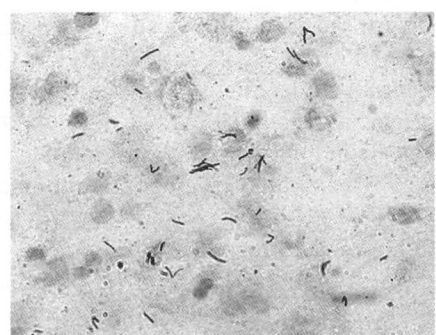

Fig. 10.1: 3+ slide of AFB stained with ZN stain.
(For color version See Color Plate 3)

Auramine-Rhodamine Method

Also referred to as Truant staining method, Auramine-Rhodamine staining method is one of the methods used for viewing and studying the acid-fast bacteria (bacilli). This method is not only easy, but also quick to use, which has made it one of the best alternatives to Ziehl-Neelsen technique today.

Principle

Auramine-Rhodamine (primary stain) is a fluorochrome dye that has affinity for acid-fast organisms. When it comes in contact with the cell wall of the bacteria, it forms a complex with the mycolic acid present in the cell wall. Heat fixing enhances this process making it difficult to decolorize when acid alcohol is used. Here, the secondary stain/counter stain used is potassium permanganate.

This stain is used to make other debris nonfluorescent so that they may not be seen when viewing under the microscope. Therefore, only the cells that take up the primary stain can be seen.

Procedure

- Using a burning stick (or wire loop) obtain and make a small smear at the center of a glass slide
- Pass the slide over the Bunsen burner flame 3 to 4 times to heat fix
- Flood the slide with auramine stain (primary stain) and allow to stand for 15 minute—cover the smear with the stain
- Rinse the smear with distilled water until no color remains—do not use chlorine water
- Flood the slide with acid alcohol (decolorizer) for about 3 minutes
- Wash the slide using distilled water
- Flood the slide with potassium permanganate (counter stain) for about 2 minutes
- Rinse with distilled water and allow to dry
- Observe under the microscope starting with low magnification and then high magnification

Observation

If acid-fast bacilli are present in the sample, it will appear as yellow or bright orange in color with a dark background.

Gram Staining

Gram staining method is used for the purposes of distinguishing between gram-positive and gram-negative bacteria. This technique has also been use for studying sputum.

Procedure

- Using a burning stick or cotton swab, obtain a small amount of the sample and make a smear at the center of the glass slide—try making a thin slide
- Place the slide on drying rack and allow to dry
- Pass the slide over the flame several times, to heat fix the smear but avoid overheating
- Flood the smear with crystal violet and allow to stand for about a minute
- Tilt the slide and rinse with distilled water
- Flood the slide with Gram's iodine for about one minute
- Tilt slide and rinse with water
- Tilt the slide and apply the alcohol drop by drop until it runs clear (95% ethyl alcohol/acetone)
- Rinse with water

- Flood the slide with safranin for about a minute
- Tilt slide and rinse with distilled water
- Blot the slide dry
- View under the microscope under high power (oil immersion)

Observation

Gram staining is aimed to observe bacterial infection. Because of the presence of various contaminating gram-positive and gram-negative microorganism deriving from throat and mouth (normal bacterial flora), Gram stained smear of sputum should be elucidated carefully.

Morphological appearance of bacterial cells on Gram stained smear is redolent of a particular microorganism as follows:
- Gram-negative diplococci: *Moraxella catarrhalis*.
- Gram-positive yeast cells with budding and pseudohyphae: *Candida*.
- Gram-positive diplococci with surrounding clear space: *Streptococcus pneumoniae*
- Gram-negative coccobacilli: *Haemophilus influenzae*.
- Gram-negative rods: *Pseudomonas spp*.
- Gram-positive cocci in grape-like clusters: *Staphylococcus aureus*.
- Large granules with center gram-negative and periphery gram-positive: *Actinomyces*.

Cytological Examination

Cytological examination of sputum is normally carried out for the diagnosis of bronchogenic carcinoma. Occasionally, it may also be useful in the identification of fungi, protozoa, asbestos bodies and viral inclusions (like those of *Cytomegalovirus* and *Herpes simplex* virus).

If asthma or other allergic condition is suspected, mix one drop of sputum with one drop of alkaline eosin solution and observe under microscope. Observe for Charcot-Leyden crystals. These are derived from eosinophils and can be seen as hexagonal, double pointed, slender crystals.

If a fungal infection is suspected, mix sputum with 10 g/dL KOH or NaOH solution and observe under microscope. Opportunistic fungi such as *Aspergillus* can be developed in patients with long-term antibiotics or steroid therapy. These can be seen as large rounded mass of cell.

To check for presence of lung cancer, a thin sputum smear is prepared on clean, sterile, grease-free glass slide from a yellowish, grayish, opaque, or blood-tinged portion, or from tissue fragments in sputum. It is then stained with Papanicolaou technique. Bronchial epithelial cells or alveolar macrophages are seen in the smear. This can be observed as nucleus with blue-violet color against pink-colored cytoplasm.

■ SPUTUM CULTURE

Sputum culture performed in microbiology laboratory is usually carried out for:
- Identification of a particular species, for the purpose of incidence, distribution, and control of diseases.
- Drug susceptibility testing.
- Diagnosis in patients who have distinctive radiological and clinical features of tuberculosis but are sputum smear-negative.

Sputum culture is more sensitive as compared to sputum smear examination. It can detect 10 to 100 microorganisms in per ml of sputum sample. Contaminating bacteria grows rapidly and digest the culture medium prior infective or tubercle bacilli begin to grow. Therefore, it is necessary to decontaminate the sputum sample by adding 4% sodium hydroxide (used as decontaminating agent). Contaminating normal flora is washed away with this step.

Cultural Procedures and Interpretation

Saline washed suspension of sputum specimen is taken and inoculated in three primary culture media. A suggested routine set of culture media is as follows:

- Blood agar for Pneumococci
- MacConkey or Eosin Methylene Blue (EMB) for gram-negative rods
- Chocolate agar anaerobic incubation for *Haemophilus influenzae*.

The blood agar and chocolate agar plates are incubated at 35-36 °C in an atmosphere containing extra carbon dioxide (e.g., in a candle jar) and the MacConkey plate is incubated in aerobic condition. Cultures should be inspected after incubation overnight (18 hours) but re-incubation for an extra 24 hours may be indicated when growth is less than expected from the microscopic findings.

Typical findings include the following:
- On blood agar, small, shiny colonies with concave centers and zones of green (alpha) hemolysis, as well as a zone of inhibition of growth around the optochin disc, may be *Streptococcus pneumoniae*.
- Tiny, water-drop, grey colonies on the chocolate agar suggest the presence of *H. influenzae*.
- Colonies on MacConkey agar suggest that *Enterobacteriaceae* or *Pseudomonas spp* or *Acinetobacter spp* are present. These organisms are usually not clinically relevant.
- Whitish, round, matt colonies on the blood agar and chocolate agar plates may be *Candida albicans*.

Confirmation of particular species from culture plate is to be done by performing specific set of biochemical tests.

For the isolation of *M. tuberculosis*, Lowenstein-Jensen medium is used. Its sensitivity for the identification of tuberculosis is 80-85%. However, this procedure is very expensive but reliable. It takes up to 6 weeks for the visible mycobacterial growth. This is very helpful for drug susceptibility testing.

Commercial Automated Culture Systems

Nowadays, rapid automated culture systems are available commercially which can give results within two weeks (instead of six weeks with standard media). However, this procedure is expensive. Examples of such systems are BACTEC™ 460TB system and BACTEC™ 9050 automatic blood culture analyzer (Becton-Dickinson Diagnostic Instruments Systems). These instruments are very sensitive and can detect *M. tuberculosis* in clinical samples. In this method, broth is used in which radiolabeled 14C-palmitate has been integrated. Mycobacteria metabolize 14C-palmitate to radiolabeled $^{14}CO_2$, which is further detected by the instrument.

CHAPTER 11

Automation in Pathology Laboratory

Learning Objectives
- The abundant and multifaceted advancements of automation technologies have also generated a profound impact on the organization of clinical laboratories, where many manual tasks have now been partially or completely replaced by automated and labor-saving instrumentation. Automation adds value to the test result with faster, improved accuracy, precision and safety.
- This chapter aims to keep readers updated with latest technologies, with its pros and cons.
- This chapter throws light on different types of analyzers which can be used in pathology laboratory, urilizers, multistix urinalysis strips and PCR. Illustration with appropriate pictures makes it easy to understand.

Keywords
Continuous flow analyzers, Discrete analyzers, Batch analyzers, Stat analyzers, Urilyzer, Multistix urinalysis strips, PCR

AUTOMATION OBJECTIVE

Advances in diagnostic methodologies and instrumentation have been impressive. This chapter tries to cover the automation required for the analysis of samples. During the past few years, in clinical pathology there has been a considerable increase in clinical demand for laboratory investigations. When the volume of work increased, there arose a need for work simplification. Monostep methods are introduced to replace multistep cumbersome and inaccurate methods like blood cell count. The efficiency of monostep methods was further increased by the introduction of automatic dispensers and diluters. Instruments designed to handle the whole analytical process in mechanized fashion have become common place in last decade. This procedure is called automation. The automation is mechanization of various duties performed by machines or analyzers which helps to lessen the workload in laboratories.

The function of autoanalyzer is to replace with automated devices the steps of:
1. Collecting, labeling, separating and preserving various specimens (such as blood, plasma, serum, etc.)
2. Pipetting reagents
3. Mixing reagent and specimen
4. Incubating reaction mixtures at specific temperatures
5. Calculating test results
6. Printing test reports
7. Increase the accuracy and precision of the methods.

The automated instruments not only save the labor and time but allow reliable quality control, reduce subjective errors and work economically by using smaller quantities of samples and reagents. There is an element of feedback which detects any tendency to malfunction.

Following are the different types of autoanalyzers used in clinical pathology (mainly chemistry) laboratories.

- *Continuous flow analyzers (CFA):* Based on continuous flow analysis, the early form of automation was introduced by Technicon Instrument Corporation. The flowing carrier solution passes through small tubes continuously. This is the main principle of continuous flow processing. Here sample is injected into a flowing carrier solution. The sample mixes with diluents and reagent and it is sent through the tubing and mixing coils. The machine prevents carry over effect between different samples by injecting bubbles of air. The air bubbles segment each sample into discrete packets and act as a barrier between packets to prevent cross contamination as they travel down the length of the tubing. The air bubbles literally create separate space for different reactions to take place inside the tubing and mixing coils. There are different apparatus for different functions, such as ion exchange, heating, incubation, and finally recording of the signal. The tubing passes the samples from one apparatus to the other. The flow conditions are regulated. When reaction is taking place, the optical density of the color formed is read and results are obtained. CFA was designed to process only colorimetric reactions, later on CFA were designed to read reactions based on ion selective electrode, flame photometry, flurometry, etc. The single channel continuous flow analyzer can perform a single estimation on a large number of specimens simultaneously, whereas, multi-channel continuous flow analyzer are large scale equipments which analyzes two or more parameters at the same time.

  There is certain disadvantages in this system:
  - Even when there is no test to be done, reagents are drawn to maintain the flow. This adds to the cost per test.
  - Maintenance of instrument is required more frequently.
  - The probe and internal tubing must be free of clogs.
  - When there is no sample the probe must be dipped in distilled water to avoid blockage or precipitation. The machine itself occupies large space.

- *Discrete analyzers:* Discrete processing: in this type of autoanalyzer, each sample is provided a discrete space. It means each analysis even for same analyte or sample takes place at different cups. This is the main principle of discrete processing. For example, if one sample is to be analyzed for 3 parameters, the sample will be sucked by the instrument and poured into 3 different cups. Then respective reagents and diluents (if needed) will be added. Mixing will be done. Cups will be read at different times to give results. Exact amount of sample and reagent is aspirated and mixed. So there is no loss of excess reagents used for flow as in continuous flow processing. As each analysis is done in different cups and read in different cuvette, there is no carry over effect at all. So literally each analysis is discrete (separate) from each other. It saves reagent cost and hence popular than continuous flow analysis. The various types of discrete autoanalyzers used in the clinical chemistry laboratories are: (A) Batch analyzers and (B) 'Stat' (means immediate reporting or emergency determination analyzers.

  A. *Batch analyzers:* This is convenient to analyze specimen in batches such as of sugar, urea creatinine, etc. state testing may not be conveniently carried out on these analyzers. The batch analyzers can be further differentiated as: (i) Semiautomated and (ii) Fully automated.
     i. *Semi-automated (batch/discrete) analyzers:* In the case of these analyzers the initial part of the procedure, i.e. pipetting of reagent and specimen, mixing and incubation is

carried out by the technician. Rest of the procedure, i.e. setting of incubation temperature (for kinetic determinations), zero setting, photometric readings, result display, automatic printing and data management and processing is carried out by the analyzer.

Advantage of semiauto analyzers:
- The semiauto analyzers are cheap and compact, compared to other fully automated analyzes.
- Specimen analysis is cheap, since volume of reagent used is 0.5 to 1.0 ml.
- Enzyme determinations by kinetic methods are performed accurately in 1 to 3 minutes.
- The enzymatic reagents are not corrosive and involve monostep testing.

ii. *Fully automated batch analyzers*: These analyzers carry out all the function of a semiautomated analyzer, in addition to the pipetting of specimen and reagents and also the mixing of the reaction mixtures. The basic working stages of these analyzers, after selecting general system parameters are as follows:
- The specimen cups are placed on the sampler.
- The required quantity of reagent is dispensed by a reagent probe, in the reaction cups.
- The respective specimens from the sample are pipetted into the appropriate reaction cups by another sample probe.
- The reaction cups are shaken mechanically to mix the contents.
- After observing the required incubation time (for delay time in the case of kinetic determinations) the reaction mixture is aspirated by a probe for photometric readings.
- The resulted values are printed and displayed in appropriate units by digital display.

B. *Stat analyzers (random access analyzers)*: In the case of these analyzers many reagents (8 to 20 or more) can be pipetted one after another, so that various biochemical determinations can be performed on one specimen, according to the number of tests ordered for the patient. Hence, these are patient (or specimen) orientated autoanalyzers.

For examples, if serum specimen no. 1 requires following tests to be performed; 1) Urea nitrogen, 2) Serum creatinine, 3) Total proteins, 4) Albumin, 5) Serum glutamic pyruvic transaminase (SGPT) and 6) Serum glutamic oxaloacetic transaminase (SGOT).
- The analyzer is programmed for these tests with respective system parameters.
- The reagents for urea nitrogen, creatinine, total proteins, albumin, SGPT and SGOT are pipetted automatically by a reagent probe in the respective reaction cups.
- The required specific serum quantities are added to the respective reaction cups by a specimen probe.
- The analyzer identifies various reagents and specimen.
- The photometric determinations are carried out by the autoanalyzer.
- The values of the respective tests are displayed on the computer screen as well as printed on a paper, after the specific test incubation periods.

The advantages of a fully automatic 'stat' (or random access) analyzers are as follows:
- The advantages the various chemistry tests from the file.
- It performs a single test, a profile, an organ panel or a 'stat' determination.
- It reduces the cost per test by utilization of micro-volumes of a reagent.

- It performs automatic monitoring of specimen and reagent volumes.
- It can perform various methodologies such as End point, kinetic, initial rate and dichromatic (readings at two different wavelengths) to eliminate errors which may arise due to haemolytic, icteric or lipemic sera.
- The analyzer can perform repetition of tests with or without automatic dilution.

Care and Maintenance of Analyzers

- On ending the working day, once the analyzer has been switched off, always empty the waste container.
- Never use detergents or abrasive products for cleaning the surface of the analyzer. Use only a damp cloth with water and pH-neutral soap.
- If a reagent or corrosive product spills or splashes onto the apparatus, clean it with a damp cloth and soap immediately.
- All the elements of the analyzer have drainage conduits leading to the exterior to enable the elimination of any liquid spilled and to prevent the apparatus from flooding. If the spillage is significant, the liquid spilled onto the table through the drainage conduits and the analyzer must be adequately cleaned.
- When not in use, close the main cover of the analyzer to protect it from dust.

Cleaning the Dispensing System

The dispensing system should be cleaned with washing solution at the start and end of each working day to ensure that it is completely free from air bubbles and is perfectly clean.

Once the wash has been performed, the analyzer asks the user to replace the container with system liquid and it automatically performs a wash and rinse of the dispensing system with system liquid. With the initial wash, the system is ready for working in optimum conditions during the entire working day, offering maximum performance. With the final wash, the analyzer cleans the needle at the end of the working day, keeping it in optimum condition for future working days. The user can also wash the dispensing system whenever he wishes by means of the dispensing system wash tool on the user program, while the analyzer is in standby mode. It is also appropriate to clean and check the filters of the system liquid container at least once every 3 months. If the needle is obstructed by solid residue and needs cleaning with the metal cleaning rod supplied with the analyzer, it can be disassembled for cleaning out of the analyzer. For this, the disassemble dispensing needle utility on the user program must be used. It is also recommendable to periodically clean the outside surface of the needle with a piece of cotton or a soft cloth dampened with alcohol. The needle must be replaced if it noticeably deteriorates.

Cleaning the semi-disposable reactions rotor: When the reactions rotor is completely full, the user must change it for one that is empty, clean and dry. The reactions rotors can be reused if they are carefully cleaned immediately after use. The procedure is as follows:
- Remove the reagents from the rotor wells and rinse abundantly with running water
- Immerse the material in a 5% wash solution (provided with analyzer) for 30 minutes.
- Rinse thoroughly with running water.
- Only deproteinize the rotor when tests for ions such as magnesium, calcium, etc., are required. Deproteinize it by adding a 3% nitric acid solution for 5 minutes.
- Rinse thoroughly with distilled water.
- Immerse in distilled water for 30 minutes and allow it to dry at room temperature.
- They must be left to dry completely before being reused. High temperature must not be used during drying.
- The rotors must be rejected if they are noticeably deteriorated.

The optical status of a rotor must be verified by means of the reactions rotor verification utility

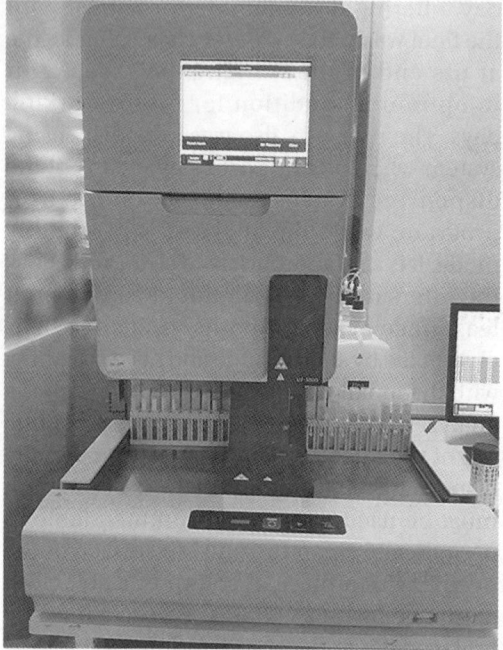

Fig. 11.1: Urilyzer

on the user program. The useful lifetime of each rotor depends drastically on its use and care.

Analyzer for Urine analysis

Urinalysis can provide the physician with important information regarding the status of a patient's health. Test results may provide information regarding the status of:
- Carbohydrate metabolism
- Kidney function
- Liver function
- Acid-base balance
- Urinary tract infection.

Pathology laboratory can have analyzer depending upon its requirement, workload, space available and budget.

Autoanalyzer for urine analysis is shown in **Figure 11.1**.

URILYZER

The Urilyzer is urine analyzer unique within the automated solutions for urine sediment, as the technology is designed to be closest to the international standardized procedure of analysing native urine by manual microscopy. An automatic benchtop urine sediment analyzer using microscopy technology and image recognition software. The urine analyzer precisely and accurately identifies and classifies a wide range of formed elements from native urine.

Features and Functions

- Throughput of up to 90 tests/hour
- Liquid level detector and minimal sample volume of 2.0 ml native urine
- Built-in bar-code reader
- Data capacity of above 200,000 records. Results are stored with high quality images-eliminating the need to repeat measurements.
- Full urinalysis quality control management system including Levey-Jennings chart.
- Automated focusing ensures sharp images.
- The use of native, non-centrifuged urine samples ensures that no particles are missing or damaged due to centrifugation.
- Real whole-field images are captured in low- and high power scan and are available for on-screen verification.

Technical Data

Measurement principle: Automatic mixing and sampling followed by an auto-identification of particles based on a morphologic analysis.

Measurement type: Microscopic measurement of native urine samples in a counting chamber (3 separate channels). Automated microscopic urine sediment particle analysis in low power (LP: 100x) and high power (HP: 400x). Identified and autoclassified particles are presented in whole field of view images (LP and HP) after being sedimentation in the counting chamber.

Automatic detected particles: Normal red blood cells, abnormal red blood cells, white blood cells, casts, epithelial cells, yeast, crystals, mucus and bacteria (further particles for sub-classification by user available).

RBC morphological analysis: Histograms with information about size, form and chroma of RBC.
- *Microscopic data*: Objective lens 10X/40X
- *Precision*: 3.2 µm (horizontal), 0.25 µm (vertical)
- *Visual field*: 4 mm × 25 mm
- *Light source*: 12V, 20W

RBC analysis: In addition to the classic auto-identification of the RBC's, the Urilyzer some urilyzer offers additional information in form of diagrams about the size, form and chroma.

Default number of images—10 for LP and HP if less than 200 particles are identified in the screening, otherwise 6 in LP and HP.
- *Throughput*: Up to 90 tests/hour
- *Detection rate*: ≥ 98% at a concentration level of 5 cells/µL
- *Sample volume*: 2.0 mL native, non-centrifuged urine (500 µL test volume)
- *Loading capacity (samples)*: Up to 50 in one batch
- *STAT*: Independent STAT sample position
- *Sample identification*: Built-in barcode reader
- *Display*: External monitor (included)
- *Printer*: External laser printer (included)
- *Memory*: 200,000 patient results including all microscope images
- *Dimensions*: 640 × 680 × 530 mm (W × D × H)
- *Weight*: 58 kg
- *Power (analyzer)*: 100–240V~ 50/60Hz 450VA

■ MULTISTIX URINALYSIS STRIPS

A standard urine test strip may comprise up to 10 different chemical pads or reagents which react (change color) when immersed in, and then removed from, a urine sample. The test can often be read in as little as 60 to 120 seconds after dipping, although certain tests require longer. Routine testing of the urine with multiparameter strips is the first step in the diagnosis of a wide range of diseases.

The analysis includes testing for the presence of proteins, glucose, ketones, hemoglobin, bilirubin, urobilinogen, acetone, nitrite and leucocytes as well as testing of pH and specific gravity or to test for infection by different pathogens.

The test strips consist of a ribbon made of plastic or paper of about 5 mm wide, plastic strips have pads impregnated with chemicals that react with the compounds present in urine producing a characteristic color. For the paper strips the reactants are absorbed directly onto the paper. Paper strips are often specific to a single reaction (e.g. pH measurement), while the strips with pads allow several determinations simultaneously.

There are strips which serve different purposes, such as qualitative strips that only determine if the sample is positive or negative, or there are semi-quantitative ones that in addition to providing a positive or negative reaction also provide an estimation of a quantitative result, in the latter the color reactions are approximately proportional to the concentration of the substance being tested for in the sample. The reading of the results is carried out by comparing the pad colors with a color scale provided by the manufacturer, no additional equipment is needed **(Fig. 11.2)**.

This type of analysis is very common in the control and monitoring of diabetic patients. The time taken for the appearance of the test results on the strip can vary from a few minutes after the test to 30 minutes after immersion of the strip in the urine (depending on the brand of product being used).

Tests performed by Multistix urinalysis strips and principles:
- *Glucose:* Glucose oxidase catalyzes the formation of gluconic acid and hydrogen peroxide from the oxidation of glucose. Peroxidase catalyzes the reaction of hydrogen peroxide with a potassium iodide chromogen to oxidize the chromogen to colors ranging from green to brown. Shades of color indicate semi-quantitative value of

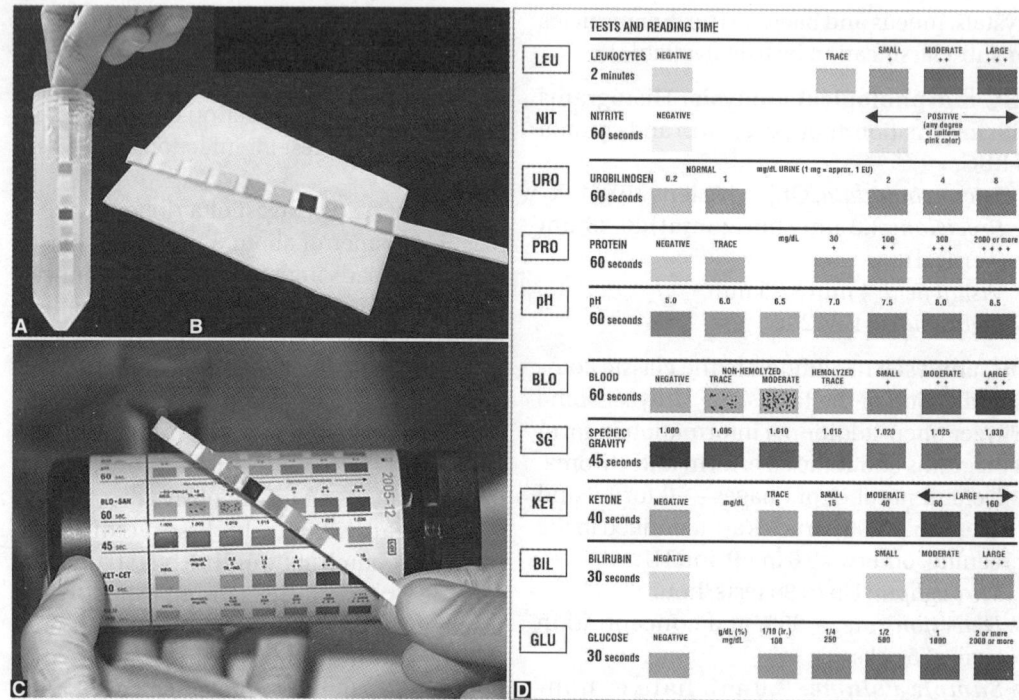

Figs. 11.2A to D: (A) Stick dipped in urine; (B) Wait for few seconds; (C) Match with the color code provided; (D) Color code for different tests with reading time.
(For color version See Color Plate 3)

glucose and are usually reported as: trace, 1+, 2+, 3+ and 4+.
- *Bilirubin:* Bilirubin couples with diazotized dichloroaniline in a strongly acid medium. Colors range through various shades of tan.
- *Ketone:* Acetoacetic acid reacts with nitroprusside. Colors range from buff-pink for a negative reading, to maroon for a positive reading.
- *Specific gravity:* pKa changes occur for certain pretreated polyelectrolytes in relation to ionic concentration. In the presence of an indicator, colors range from deep blue-green in urine of low ionic concentration through green and yellow-green in urines of increasing ionic concentration.
- *Blood:* Hemoglobin catalyzes the reaction of diisopropylbenzene dihydroperoxide and 3,3′,5,5′-tetramethylbenzidine. Colors range from orange through green; very high levels of blood may cause the color development to continue to blue.

- *pH:* The double indicator principle gives a broad range of colors covering the entire urinary pH range. Colors range from orange through yellow and green to blue.
- *Protein:* At a constant pH, the development of any green color is due to the presence of protein (protein error-of-indicators principle). Colors range from yellow for "Negative" through yellow-green and green to green-blue for "Positive" reactions.
- *Urobilinogen:* In a modified Ehrlich reaction, p-diethylaminobenzaldehyde in conjunction with a color enhancer reacts with urobilinogen in a strongly acid medium to produce a pink-red color.
- *Nitrite:* Nitrate (derived from the diet) is converted to nitrite by the action of gram negative bacteria in the urine. At the acid pH of the reagent area, nitrite in the urine reacts with p-arsanilic acid to form a diazonium compound. This diazonium compound

couples with 1,2,3,4-tetrahydrobenzo(h) quinolin-3-ol to produce a pink color.
- *Leukocytes:* Esterases in granulocytic leukocytes catalyze the hydrolysis of the derivatized pyrrole amino acid ester to liberate 3-hydroxy-5-phenylpyrrole. This pyrrole then reacts with a diazonium salt to produce a purple product.

■ POLYMERASE CHAIN REACTION

Polymerase chain reaction (PCR) is a cyclic temperature-dependent reaction used to amplify the gene of interest. Enzyme *Taq* DNA **P**olymerase is used in this technique, which generates the **C**hain of **R**eaction to produce multiple copies of the DNA. Hence the name **P**olymerase **C**hain **R**eaction.

PCR was developed in 1983 by Kary B Mullis, an American biochemist who won the Nobel Prize for Chemistry in 1993 for his invention.

Requirements

Chemicals

1. *dNTPs*: The dNTP stands for Deoxyribose Nucleotide Triphosphate. These artificially synthesized nucleotides are made up of pentose sugar, phosphate and nitrogenous base. The adenine and guanine cytosine and thymine are nitrogenous bases. These are used as building blocks for DNA synthesis.
2. *Enzyme Taq DNA polymerase*: In the extension step, this enzyme helps in the binding of dNTPs at growing DNA strand. *Taq* DNA **polymerase**, is named after the heat-tolerant bacterium *Thermus aquaticus* from which it was isolated. *T. aquaticus* lives in hot springs.
3. *Primers:* Two artificially synthesized "primers" are needed. These are short single-stranded DNA sequences which correspond to the beginning and ending of the template DNA stretch to be copied. The primers bind, or anneal, to the template at their complementary sites and serve as the starting and ending point for copying.
4. *Template DNA:* It is DNA sample which is to be copied. It contains few nucleotide sequences. It can be obtained from blood, hair, pus, skin scraping, parasites, virus, bacteria, etc., depending upon aim to do PCR.
5. *PCR buffer:* PCR buffer is yet another important ingredient in the polymerase chain reaction. It contains all the enhancer which helps in proper amplification. Also, the PCR buffer maintains the constant pH of the reaction nearly 7.9 to 8.5 by maintaining the constant chemical environment for the PCR reaction.

Instruments

The PCR machine is called a thermocycler. This machine is simply a heating block which provides the constant temperature and even rapidly changes between two temperature states. The machine has a lower block of metal having deep wells for putting PCR tubes. Also, the temperature of the inner environment is maintained by the heating block present on the upper side of the lead. Further, the machine contains the display, power on and off switch and cooling assembly. The machine has the ability to heat and cool the PCR tube in a short period of time.

Other Utilities

PCR tubes, stands, pipettes, etc.

Principle

PCR uses the enzyme Taq DNA polymerase that directs the synthesis of DNA from deoxynucleotide substrates on a single-stranded DNA template. DNA polymerase adds nucleotides to the 3` end of a custom-designed oligonucleotide (primer) when it is binded to a longer template DNA. Repetition of this result in formation of double-stranded DNA.

Procedure (Fig. 11.3)

The entire PCR reaction is basically governed by the temperature, different temperature zone

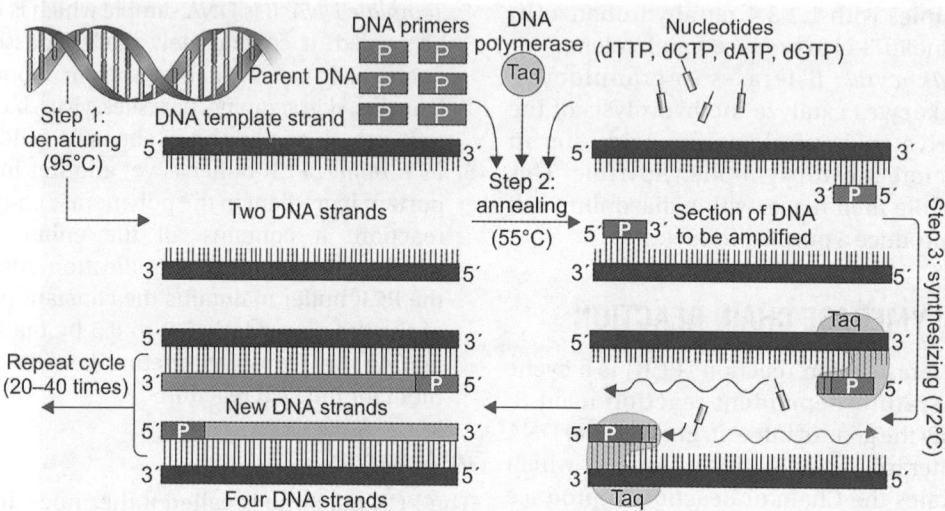

Fig. 11.3: PCR mechanism.
(For color version See Color Plate 4)

facilitates different reactions. Denaturation, annealing and extension are three PCR steps. Cyclic repetitions of these results in formation of millions of copies of required DNA.

1. *Denaturation:* The denaturation is the process in which the double-stranded DNA becomes single-stranded. The DNA template is heated to 94°C. This breaks the weak hydrogen bonds that hold DNA strands together in a helix, allowing the strands to separate creating single-stranded DNA. This step takes 30 seconds to 90 seconds of time to complete.

2. *Annealing:* The mixture is cooled to anywhere from 50°C to 70°C. This allows the primers to anneal (bind) to their complementary sequence in the template DNA. Each primer has its own annealing temperature, at that particular temperature; the primer binds to its complementary sequence. Generally, the annealing temperature is ranging from 55°C to 65°C.

   Maintaining time and temperature is very important in this step. Lower annealing temperature leads to non-specific bindings while higher temperature leads to failure in amplification.

   It should last for 45 seconds. If the annealing step is performed for more than 45 seconds, it can cause non-specific bindings and weakening of primer.

3. *Extension:* After the binding of the primer, its time to expand the DNA strand. Here in extension step the Taq DNA polymerase comes in action and adds dNTPs to the growing DNA strand. The temperature for the extension is 72°C for 45 seconds.

With one cycle, a single segment of double-stranded DNA template is amplified into two separate pieces of double-stranded DNA. These two pieces are then available for amplification in the next cycle. There are many copies of the primers and many molecules of *Taq* polymerase floating around in the reaction, so the number of DNA molecules can roughly double in each round of cycling.

RT-PCR

RT-PCR is Reverse Transcriptase PCR test that is designed to detect and measure RNA. RT-PCR differs from conventional PCR by first taking RNA and converting the RNA strand into a DNA strand. This is done by essentially the same method for PCR described above with the exception of using an enzyme termed reverse transcriptase instead of the *Taq* DNA polymerase. The reverse transcriptase allows a single-strand of RNA to be translated into a complementary strand of DNA. Once that reaction occurs, the routine PCR method can then be used to amplify the DNA. RT-PCR has been used to detect and study many RNA viruses.

Analysis of PCR

The PCR enables investigators to obtain the large quantities of DNA that are required for various experiments and procedures in molecular biology, forensic analysis, evolutionary biology, and medical diagnostics.

The key to understanding PCR is to know that every human, animal, plant, parasite, bacterium, or virus contains genetic material such as DNA (or RNA) sequences that are unique to their species. PCR amplification is only part of the identifying test, however once the amplification is done, the amplified segments need to be compared to other nucleotide segments from a known source for example, a specific person, animal, or pathogenic organism. This comparison of unique segments is often done by placing PCR-generated nucleotide sequences next to known nucleotide sequences from humans, pathogens, or other sources in a separating gel.

Gel Electrophoresis

Gel electrophoresis is a technique used to separate DNA fragments (or other macromolecules, such as RNA and proteins) based on their size and charge.

As the name suggests, gel electrophoresis involves a gel—a slab of jello-like material made out of a polysaccharide called agarose, placed in a gel box. One end of the box is hooked to a positive electrode, while the other end is hooked to a negative electrode. The main body of the box, where the gel is placed,

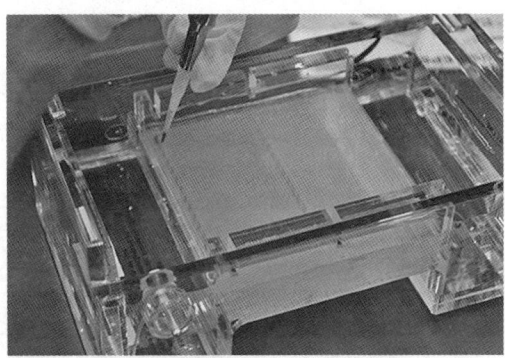

Fig. 11.4: Sample loading in wells.

is filled with a salt-containing buffer solution that can conduct current. Buffer should be filled up in the gel box to a level where it just barely covers the gel.

At one end of the box, it has wells to hold DNA samples to be examined **(Fig. 11.4)**. One well is reserved for a DNA ladder, a standard reference that contains DNA fragments of known lengths. The end of the gel with the wells is positioned towards the negative electrode. The end without wells is positioned towards the positive electrode. Next, the power to the gel box is turned on, and current begins to flow through the gel. The DNA molecules have a negative charge because of the phosphate groups in their sugar-phosphate backbone, so they start moving through the matrix of the gel towards the positive electrode. When the power is turned on and current is passing through the gel, the gel is said to be running.

As the gel runs, shorter pieces of DNA will travel through the pores of the gel matrix faster than longer ones. After the gel has run for awhile, the shortest pieces of DNA will be close to the positive end of the gel, while the longest pieces of DNA will remain near the wells **(Fig. 11.5)**.

Visualizing the DNA Fragments

Once the fragments have been separated, different sizes of bands are found on it. When a gel is stained with a DNA-binding dye and

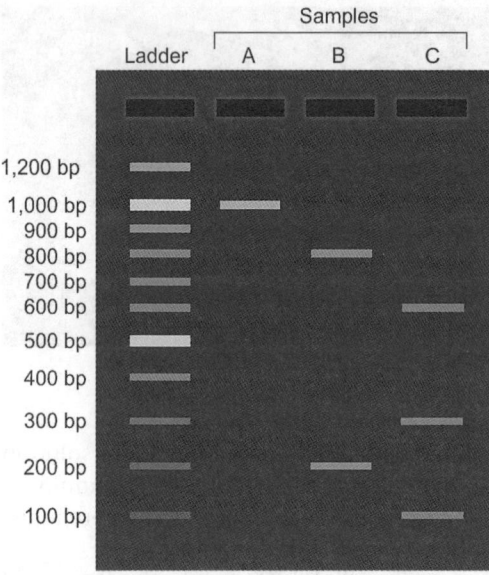

Fig. 11.5: Bands of electrophoresis.

placed under UV light, the DNA fragments will glow, allowing us to see the DNA present at different locations along the length of the gel.

This well-defined "line" of DNA on a gel is called a band. Each band contains a large number of DNA fragments of the same size that have all traveled as a group to the same position. By comparing the bands in a sample to the DNA ladder, we can determine their approximate sizes. Reference sample is called ladder as it contains various nucleotide sequences that form bands which resemble a "ladder". Commercial DNA ladders come in different size ranges; one with good "coverage" of the size range of our expected fragments is to be chosen.

Advance PCR

Real-Time PCR is a variation of PCR that allows analysis of the amplified DNA during the usual 40 cycles of the procedure. Although the procedure is similar to conventional PCR with cycling, real-time PCR uses fluorescent dyes attached to some of the building blocks or small nucleotide strands. Depending on the method used, fluorescence occurs when the amplified DNA strands are formed. The amount of fluorescence can be measured throughout the 40 cycles and allows the investigators to measure specific products and their amounts during the amplification cycles. This often allows investigators or lab technicians to skip the gel electrophoresis or other secondary procedures needed for analysis of the PCR products, thus producing more rapid results.

Real-time PCR and Reverse Transcription PCR are variations or modifications of the original PCR test. However, there are many more variations (at least 25) that exist and are used to solve specific problems. They all have different names such as Assembly PCR, Hot-start PCR, Multiplex PCR, Solid-phase PCR and many others.

Applications of PCR

- PCR is used in analyzing clinical specimens for the presence of infectious agents, including HIV, hepatitis, malaria, anthrax, etc.
- PCR can provide information on a patient's prognosis, and predict response or resistance to therapy. Many cancers are characterized by small mutations in certain genes, and this is what PCR is employed to identify.
- PCR is used in the analysis of mutations that occur in many genetic diseases (e.g. cystic fibrosis, sickle cell anemia, phenylketonuria, muscular dystrophy).
- PCR is also used in forensics laboratories and is especially useful because only a tiny amount of original DNA is required, for example, sufficient DNA can be obtained from a droplet of blood or a single hair.
- PCR is an essential technique in cloning procedure which allows generation of large amounts of pure DNA from tiny amount of template strand and further study of a particular gene.
- The Human Genome Project (HGP) for determining the sequence of the 3 billion base pairs in the human genome, relied heavily on PCR.
- PCR has been used to identify and to explore relationships among species in the field of evolutionary biology.

Section 2

Hematology

CHAPTER 12

The Blood

Learning Objectives
- Blood plays an important role in regulating the body's systems and maintaining homeostasis. Hematology involves the diagnosis and treatment of patients who have disorders of the blood and bone marrow.
- This chapter describes composition and functions of blood.
- Study of blood cells becomes easy and interesting with clear, colorful diagrams and table of comparison of blood cells.

Keywords
Erythrocyte, Leukocyte, Neutrophil, Basophil, Eosinophil, Lymphocyte, Thrombocyte, Plasma

Hematology is the study of blood, and its different components. The hematological laboratory routinely reports number of cells in blood, hemoglobin concentration, erythrocyte sedimentation rate (ESR), packed cell volume (PCV), etc.

■ BLOOD

Blood is a red vascular connective tissue. It forms 6 to 10% of body weight. Generally, 90 mL/kg of blood is present in human body. It is somewhat sticky and slightly heavier than water. It is slightly alkaline, having pH 7.4.

Blood transports vital requirements and waste products of the body. Blood consists of two types of components:

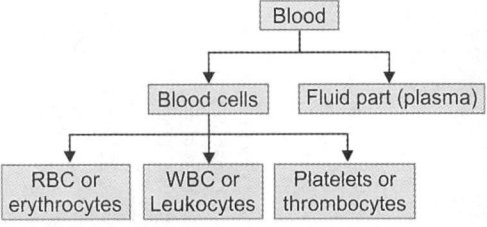

1. Blood cells,
2. Plasma.

■ BLOOD CELLS

There are three types of blood cells (**Table 12.1**):
1. *RBC:* Red blood cells/corpuscles or erythrocyte.
2. *WBC:* White blood cells/corpuscles or leukocyte.
3. Platelets or thrombocytes.

Erythrocyte (RBC)

Erythrocytes are red blood cells.

These are bi-concave, non-nucleated, disks like cells. The central area is thin, while edges are thick. The edges contain hemoglobin, which transports respiratory gases, i.e. oxygen (O_2) and carbon dioxide (CO_2). The shape favors flexibility for absorbing and releasing of gases quickly. The size of RBC is 7.2 micron (μ). In a mature male, about 5 to 5.5 million per cubic mm of blood, and in females, about 4 to

Section 2: Hematology

TABLE 12.1: Brief description of blood cells.

About cells	Neutrophil	Eosinophil	Basophil	Monocyte	Small lymphocyte	Large lymphocyte	Red blood cell	Thrombocytes or platelets
Shape of nucleus	3 to 7 lobes connected with chromatin strand	Bilobed connected with chromatin strand looks like spectacle	Kidney shaped and granules are centrical and overlap nucleus	Kidney shaped and eccentric	Large and rounded in shape	Small and rounded in shape	Biconcave, oval, disk like non-nucleated	Cell is spindle shape, and smallest with granules. Nucleus is absent
Number in percentage	65 to 70% of total WBCs	1 to 6% of total WBCs	0.005 to 1% of total WBCs	2 to 6% of total WBCs	50% in children upto 1 year 35% upto 15 year and 20 to 30% in adults	5 to 10% of total WBCs	—	—
Number in cells per cu. mm of blood	3000 to 7000 cells	15 to 400 cells	0 to 50 cells	200 to 600 cells	1000 to 3000 cells	500 to 1000 cells	4 to 4.5 million cells per cu. mm in females and 5 to 5.5 million per cu. mm in males	1.5 to 4 lakhs cells
Diameter	12 to 15 μ	10 to 12 μ	8 to 10 μ	15 to 18 μ	8 to 10 μ	15 to 18 μ	7.2 μ (Approximate 6 to 8 μ)	2 to 3 μ
Life period	12 to 15 days	10 to 12 days	8 to 10 days	1 to 2 days	Less than 24 hours	Few hours	90 to 120 (Approximate 100 days)	Few days
Function	It is phagocytic in nature. It protects the body against foreign particles	It protects the body by releasing a chemical substance histamine	It prevents the clotting of blood inside the blood vessels by secreting heparine	It is phagocytic in nature	It produces antibody	It produces antibody	It transports respiratory gases—O_2 and CO_2 with the help of hemoglobin	It helps in the process of blood clotting
	(See Fig. 12.2)	(See Fig. 12.4)	(See Fig. 12.3)	(See Fig. 12.6)	(See Fig. 12.5)	(See Fig. 12.5)	(See Fig. 12.1A)	(See Fig. 12.7)

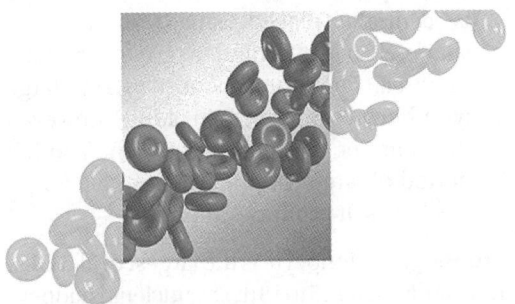

Fig. 12.1A: The red blood cells.

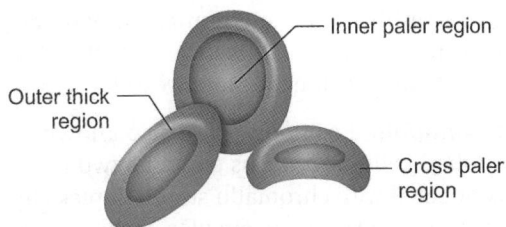

Fig. 12.1B: Erythrocyte.

4.5 million per cubic mm of blood are present. The life period of RBC is about 90 to 120 days (Figs. 12.1A and B).

Leukocyte (WBC)

These are colorless, nucleated cells. Normally, 4,000 to 10,000 WBC per cu mm of blood are present. There are two different types of WBCs, classified on the basis of presence of granules in their cytoplasm (Flowchart 12.1).
a. Granulocyte
b. Agranulocyte

Granulocyte

These are characterized by presence of granules in their cytoplasm. These cells are produced in bone marrow.

Granulocytes are classified on the basis of shape of nucleus and the dye, which they take. These are:
a. Neutrophil
b. Basophil
c. Eosinophil.

Neutrophil: Neutrophil is also known as polymorph or microphage. There are about 65 to 70% neutrophils present of total WBC. The cytoplasm is full of granules that picks up, both, acidic as well as basic dye. The nucleus has about 3 to 7 lobes connected by chromatin strand or thread. The life period of neutrophil is about 3 to 5 days. It is a large cell, having diameter 12 to 15 m. Neutrophils are phagocytic in nature (Fig. 12.2).

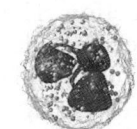

Fig. 12.2: Neutrophil.

Basophil: Cytoplasm of basophil contains small rounded granules, which takes up basic stain. The size is somewhat small with diameter 8 to 10 µ. The nucleus is usually kidney-shaped or slightly lobulated. The cytoplasmic granules are central and overlap the nucleus. The life period of basophil is 8 to 12 days. Normally, about 0.005 to 1% basophils are present (Fig. 12.3).

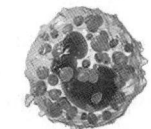

Fig. 12.3: Basophil.

Flowchart 12.1: Types of WBC.

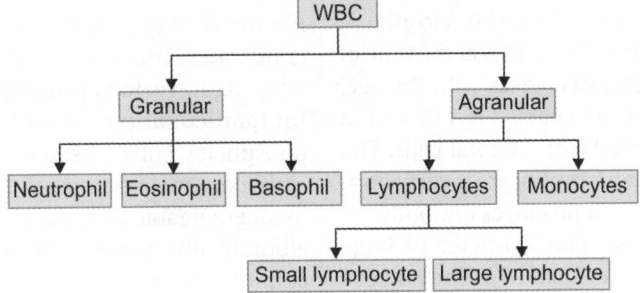

Basophil secrets a chemical substance, known as heparine, which prevents the clotting of blood inside the blood vessel.

Eosinophil: Eosinophils are also known as bilobed cells, as nucleus contains two lobes connected with chromatin strand. It picks up acidic stain. These are circular in shape with diameter 10 to 12 µ. Normally, about 15 to 400 cells, i.e. about 1 to 6% of blood is present. Life period of eosinophil is 8 to 10 days. It protects the body by releasing a chemical substance, called as histamine. Histamine sets off a chain of reactions that ultimately leads to an inflammatory response at the site of infection. Therefore, in case of allergic conditions the number of eosinophil increases **(Fig. 12.4)**.

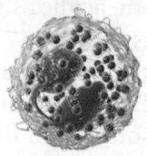

Fig. 12.4: Eosinophil.

Agranulocyte

These are characterized by the absence of granules in the cytoplasm.

These cells are manufactured in lymph gland and spleen. These are of two types:
1. Lymphocytes
2. Monocytes

Lymphocytes: There are two types of lymphocytes on the basis of area of cytoplasm **(Fig. 12.5)**.

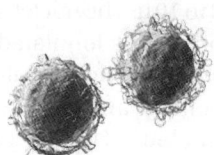

Fig. 12.5: Lymphocytes.

i. *Small lymphocyte:* In small lymphocyte, the nucleus is relatively large in size and rounded in shape, which occupies a major part of the cell, leaving behind small cytoplasmic area. The diameter of the cell is 8 to 10 µ. It is about 50% of the total WBCs at the time of birth. The number decreases with the age, at the age of 10 to 15 years, it is 35% and in adults, it is 20 to 30% of the total cells. The life period of small lymphocyte is very short, less than 24 hours. It produces antibody.

ii. *Large lymphocyte:* The diameter of large lymphocyte is about 15 to 18 µ. The nucleus is centrally placed, small, rounded in shape, leaving behind a large cytoplasmic area. There are about 5 to 10% large lymphocytes presents in adult, however, the number is more in children. The life period of large lymphocyte is small, about few hours. It produces antibody.

Monocyte: Monocyte is the largest of all WBC, having diameter 15 to 18 µ. The nucleus is kidney-shaped. It can be differentiated from basophil, as the nucleus of monocyte is eccentric. The monocytes are about 2 to 6% of total WBCs, i.e. about 100 to 600 cells per cu. mm. The life period of monocyte is about 1 to 2 days. The monocytes are phagocytic in nature **(Fig. 12.6)**.

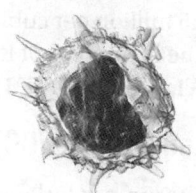

Fig. 12.6: Monocyte.

Platelets or Thrombocytes

These are the smallest of all blood cells. Platelets are spindle-shaped cells, having diameter 2 to 3 µ. These are also known as thrombocytes. Along with another coagulation factors, it helps in the process of clotting of blood. Thrombocytes are having very short life-span, it is of few hours. Normally, 1.5 to 4 lakh platelets per cu. mm of blood are present. These are non-nucleated cells containing very fine granules **(Fig. 12.7)**.

A brief description of blood cells given in **Table 12.1**.

■ PLASMA

Plasma is a liquid (fluid) part of blood. It contains about 90 to 91% of water. Plasma contains fats, sugar, various proteins and hormones. Inorganic components of plasma includes phosphates, sulfates, sodium chloride, sodium carbonate, magnesium, etc. These are dissolved in water. Organic components of plasma include albumin, fibrinogen, globulin, etc. Plasma also contains digestive nutrients like glucose, fatty

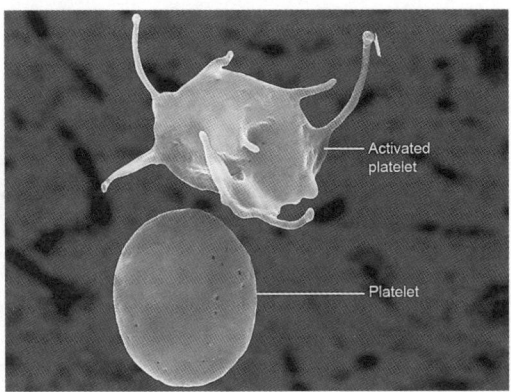

Fig. 12.7: Platelets.

FUNCTIONS OF BLOOD

- Transport of oxygen from the lungs to the tissues and of carbon dioxide from tissues to the lungs.
- Transport of metabolic wastes to the lungs, kidneys, skin and intestines for removal.
- Maintenance of normal acid-base balance.
- Transport of absorbed fatty acids, monosaccharides and amino acids.
- Regulation of water balance.
- Regulation of body temperature.
- Transport of hormones, vitamins and salts which contain cations such as sodium, potassium, calcium, etc. and anions such as chlorides, phosphates, sulfates and carbonates.
- Transport of metabolites.
- Defense against infection by the white cells and by the antibodies.
- To stop bleeding by clotting.

acids, glycerol and calcium, etc. Excretory substances like urea, uric acid are also present in plasma. The other substances present in plasma include antigen, antibodies, vitamins, etc.

Chemical composition of plasma is not constant because continue exchange of various substances from plasma to different organs is going on. In this way, plasma is acting as a transport medium in body.

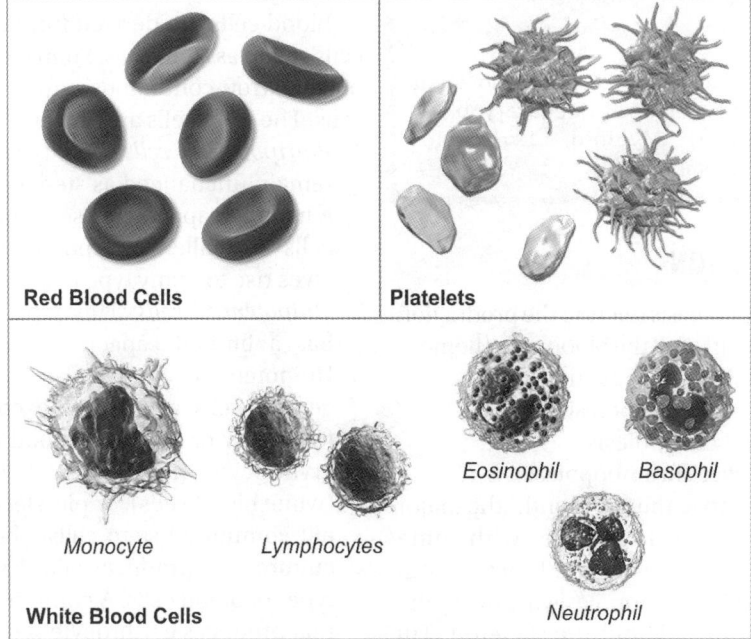

Fig. 12.8: Elements of blood.
(For color version See Color Plate 4)

CHAPTER 13

Hemopoiesis

Learning Objectives
- Studying hemopoiesis can help clinicians to understand the processes behind blood disorders and cancers.
- This chapter explains different stages of formation of blood cells and other requirements for the same. Flowchart represented here is a valuable tool in understanding the theory through visual perception.
- It also throws light on role of spleen in hemopoiesis.

Keywords
Erythropoiesis, Leukopoiesis, Myeloid stem cell, Lymphoid stem cell, Megakaryoblast, Proerythroblast, Myeloid, Lymphoid, Reticulocyte, Thrombopoiesis

INTRODUCTION

The word hemopoiesis refers to the production and development of all the blood cells (heme—blood cells, poiesis—production).
- *Erythrocytes*: Erythropoiesis
- *Leukocytes*: Leukopoiesis
- *Thrombocytes*: Thrombopoiesis

In fetal life (up to the 3rd month) the major site of hemopoiesis is the liver with some contribution from the spleen. From the 4th month of fetal life hemopoiesis begins in the bone marrow throughout the skeleton. Till puberty hemopoiesis is actively seen in all bones but in adults, it is confined to the axial skeleton mainly to the ends of long bones and the flat bones such as ribs, sternum and pelvis.

Bone marrow is the spongy tissue that fills the cavities inside bones. It fills the shafts of the long bones, the trabeculae (spaces within cancellous tissue), and even extends into the bony canals that hold the blood vessels. The marrow contains fat cells, fluid, fibrous tissue, blood vessels, and hematopoietic, or blood-forming, cells. It is one of the largest organ of the body.

Blood cells are derived from hemopoietic cells called as stem cells. Stem cells within the bone marrow continuously divide to form new cells. The stem cells are of two types:

1. *Pluripotential cells*: This type of new cell remain unchanged as stem cells and have a lifelong capacity for self-renewal. These cells are called pluripotential cells as it gives rise to many type of cells.

2. *Unipotential cells*: This type of stem cell has a limited capacity for self-renewal. Unipotential cells are also known as progenitor cells and become committed to form only one type of blood cell such as erythrocytes (red blood cells), leukocytes (white blood cells), or platelets. The different committed stem cells when grown in culture will produce colonies of specific types of blood cells. A committed stem cell that produces erythrocyte is called Colony Forming Unit—Erythrocyte (CFU-E) is used to designate this type of stem cell.

Likewise colony forming units that form granulocytes and monocytes have the designation CFU-GM.

The stem cells are stimulated to proliferate by growth factors, e.g. interleukin-3, which promotes the proliferation of both pluripotent stem cells and unipotent progenitor cells. There are other growth factors that only induce specific committed progenitor cells. Another important regulator is the level of tissue oxygenation.

Flowchart 13.1 lists the stages in production of blood cells.

ERYTHROPOIESIS

The principal factor that stimulates red blood cell production is erythropoietin, which stimulates CFU-E to differentiate into proerythroblasts. This 'blast cell' undergo following steps to form erythrocyte.

i. *Proerythroblast:* Erythroblast is a term used for all forms of nucleated RBC. The least mature erythroid precursor cell is called a proerythroblast. It is a large cell with a rim of basophilic cytoplasm, a large nucleus which occupies most of the cell. Nuclear chromatin is coarse and prominent multiple nucleoli are seen. Hemoglobin is absent, 15–20 microns in size. Mitosis is there.

ii. *Basophilic/early normoblast:* This is smaller than the proerythroblast with a smaller nucleus but a more basophilic cytoplasm due to increased numbers of ribosomes in the cytoplasm. These ribosomes are involved in the production of hemoglobin. Nucleoli are not seen at this stage. It contains little hemoglobin, 14–17 microns in size. Active mitosis is observed.

iii. *Polychromatic/intermediate normoblast:* This is the last precursor cell capable of mitosis and is smaller than the basophilic

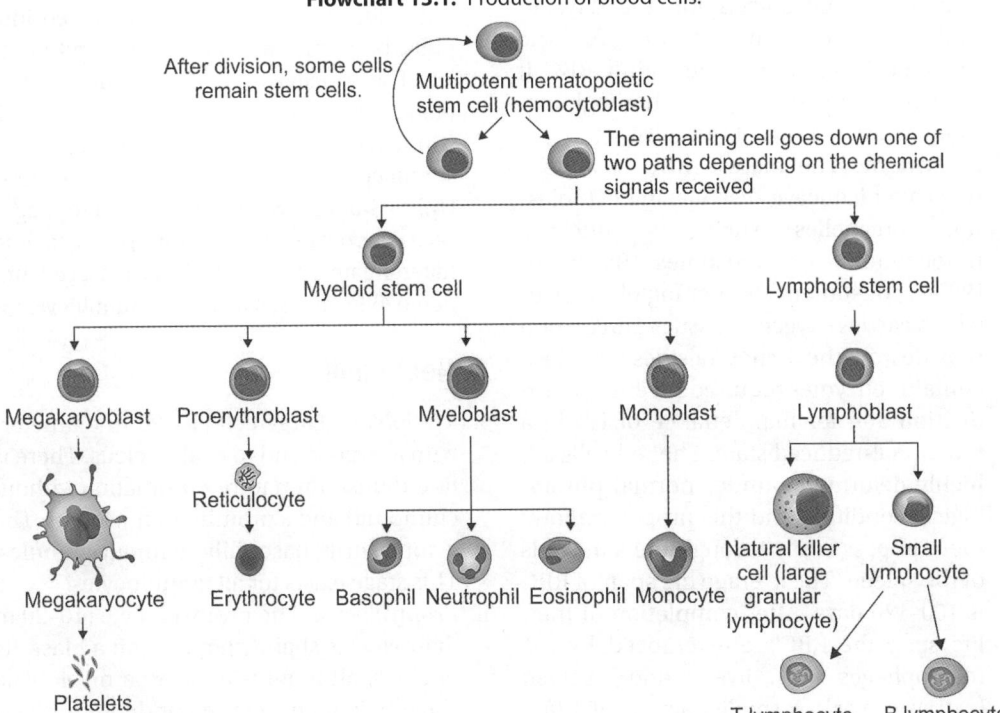

Flowchart 13.1: Production of blood cells.

erythroblast. Its cytoplasm appears grayer due to the increased acidophilic staining caused by the presence of hemoglobin. Nuclear chromatin undergoes condensation, 10–15 microns in size.

iv. *Orthochromatic or late normoblast:* It is the smallest of the precursors and only slightly larger than a mature erythrocyte. Hemoglobinization is complete and so the cytoplasm appears eosinophilic. The nucleus shrinks and the chromatin is greatly condensed giving the nucleus a homogeneous appearance. The nucleus becomes smaller and dark staining (pyknotic). It is ejected to become a reticulocyte, 7–10 microns in size.

v. *Reticulocyte:* The cell is larger than a mature RBC, does not have a nucleus and has remnants of cytoplasmic ribosomal RNA which appear as a fine reticulum when stained with dyes such as new methylene blue and brilliant cresyl blue. After its release from the marrow it remains in the spleen for 1–2 days to undergo further maturation. As the reticulocyte matures to an adult RBC it loses its ability to synthesize hemoglobin. Blood count is 1–2% of red cells.

vi. *Erythrocyte:* The mature RBC is a non-nucleate biconcave disk lacking cytoplasmic organelles such as nucleus, mitochondria or ribosomes. Its major (90%) constituent is hemoglobin (Hb) which carries oxygen to tissues and carbon dioxide from the tissues. Besides Hb, it also contains enzymes required for energy production and for maintenance of Hb in a functional-reduced state. The red cells are highly deformable under normal physiological condition and this property allows them to pass easily through the sinusoids of the spleen. The average life span of RBC is 100–120 days. After completion of their life span the RBC's are removed by the macrophages of liver and spleen (extravascular). A small fraction of RBCs may undergo destruction within the circulation (intravascular).

Requirements for Red Blood Cell Maturation

- Amino acids
- Iron, Fe^{2+}—important component of hemoglobin as it binds oxygen
- Vitamin B_{12} and folic acid—it regulates the synthesis of DNA by increasing the speed of erythroblast proliferation (deficiency causes a decrease in the speed and causes the erythrocytes to develop into larger and weaker megaloblasts).

■ LEUKOPOIESIS

It is the formation of white blood cells. Leukopoiesis involves differentiation of pluripotential stem cells along two pathways: myeloid and lymphoid stem cells.

A. **Myeloid** ('my-loid') stem cells develop into red cells, white cells (neutrophils, eosinophils, basophils and monocytes) and platelets. The principal factor that stimulates white blood cell production is cytokines growth stimulating factor and interlukin-3, which stimulates CFU-GEMM (Colony Forming Unit—Granulocyte–Erythroid–Macrophage–Megakaryocyte, a common precursor) to differentiate into CFU-G. This 'blast cell' undergo following steps to form granulocytes.

1. Neutrophil

i. *Myeloblast*: Large cell (10–20 m diameter) with a large round to oval nucleus. There is fine diffuse immature chromatin (without clumping) and a prominent nucleolus. The cytoplasm is basophilic without granules. This stage exists for all granulocytes.

ii. *Promyelocyte*: The promyelocyte (10–20 m diameter) is slightly larger than a blast. Its nucleus, although similar to a myeloblast shows slight chromatin condensation and less prominent nucleoli. The cytoplasm contains striking primary (azurophilic—a small red or reddish-purple granule that easily takes a stain with azure dyes) granules or primary granules. This stage exists for all granulocytes.

iii. *Neutrophilic myelocyte*: Myelocytes (10-18 m) are slightly smaller than promyelocytes and have eccentric round-oval nuclei, often flattened along one side. The chromatin is fine, but shows evidence of condensation. Nucleoli may be seen in early stages but not in the late myelocyte. Primary azurophilic granules are still present, but secondary granules predominate. Secondary granules (neut, eos, or baso) first appear adjacent to the nucleus. The developing neutrophil can now be differentiated from basophils and eosinophils as neutrophil-specific granules are now being formed.

iv. *Neutrophilic metamyelocyte*: Metamyelocytes (10-18 m) are slightly smaller than myelocytes. At this stage, mitosis can no longer occur. The nucleus elongates, becomes heterochromatic and has a kidney like shape. Differentiation is now much clearer from other granulocytes as the specific granules are in a far greater number than the primary granules formed in the promyelocyte stage.

v. *Band cell*: Nucleus elongates further and represents a horseshoe shaped. Nucleus starts to segment.

vi. *Neutrophil*: Mature neutrophil (average 14 m diameter) is formed and the nucleus is segmented and has 3 to 5 lobes. This lobular structure of the nucleus gives rise to the name polymorphonuclear neutrophil. The chromatin of the segmented neutrophil is coarsely clumped and the cytoplasm is pink due to large numbers of secondary granules.

2. Basophils

Under the stimulation of GM-CSF and IL-3, the CFU-GEMM differentiates into Colony Forming Unit—Basophils.

Stages

i. *Myeloblast and promyelocyte*: These stages are common to all granulocytes and no distinction can be made between different cell lines.

ii. *Basophilic myelocyte and metamyelocyte*: Specific granules start to appear in the myelocyte stage, and as the cell develops into the metamyelocyte stage, mitosis ceases.

iii. *Basophil*: Final nuclear shape is masked by the high density of cytoplasmic granules.

3. Eosinophils

Under the stimulation of GM-CSF, IL-3 and IL-5 the CFU-GEMM differentiates into the Colony Forming Unit—Eosinophils.

Stages

i. *Myeloblast and promyelocyte*: These stages are common to all granulocytes and no distinction can be made between different cell lines.

ii. *Eosinophilic myelocyte and metamyelocyte*: Specific granules start to appear in the myelocyte stage and once the cell has reached the metamyelocyte stage it cannot undergo further mitosis.

iii. *Eosinophil*: Mature cell has a bilobed nucleus. There are species specific variations in granule size once stained.

4. Monocytes

Monocytes develop from the same precursor as neutrophils—the CFU-GM. This then differentiates into the CFU-M under the influence of GM-CSF, IL-3 and M-CSF.

Stages

i. *Monoblast*: This is the first stage after cell has differentiated into the Colony Forming Unit—Monocyte.

ii. *Promonocyte:* Cell has a large nucleus and basophilic cytoplasm and consists of two populations: One rapidly dividing and the other slowly dividing, which acts as a reservoir.

iii. *Monocyte*: Monocytes are incapable of mitosis and enter the circulation. They have a large kidney-shaped nucleus with a slightly basophilic cytoplasm, which is often vacuolated.

iv. *Macrophage*: Once the monocyte has entered tissue it differentiates into a macrophage.

B. **Lymphoid** ('lim-foid') stem cells develop into two other types of white cells called T-progenitor cells and B-progenitor cells. Those destined to become T-cells leave the bone marrow and migrate to the thymus, and those destined to be B-cells migrate to the spleen and Gut-Associated Lymphoid Tissue (GALT) or proliferate directly from the bone marrow.

B-cell

The lymph nodes are arranged along the route of large blood vessels and are concentrated in areas such as the abdomen, underarms, groin, and neck. Small sacs called follicles within the lymph nodes contain B lymphocytes (B-cells). B-cells eventually mature into plasma cells that produce antigen-specific antibody, which is an immune system chemical that is directed against a specific foreign substance.

T-cell

The thymus gland is, to some extent, an "age-dependent" organ. It functions to create T lymphocytes (T-cells) in the developing fetus, attains its full size after a child is 2 years of age, and then shrinks to a nearly undetectable size by puberty (adolescence). Although the thymus shrinks with age, it continues to aid immune system function throughout a person's lifetime.

The thymus is located in front of the heart. It has two lobes and contains thymocytes (immature lymphocytes), epithelial cells (cells that cover the internal and external body surfaces, including the lining of blood vessels, etc.) and macrophages (large cells that ingest microorganisms and other foreign substances). T-cells primarily are responsible for cell-mediated immunity and immune system regulation. Within the thymus, immature pre-T cells develop and are able to recognize antigens (substances capable of starting a specific immune system response, e.g. bacteria, foreign proteins, etc.). The immature pre-T cells then migrate to other lymphoid tissues, such as the spleen and lymph nodes, where they mature and undergo additional differentiation.

Role of Spleen in Hemopoiesis

The spleen is a vital organ that is located on the left side of the body under the lower rib cage. It is a "ductless gland" that is closely associated with the circulatory system. The spleen contains a white pulp of lymphoid tissues and a red pulp that contains red blood cells and hollow cavities called sinuses. Both red and white pulps are abundant in phagocytes, the cells that consume foreign substances within the body. The spleen manufactures lymphocytes and other immune system cells to combat infection. It is a storehouse for healthy blood cells, and its lymphatic tissue filters out old and damaged blood cells, microorganisms, and cell waste. In case of bone marrow malfunction, the spleen may assume the role of blood cell formation.

■ THROMBOPOIESIS

Platelets are produced in the bone marrow, the same as the red cells and most of the white blood cells. Platelets are produced from very large bone marrow cells called megakaryocytes. As megakaryocytes develop into giant cells, they undergo a process of fragmentation that results in the release of over 1,000 platelets per megakaryocyte. The dominant hormone controlling megakaryocyte development is thrombopoietin (often abbreviated as TPO).

Platelet Structure

Platelets are actually not true cells but merely circulating fragments of cells. But even though platelets are merely cell fragments, they contain many structures that are critical to stop bleeding. They contain proteins on their surface that allow them to stick to breaks in the blood vessel wall and also to stick to each other. They contain granules that can secrete other proteins required for creating a firm plug to seal blood vessel breaks. Also platelets contain proteins similar to muscle proteins that allow them to change shape when they become sticky.

CHAPTER 14

Collection of Blood

Learning Objectives
- Collection of blood is the first and foremost step in acquiring quality test results. It requires both knowledge and skill to perform. Several essential steps that are required for three types of collection procedure—arterial blood collection, capillary blood collection and venous blood collection are discussed here.
- Choice of appropriate anticoagulant and correct form of labeling is interpreted in this chapter. Latest technique, such as use of evacuated tube for vein punctures is described with suitable picture.
- At times, blood does not come in needle immediately; different possible reasons for this situation are illustrated with diagram. Different sample rejection criteria are mentioned in this chapter.

Keywords
Vascular access device (VAD), Median cubital, Cephalic and Basilic veins, Tourniquet, Phlebotomist, Anticoagulant, Evacuated tube, Hemolysis

■ INTRODUCTION

The first step in acquiring a quality laboratory test result for any patient is the specimen collection procedure. Blood has to be tested in most of the blood-related disorders, metabolic disorders and various infections. The act of drawing or removing blood from the circulatory system through a cut (incision) or puncture in order to obtain a sample for analysis and diagnosis is called as Phlebotomy. *Phlebotomist is a* person who draws blood for diagnostic tests or to remove blood for treatment purposes.

Depending upon the site of collection, there are three popular methods of blood collection:
1. Arterial blood collection
2. Capillary blood collection
3. Venous blood collection

■ ARTERIAL BLOOD COLLECTION

This form of blood collection most commonly takes place within a hospital environment. The most common reason for collection of arterial blood is the evaluation of arterial blood gases. Arterial blood may be obtained directly from the artery (most commonly, the radial artery) by personnel who are trained to perform this procedure and are knowledgeable about the complications that could occur as a result of this procedure. Arterial blood may also be obtained from a vascular access device (VAD) inserted in an artery such as a femoral arterial line or Swan-Ganz catheter.

■ CAPILLARY BLOOD COLLECTION

Capillary blood is obtained from capillary beds that consist of the smallest veins (venules) and arteries (arterioles) of the circulatory system. The venules and arterioles join together in capillary beds forming a mixture of venous and arterial blood. Capillary blood is often the specimen of choice for infants, very young children, elderly patients with fragile veins, and severely burned patients. Point-of-care testing is often performed using a capillary blood specimen.

Capillary blood is obtained by pricking the tip of finger, lobe of ear, from the toe, and in infants, it is obtained from the heel.

However, the most convenient place to prick is finger. It is to be pricked from about half (½) cm from the nail. It is to be pricked about 3 mm deep. The area to be punctured should not be cold. If it is cold, warm it by massaging. Disinfect the site of puncture by using spirit or 95% alcohol. Wipe-off the first drop of blood, and use the next drop for testing. After obtaining sufficient amount of blood, let the patient apply slight pressure by using spirit with sterile swab.

This way of blood collection can be used when the amount of blood required is only few drops, like Hb, total leukocyte count (TLC), differential leukocyte count (DLC), etc. For capillary puncture, sterile needle or sterile lancet should be used.

Generally, nowadays, disposable needles are used. If, reusable needles are used, it should be sterile one.

VENOUS BLOOD COLLECTION (VENOUS PUNCTURE)

This is most common site of blood collection. With introduction of analyzers (automation), quantity of blood required is quite more. For venipuncture use the large veins of the arm which are the median cubital, cephalic or basilic veins. The basilic vein changes its direction toward the anterior surface of the arm and is joined to the cephalic vein by the median cubital vein. These veins are ideal for venipuncture due to their fairly large size and the fact that most are well anchored in tissue and will not "roll".

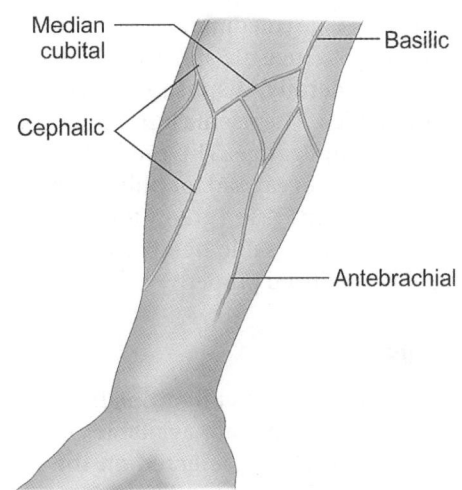

Fig. 14.1: Veins of the anterior forearm.

The correct order of vein selection is **(Fig. 14.1)**:
1. Median cubital
2. Cephalic
3. Basilic

To determine if the vein is adequate use the tip of the index finger to palpate the veins to determine their direction, depth and size. Choose the veins that are large and accessible.

First of all, assemble all the necessary equipments such as:
1. Needle
2. Syringe
3. Tourniquet
4. Disinfectant
5. Cotton swab
6. Tray of water
7. Collection bottle

Needle

There are several sizes of needles available; the size depends on the length and gauge of the needle that goes into the vein. Blood collection needle lengths range from 1 to 1½ inches. One-inch needles are used for routine venipuncture, 1½ inch needles are used for patients with very deep veins. The gauge of a needle is a number that indicates the diameter of its lumen; the lumen, also called the bore, is the circular hollow space inside the needle. Higher is the number of gauge, smaller is the lumen. Sterilized sharp needles of bore size of 18 to 20 gauge (medium, 1.2 to 0.9 mm) for adults and 23 gauge (0.5 mm) for children are needed. Generally, disposable needles are recommended. The needle top is color coded to indicate the gauge. The most frequently used needle gauges used for phlebotomy are: 20g (yellow top), 21g (green top), and 22g (black top). If reusable needles are used, it should be sterilized properly.

Syringe

Syringe of different capacities like 2 mL, 5 mL, 10 mL, 20 mL, are available. The size of syringe should be selected on the basis of amount of blood required for testing. Generally, disposable syringes are used if reusable syringes are used, it should be washed immediately and then sterilized before using.

Tourniquet

It may be soft rubber tube or belt. It is applied to arm about three inches above the elbow. It helps to slow the blood flow and makes vein more prominent, so that the puncture site is selected. Velcro tourniquets are also available. The tourniquet is tied in such a way that it can be removed with one hand.

Disinfectant

Clean the puncture site with 70% isopropyl alcohol with cotton swab. Vigorous back and forth friction is suggested. Use enough pressure to remove all perspiration and dirt from the puncture site. Allow the site to air dry. This serves two purposes: 1) drying allows for optimal site decontamination and 2) the site will not burn when the needle is inserted. After cleansing, do not touch the site.

Water Bath or Water Tray

Water tray should be used in case, if reusable syringes are used. If any small amount of blood is present inside the syringe after pouring in a container, the blood will be dried and clotted. This will be difficult in cleaning and in the movement of piston to reuse. Therefore, water tray is used for rinsing the syringe immediately. It is ready to reuse only after proper sterilization is done.

Collection Bottle/Tubes

The bottle should be sterilized and with cap. If anticoagulant is required, it should be added within the bottle in proper amount before blood collection. Now-a-days ready to use collection tubes are available. These are mostly made of plastic. These tubes are provided with additives. An additive is any substance added to a tube by the manufacturer. Different additives serve different purposes.

For example, an anticoagulant is the most common additive found in tubes. It prevents the blood from clotting by binding or inactivating one of the elements necessary for clotting to occur. With anticoagulated blood, we get plasma specimen. The most common anticoagulants used include sodium citrate, heparin, Ethylenediaminetetraacetic acid (EDTA), and potassium oxalate (Refer Chapter 15—Anticoagulants).

A clot activator is another type of additive found in most plastic tubes. Clot activators help the clotting process start and go to completion. The clot settles down and the liquid part that comes as supernatant is called serum.

For easy identification, standard colored stopper is provided for tubes which are indicative of the additives is summarized in **Table 14.1**.

Procedure

- First of all decide the amount of blood required and select the container according to the test to be done.
- Now ensure the patient what is to be done.
- Lay the arm of the patient on the table.
- Apply the tourniquet and select the prominent vein of the patient.

TABLE 14.1: Stopper color, additives and usage of blood sample.

Stopper Color	Additive	Specimen Usage
Yellow Blood culture bottles	<ul><li>Sodium polyanetholesulfonate (SPS)</li><li>Additives to keep microorganisms alive</li></ul>	Whole blood for blood cultures
Light blue	<ul><li>Sodium citrate</li><li>Ratio: 1 part anticoagulant to 9 parts of blood</li></ul>	Plasma for coagulation studies: PT, PTT and fibrinogen
Red	<ul><li>Clot activator</li><li>No anticoagulant/no additive</li></ul>	<ul><li>Serum for chemistry and serology tests</li><li>Chemistries: Cholesterol, glucose, BMP, CMP</li><li>Serologies: Hep B antibody, RPR, CRP</li></ul>
Green	<ul><li>Sodium heparin OR</li><li>Lithium heparin OR</li><li>Ammonium heparin</li></ul>	<ul><li>Plasma for chemistry tests</li><li>Often used for STAT chemistry tests</li></ul>
Lavender (purple)	K_2 EDTA (ethylenediaminetetraacetic acid)	Whole blood for hematology studies: CBC, WBC count, hemoglobin and hematocrit, platelet count, reticulocyte count, ESR
Pink	K_3 EDTA	Plasma and red blood cells for blood bank testing using gel system
Gray	<ul><li>Potassium oxalate and sodium fluoride (plasma)</li><li>Na_2 EDTA and sodium fluoride (plasma)</li><li>Sodium fluoride (serum)</li></ul>	Glucose, blood alcohol (ethanol) levels, lactic acid
Royal blue	Color of tube label indicates additive:<ul><li>Purple – EDTA (plasma)</li><li>Green – heparin (plasma)</li><li>Red – none (serum)</li></ul>	Nutrients, toxicology and trace metal analysis. Examples: antimony, arsenic, cadmium, chromium, copper, lead, magnesium, manganese, zinc
Black	Buffered sodium citrate	Whole blood for Westergren, erythrocyte sedimentation rate (ESR)
Yellow	Acid citrate dextrose (ACD)	Whole Blood for genetic and tissue test

- With cotton swab, disinfect the puncture site.
- The cotton swab should be previously soaked in the disinfectant.
- Assemble needle and syringe, check that, it is sharp and unblocked, and it is moving smoothly. This can be checked by passing air through the syringe. But there should not be any air present in the syringe at the time of blood collection.
- With the left hand, hold patients arm, so that skin over vein is tightened. Ask the patient to open and close the wrist.
- Take the syringe in right hand, holding index finger against the base of the needle, keep the point of needle to upper side and push firmly and steadily without any hesitation into the center of vein.
- The angle between skin and needle should not be more than 30°. The moment needle enters in vein, blood flows back into syringe.
- With your left hand, slightly pull back the piston till required amount of blood is obtained in the syringe.
- Now, remove the tourniquet, place cotton swab over the needle and wound. Withdraw the needle slowly, and ask the patient to place a cotton swab over the wound. This stops bleeding from wound.
- Remove the needle from the syringe and gently expel the blood into appropriate container.

- If anticoagulant is used, gently shake the bottle for proper mixing. Or gently invert at least five times to ensure proper mixing of additive.
- Discard the needle and syringe properly. If reusable syringe is used immediately wash it with water using water tray.

Specimen Labeling

Each blood sample must be labeled immediately following collection in the presence of the patient. The minimum amount of information required is:
- Patient's full name (last name first, first name second)
- Identification number (may be the patient's Date of Birth or other unique number)
- Date and time of collection. Many laboratories require the use of military time.
- Phlebotomist's initials.

Note: Never label tubes before collecting the sample, never take the tubes to another location to label them.

USE OF EVACUATED TUBE FOR VEIN PUNCTURES (VACUUM BLOOD COLLECTION SYSTEM)

Blood collection using the evacuated tube provides blood samples for analysis. The blood goes directly from the patient's vein into the appropriate test tube. The vacuum system consists of a double-pointed needle, a tube holder, and a series of vacuum tubes with rubber stoppers of various colors. The tube stopper color indicates the type of additive present (as discussed in **Table 14.1**).

Needle

The needle for vacuum blood collection is pointed at both ends, with one end shorter than the other. The long end of the needle is used for insertion into the vein; the shorter end is used to pierce the rubber stopper of the vacuum tube and is usually covered by a rubber sheath. The sheath makes it possible to draw several tubes of blood by preventing leakage of blood as tubes are changed; this is called a multi-draw needle. Most frequently used needles are of gauge 21 to 23.

Holder

The shorter end of needle which is covered by a rubber cuff is screwed into the holder. A thread separates the two ends, and this is where the holder is screwed into place. Thus holder has needle on each end. This holds the sample collection tube in place and protects the phlebotomist from direct contact with blood. Holders are available in two sizes, one for adult venipuncture and one for pediatric procedures. The mostly all holders are for single use only.

Vacuum Collection Tubes

Vacuum collection tubes are glass or plastic tubes sealed with a partial vacuum inside by rubber stoppers. The air pressure inside the tube is negative, less than the normal environment. After inserting the longer needle into the vein, the phlebotomist pushes the tube into the holder so that the shorter needle pierces the stopper of tube. The difference in pressure between the inside of the tube and the vein causes blood to fill the tube. Multiple vacuum tubes (as per type of sample needed) can be attached to and removed in turn from a single needle, allowing multiple samples to be obtained from a single procedure. This is possible due to the multiple sample sleeve, which is a flexible rubber fitting over the posterior end of the needle which seals the needle until it is pushed out of the way. This keeps blood from freely draining out of the back of the needle inserted in the patient's vein, as each test tube is removed and the next impaled. This is called a multi-draw or multi sample needle.

The tubes are available in various sizes for adult and pediatric phlebotomies. Adult tubes have volumes of 5, 7, 10 and 15 mL and pediatric tubes are available in volumes of 2,

3 and 4 mL. The color of the stopper on each tube indicates additives in the tube (Refer **Table 14.1**). Because the additives from each tube can be left on the needle used to fill the tubes, they must be drawn in a specific order to ensure that cross contamination will not negatively affect testing of the samples if multiple tubes are to be drawn at once. The "order (sequence) of draw" suggested for evacuated tube collection method is:

- Blood cultures and sterile collections (culture bottles)
- Sodium citrate (light blue)
- No additive/silica clot activator (red)
- Lithium heparin (green)
- Sodium heparin (green)
- K_2 and K_3 EDTA (purple/lavender)
- Sodium fluoride and potassium oxalate (gray)
- Tube containing EDTA or clot activator or no additive used for testing trace elements (navy/royal blue)
- Acid citrate dextrose (ACD) (yellow) and any other tubes.

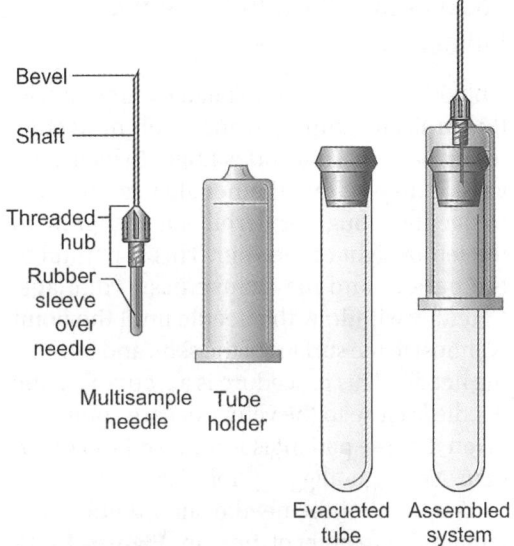

Fig. 14.2: Evacuated tube assembly system.

Procedure (Fig. 14.2)

- Assemble equipment and supplies.
- Prepare the vacuum system by attaching the needle to the hub and positioning a tube in the holder.
- Apply the tourniquet and examine the arm for palpable veins.
- Cleanse the chosen site with a 70% alcohol swab. Allow the site to air dry.
- Ask patient to clench fist tightly.
- Position the holder in the palm of your hand between your thumb and index finger.
- Uncap the needle. Inspect the needle for manufacturer's defects.
- Anchor the vein selected, using the thumb and index finger.
- Position the needle in the same direction as the vein selected. Insert the needle, bevel up, at a 15° angle. The needle should be inserted in one smooth motion. Only the index finger and thumb should move forward to guide the needle into the vein.
- Release the vein and push the evacuated tube onto the back of the needle. This will puncture the tube and it will get filled up with blood to due pressure difference.
- Allow the tube to fill, when the vacuum has been exhausted, blood will no longer enter the tube.
- Keeping the holder absolutely still, pull the evacuated tube of the back of the needle and replace it with the second tube (if the first tube contained an additive, gently invert it while waiting for the second tube to fill).
- Once blood begins to enter the second tube, release the tourniquet within one minute of application.
- Pull the evacuated tube off of the needle. Allow it to rest in the holder.
- Place a piece of gauze or a cotton ball over the puncture site.
- Remove the needle from the patient's arm and immediately apply pressure with the gauze.
- Withdraw needle and immediately activate the needle safety device and place the needle assembly in disposal container.
- Label the tubes collected immediately as discussed above.

Possibilities of Failure in Blood Collection

If blood does not come in needle immediately, this indicates improper insertion of needle. In this case, use free index finger to locate the vein. It may be that the needle has not gone in deeply enough or perhaps it is slightly to the left or right of the vein. This is painful to the patient and may cause tissue damage. Carefully withdraw the needle until the point is almost to the surface of the skin, and redirect the needle. This procedure is acceptable if the needle is close to the vein, but care should be taken that the patient is not caused too much pain. Never go "digging" for veins.

The bevel of the needle should enter and remain in the center of the vein. **Figures 14.3A to F** are shown proper and improper needle positioning.

Rejection of Sample

The quality of laboratory results are directly affected by the quality of the blood sample obtained from the patient. Samples may need to be rejected as unacceptable for the following reasons:

- Hemolysis—is usually caused by a procedural error such as using too small of a needle or pulling back to hard on the plunger of a syringe used for collecting the sample. The red cells rupture resulting in hemoglobin being released into the serum/plasma, making the sample unsuitable for many laboratory tests. The serum/plasma will appear red instead of straw-colored.
- Clotted—failure to mix or inadequate mixing of samples collected into an additive tube. In this case, the red cells clump together making the sample unsuitable for testing.
- Insufficient sample (quantity not sufficient)—certain additive tubes must be filled completely. Incorrect blood to additive ratio will adversely affect the laboratory test results. When many tests are ordered on the same tube, be sure to know the amount of sample needed for each test.
- Wrong tube collected for test ordered.
- Improper storage—for certain tests, once blood is collected, it must be placed in ice, protected from light, or be kept warm after collection.
- Improperly labeled.

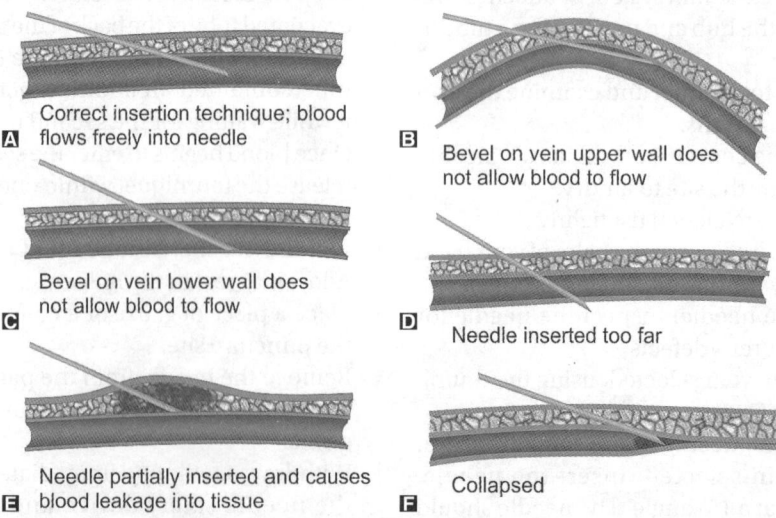

Figs. 14.3A to F: Proper and improper needle positioning. (A) Proper needle position; (B) Needle bevel against the upper wall of a vain; (C) Needle bevel against or embedded in opposite wall of vein; (D) Needle inserted all the way through a vein; (E) Needle partially inserted into vein; (F) Needle in collapsed vein.

CHAPTER 15

Anticoagulants

Learning Objectives
- Choice of correct anticoagulant for a particular blood test is very crucial.
- This chapter has brief description of chemical and biological anticoagulant.
- Preparation and use of different anticoagulants are mentioned in this chapter.

Keywords
Citrate, EDTA, CPD, Oxalate, Heparine

■ INTRODUCTION

Anticoagulant prevents clotting from blood. It is used in hematological laboratory where complete blood or plasma is required; depending upon the test to be done, the type of anticoagulant is decided. Most of the anticoagulants prevent clotting by removing calcium, or iron which are necessary for clotting process. Every anticoagulant is added in fixed proportion to blood. Anticoagulants are of following types:

■ CHEMICAL ANTICOAGULANTS

These anticoagulants are prepared in laboratory. These are as follows:
i. Citrate:
   a. Trisodium citrate
   b. Disodium citrate
ii. Ethylenediaminetetraacetic acid (EDTA)
iii. Citrate phosphate dextrose (CPD)
iv. Oxalate

i. **Citrate**
   a. *Trisodium citrate*: This anticoagulant is prepared by dissolving 3.8 g of trisodium citrate in 100 mL of distilled water. About 0.4 mL of anticoagulant is required for 2 mL of blood. Addition of dextrose to anticoagulant provides nutrition to the red cells and helps in longer storage. Such anticoagulant is known as acid citrate dextrose (ACD) because along with citric acid, trisodium citrate and dextrose are mixed in this anticoagulant. This anticoagulant is used in the solution form, as it is in blood bank. The storage of blood with this anticoagulant is maximum up to 21 days.
   b. *Disodium citrate*: This itself provides the buffering action along with nourishment provided by dextrose. This is used in solution form. Maximum period of storage with this anticoagulant is 21 days.
ii. **Ethylenediaminetetraacetic Acid (EDTA)**: It can be prepared by dissolving 10 g of EDTA in 1000 mL of distilled water. About 0.4 mL of anticoagulant is required for 2 mL of blood. This anticoagulant does not

disturb the cellular structure. Therefore, it can be used for blood cell count, ESR, prothrombin estimation, etc.

EDTA however, cannot be used for biochemical tests. This anticoagulant is dried in the container by keeping in an incubator or hot air oven for overnight period, i.e. for 12 hours. The storage period with EDTA is 2 to 3 days.

iii. **Citrate Phosphate Dextrose (CPD):** In this anticoagulant, the citrate is dissolved in phosphate buffer, which maintains pH more accurately than ACD solution. The dextrose present in this provides nutrition to other cells. The storage period of CPD is 21 days. The disadvantage is that, it is costly and difficult to prepare and adjust pH.

iv. **Oxalate:** It is prepared by dissolving 1.2 g of ammonium oxalate and 0.8 mL of potassium oxalate to 100 mL of distilled water. About 0.2 mL of anticoagulant is required for 2 mL of blood. This anticoagulant may disturb cellular structure if kept for longer period, however, if used immediately, it can be used for estimation of bilirubin, and prothrombin time and estimation of blood cells, PCV (packed cell volume). This anticoagulant is dried in a container by keeping it for overnight period in hot air oven. It is also called as double oxalate.

BIOLOGICAL ANTICOAGULANT: HEPARINE

Heparine is the only biological anticoagulant which can not be prepared in a laboratory. It is obtained from leech. It is a good anticoagulant and does not alter size of RBC. It is used in concentration of 10–15 units/mL blood. This anticoagulant act by destroying thrombin or thromboplastin required for clotting.

Heparine is used to determine the blood gases. It can be used for erythrocyte sedimentation rate (ESR), packed cell volume (PCV) osmotic fragility and other hematological tests.

Anticoagulant should be sterilized before use, then blood is added to the anticoagulant, it should be mixed gently by inverting it 10 to 15 times or shacking it gently.

CHAPTER 16

Total RBC Count

Learning Objectives
- Red blood cells are very important constituent of blood, as it carries oxygen throughout the body. Total RBC count is one of the several tests that are included in complete blood count (CBC).
- This chapter has description of counting red blood cells by using hemocytometer.
- It also discusses clinical significance of red blood cells.

Keywords
RBC diluting fluid, RBC pipette, Neubauer chamber, Anemia polycythemia, Pulmonary fibrosis, Erythrocytopenia, Erythrocytosis, Hemolysis, Leukemia

INTRODUCTION

The counting of blood cells, manually with the help of microscope, is not possible. Therefore, to count the cells, blood is diluted and placed in a special type of counting chamber. This technique is called hemocytometeric counting. The cells often counted by this method are red cells, white cells, platelets, and eosinophils.

Red Cell Count

For total red cell count following equipment are required:
1. RBC diluting fluid
2. RBC pipette
3. Hemocytometer
4. Microscope
5. Blood sample

RBC Diluting Fluid

RBCs are about 5 millions/cu. mm of blood. Counting this much number is highly impossible. Therefore, the blood sample is diluted with the help of RBC diluting fluid. It fixes and preserves RBC. It is isotonic to red cells.

Following two types of RBC diluting fluid are commonly used:

Formalin citrate diluting fluid

Composition:
- Trisodium citrate: 3 g
- Formalin: 1 mL
- Distill water: 99 mL

This diluting fluid is cheap and commonly used.

Haym's diluting fluid

Composition:
- Sodium chloride: 0.5 g
- Sodium sulfate: 2.5 g
- Mercuric chloride: 0.25 g
- Distilled water: 100 mL

The RBC diluting fluid prevents hemolysis and removes unwanted blood cells.

RBC Pipette

RBC pipette is graduated to give dilution 1 : 100 or 1 : 200. It has bottom marked with 0.5

and 1 and the top is marked with 101. It has a round bulb containing red bead. A rubber tube is attached to the top for sucking. Blood sucked up to 0.5 mark gives dilution 1 : 200. In case of anemic patient, it is sucked up to 1 mark to give dilution 1 : 100. After blood, RBC diluting fluid is sucked up to 101 mark and mixed gently.

■ HEMOCYTOMETER

This is a chamber used for cell count. Generally improved Neubauer chamber is used **(Fig. 16.1)**. Other chambers like Burgers and Fuchs-Rosenthal may also be used. The Neubauer chamber has ruled area of total 9 sq. mm and the depth is 0.1 mm. The central one square is highly ruled. The central square is divided into 25 squares. Each square is further subdivided in 16 small squares. For RBC count, count the cells in each corner and one central square, i.e. total 5 squares. As each square is further divided into 16 small squares, the area to be counted is, 16 × 5 = 80 small squares.

Microscope

Generally, for total red cell count a conventional microscope, with an objective of the magnification power of 40x is used.

Blood Sample

Capillary blood or EDTA anticoagulated blood may be used.

Principle

The blood specimen is diluted (usually 200 times) with red cell diluting fluid. This diluted blood is placed in hemocytometer. The cells are counted under proper magnification over the specified area of hemocytometer. The known factors are:
1. Number of cells counted
2. Volume of fluid inside the counting chamber
3. Dilution of blood

With the help of these known factors, the number of RBC/cu. mm of undiluted blood can be calculated.

■ PROCEDURE

Assemble all the equipment; draw the blood directly from finger or collected sample into RBC pipette up to 0.5 mark **(Fig. 16.2)**. Wipe off the tip of pipette to remove extra blood, if present. Then immediately draw up the diluting fluid up to 101 mark. Now rotate the pipette gently, so that the diluting fluid gets

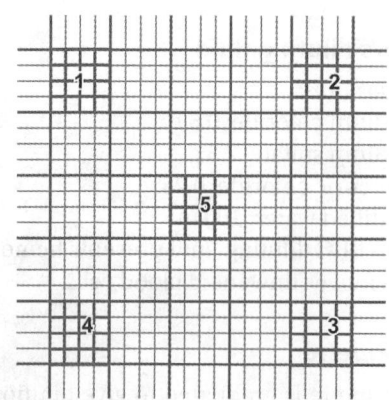

Fig. 16.1: Central square of Neubauer chamber.

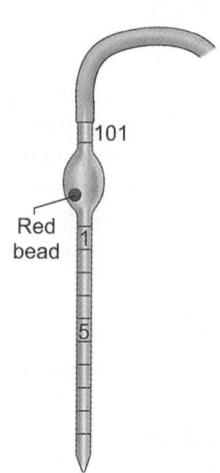

Fig. 16.2: RBC pipette.

mixed properly. This will give dilution 1 : 200. Place the coverslip in position over the ruled area of chamber. Once again mix the solution thoroughly by rotating the pipette. Now apply slight pressure on the rubber tube of pipette, so that the second drop of fluid is in hanging position. Touch the tip of pipette (hanging drop) against the edge of coverslip. The angle between pipette and coverslip is 45°. With this process, chamber gets filled with the fluid. This is known as charging of the chamber.

The care should be taken that, no air bubble is present inside the chamber and there is no over filling beyond the ruled area.

Leave the counting chamber as it, without disturbing for about 3 minutes. This will allow the settling down of RBCs. Place the chamber on stage of microscope. Adjust the light and ruled area. Make sure that, the distribution of RBC over the chamber is uniform.

Now count the RBC in Central Square (Fig. 16.1). The central square is subdivided into 25 squares. Out of 25 squares, count four at each corner and one at center. Each of these five squares is subdivided into 16 small squares. Thus, RBCs are counted in 16 × 5 = 80 small squares. In case of marginal cells, count the cells on 'L' line, i.e. either right and lower or left and upper margin. Make the total of cells counted in 5 squares and repeat the procedure to another side of the chamber.

▮ CALCULATIONS

Thus, the known things are:
1. Number of cells counted:
   Suppose the number of cells counted is 'N'.
2. The volume of fluid inside the chamber.
   i.e. Area × depth

   Area = Central 1 sq. mm
        = 25 sq.
   Out of which, 5 are counted.
   $\therefore$ 25 = 1. sq. mm.
   5 = ?
   $$\frac{5}{25} = \frac{1}{5}$$

$$\text{Total RBC count} = \frac{N \times \text{Dilution}}{\text{Area} \times \text{Depth}}$$

$$= \frac{N \times 200}{\frac{1}{5} \times 0.1}$$

$\therefore$ Total RBC count = N × 10,000.

Thus, with the help of this formula, we can calculate the total number of RBC present in blood.

For example, total number of RBCs counted in five squares are 452.

Therefore N = 452

Total RBC count is 452 × 10,000 = 4,520,000 = 4.52 million

▮ CLINICAL SIGNIFICANCE

RBCs are the most common component of human blood. The cells contain hemoglobin, which is a protein that carries oxygen around the body. Hemoglobin is also responsible for blood's red color. RBCs circulate the body for an average of 110 days. After this, the cells go to the liver, where they breakdown. The body recycles their nutrients back into the cells.

The bone marrow continuously produces RBCs. If the body does not receive a regular supply of necessary nutrients, the RBCs may become malformed or die off at a faster rate than the body can replace them.
- The normal RBC range for men is 4.7 to 5.9 million cells per microliter (mcL).
- The normal RBC range for women who are not pregnant is 4.2 to 5.4 million per mcL.
- The normal RBC range for children is 4.0 to 5.5 million per mcL.

These ranges may vary depending on the laboratory or doctor.

Conditions associated with higher RBC count (erythrocytosis):
- Cigarette smoking
- Congenital heart disease
- Dehydration
- Renal cell carcinoma, a type of kidney cancer

- Pulmonary fibrosis
- Polycythemia vera, a bone marrow disease that causes overproduction of RBCs and is associated with a genetic mutation
- At higher altitude, your RBC count may increase for several weeks because there is less oxygen in the air.
- Certain drugs like gentamicin and methyldopa can increase RBC count. Gentamicin is an antibiotic used to treat bacterial infections in the blood. Methyldopa is often used to treat high blood pressure. It works by relaxing the blood vessels to allow blood to flow more easily through the body.
- A high RBC count may be a result of sleep apnea, pulmonary fibrosis, and other conditions that cause low oxygen levels in the blood.
- Performance-enhancing drugs like protein injections and anabolic steroids can also increase RBCs.

Conditions associated with lower RBC count (erythrocytopenia):
- Anemia
- Bone marrow failure
- Erythropoietin deficiency, which is the primary cause of anemia in patients with chronic kidney disease
- Hemolysis or RBC destruction caused by transfusions and blood vessel injury
- Internal or external bleeding
- Leukemia
- Malnutrition
- Multiple myeloma, a cancer of the plasma cells in bone marrow
- Nutritional deficiencies, including deficiencies in iron, copper, folate, and vitamins B_6 and B_{12}
- Pregnancy
- Thyroid disorders
- Certain drugs can also lower your RBC count, especially, chemotherapy drugs, chloramphenicol, which treats bacterial infections, quinidine, which can treat irregular heartbeats and hydantoins, which are traditionally used to treat epilepsy and muscle spasms.

CHAPTER 17

Total White Cell Count

Learning Objectives
- White blood cells are very important constituent of blood, as these are immunity cells and can detect hidden infections of the body. Total WBC count is one of the several tests that are included in complete blood count (CBC).
- This chapter has description of counting white blood cells by using hemocytometer.
- It also discusses clinical significance of white blood cells.

Keywords
WBC diluting fluid, WBC pipette, Neubauer chamber, Autoimmune disorders, Leukopenia, Leukocytosis

■ INTRODUCTION

The normal white cell count is 4,000 to 10,000/cu mm of blood. These cells can be counted with the help of hemocytometer.

Principle

The whole blood is used for total white cell count. With the WBC diluting fluid, it is diluted 20 times and placed in hemocytometer. The cells are counted under proper magnification over specified area. Thus, the known factors are:
1. The number of cells counted.
2. The volume of fluid inside the chamber (i.e. the counting area × depth).
3. Dilution of blood.

With the help of these known factors, the number of WBC/cu mm of undiluted blood can be calculated.

Equipments Required

For total WBC counting following equipments are required:
1. WBC diluting fluid
2. WBC pipette
3. Hemocytometer
4. Microscope
5. Blood sample.

WBC Diluting Fluid

WBCs are about 4000 to 10,000 per cu. mm of blood. Counting this much number is highly impossible. Therefore, the blood sample is diluted with the help of diluting fluid or Türk's fluid.

Türk's solution is a hematological stain (crystal violet or aqueous methylene blue) in 1-2% acetic acid and distilled water. The solution destroys the membrane of WBCs, RBCs and platelets within a blood sample, and stains the nuclei of the white blood cells, making them easier to see and count.

Composition
- Glacial acetic acid: 3 mL
- Aqueous gentian violet: 1%
- Distilled water: 97 mL

Acetic acid of diluting fluid removes red cells, and gentian violet stains the nucleus of WBC to facilitate the WBC counting.

WBC Pipette

WBC pipette is graduated to give blood dilution 1 : 20. It has rubber tube, containing white bead. The bottom of pipette is marked with 0.5 and on top, it is 11. It has rubber tube attached for sucking.

■ HEMOCYTOMETER

It is a chamber used for cell count. Generally, improved Neubauer chamber is used. Other chambers like Burgers and Fuchs-Rosenthal may also be used. Neubauer chamber consists of 9 square mm area marked and ruled. It has four squares, each with 1 mm. The outer four squares are divided into 16 small squares (**Fig. 17.1**).

∴ 16 × 4 = 64 small squares.

The depth of Neubauer chamber is 0.1 mm. It has a special coverslip.

Microscope

Generally, for total leucocyte count a conventional microscope, with an objective of the magnification power of 10X (0.25 NA) is used.

Blood Sample

Capillary blood or EDTA anticoagulated blood is used for WBC counting.

■ PROCEDURE

Assemble all the equipment. Draw the blood directly into WBC pipette up to 0.5 mark. Wipe off the tip of pipette to remove extra blood present at the tip. Then immediately draw up the WBC diluting fluid up to 11 mark. Now rotate the pipette gently, so that the fluid and the blood get properly mixed. This will give dilution 1 : 20. Place coverslip in position over the ruled area. Once again mix the solution thoroughly by rotating the pipette. Expel one drop of fluid from the pipette. Now the second drop is allowed to hang from the pipette. This can be done by applying slight pressure on the rubber tube of the pipette. Immediately when the drop is in hanging position, touch the tip against the edge of coverslip.

The angle between the pipette and Neubauer chamber is about 45°. With this process, the fluid gets inside the chamber. This is known as charging of the chamber. The care should be taken during charging, so that there should not be any air bubble present inside the chamber and there is no over filling beyond the ruled area.

Leave the counting chamber as it is without disturbing for about 2 to 3 minutes. This will allow settling down the WBCs in the counting chamber. Place the counting chamber on the stage of microscope, adjust the light and the ruled area.

The difference between the two square cell count should not be more than 10 WBC. Now, count the WBC in all four outer squares. Make the total and repeat the same procedure on the another side of the chamber. Take average of the two sides.

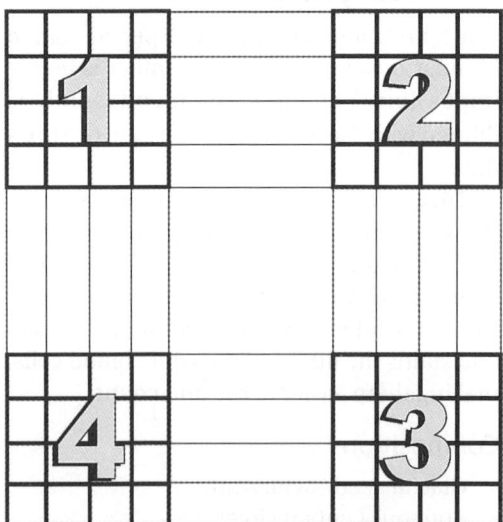

Fig. 17.1: Corner squares of Neubauer chamber.

In case of marginal cells, count the cells on the margin of 'L' shape, i.e. either right and lower or left and upper side.

■ CALCULATIONS

The known factors are:
1. The volume of fluid inside the chamber
$$= \text{Area} \times \text{depth}$$
$$= 4 \times 0.1$$
$$= 0.4$$
2. Dilution of blood $= 20$
3. The number of cells counted in four squares
Suppose, it is $= N$

$$\therefore \text{TLC} = \frac{N \times 20}{\text{Area} \times \text{Depth}}$$

$$= \frac{N \times 20}{4 \times 0.1} = \frac{N \times 20}{0.4}$$

$$\therefore \text{TLC} = N \times 50$$

With the help of this formula, we can calculate the total number of leucocytes in blood.

For example, total number of WBCs counted in outer four squares are 168

Therefore $N = 168$

Total WBC count is $168 \times 50 = 8,400$ (per mcL of blood)

Normal Value

Age range for WBC count (per mcL of blood)
Newborns: 9,000 to 30,000
Children under 2: 6,200 to 17,000
Children over 2 and adults: 5,000 to 10,000

■ CLINICAL SIGNIFICANCE

A WBC count can detect hidden infections, such as autoimmune diseases, immune deficiencies, and blood disorders. This test also help doctors monitor the effectiveness of chemotherapy or radiation treatment in people with cancer.

Conditions associated with lower WBC count (Leukopenia):
- HIV
- Autoimmune disorders
- Bone marrow disorders or damage
- Lymphoma
- Severe infections
- Liver and spleen diseases
- Lupus
- Radiation therapy
- Some medications, such as antibiotics

Conditions associated with higher WBC count (Leukocytosis):
- Smoking
- Infections such as tuberculosis
- Tumors in the bone marrow
- Leukemia
- Inflammatory conditions, such as arthritis and bowel disease
- Stress
- Exercise
- Tissue damage
- Pregnancy
- Allergies
- Asthma
- Some medications, such as corticosteroids

CHAPTER 18

Differential Leukocyte Count

Learning Objectives
- A differential leukocyte count gives the relative percentage of each type of white blood cell and also helps to reveal abnormal white blood cell.
- This chapter reveals preparation, staining and microscopic examination of blood smear for DLC.
- It also contains information of different leukocytes on clinical significance, normal values and their role in immune system.

Keywords
Blood smear, Leishman stain, Giemsa's stain, Wright's stain, Neutrophilia, Lymphocytopenia, Lymphocytic leukemia, Aplastic anemia, Lymphocytosis, Myelofibrosis, Monocytosis

1. Preparation of blood smear
2. Staining of blood
3. Staining of smear
4. Microscopic examination

■ PREPARATION OF BLOOD SMEAR

Take a clean grease free slide. Obtain capillary blood directly from the finger or EDTA anticoagulated blood. Place it on a corner of a slide. Take a spreader [spreader is a slide with sharp edges **(Fig. 18.1)**]. Touch the edge of the spreader to blood drop on slide. Slightly push it backward so that, the drop is spread evenly

■ INTRODUCTION

Differential leukocyte count (DLC) is important for the diagnosis of various blood-related disorders, involving white cell or red cell. Generally, it is performed to check the normal number or distribution of different leukocytes. It also gives the morphology of different cells.

The blood specimen to be used for differential leukocyte count is capillary blood or ethylenediaminetetraacetic acid (EDTA) anticoagulated blood.

There are three major steps involved in differential cell count:

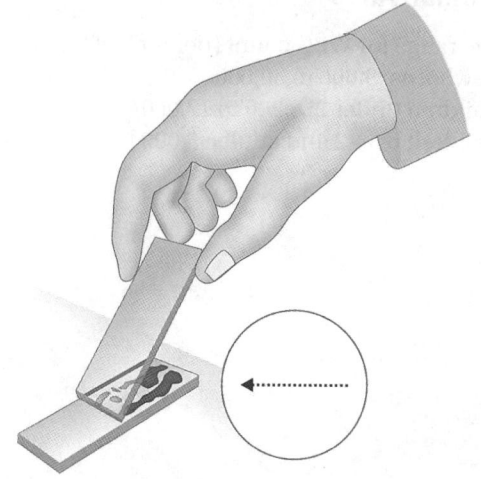

Fig. 18.1: Smear preparation.

to the edge of the spreader. Now, spread blood with the help of a spreader across clean grease free slide.

The angle between spreader and slide should be about 45°. With a quick movement, push the spreader towards the other end of the slide. Blood film should not be too thick. It should be 1 cm from the edge of slide and 5 mm in width.

■ STAINING OF BLOOD SMEAR

Blood cells have different structures, which take different stains. Some are basophilic, others are acidophilic while some cells accept neutral stain. Therefore, the blood smear is stained with a combination of three stains. These are called as 'Romanowsky stain'.

The three different types of Romanowsky stains are commonly in use.
1. Leishman stain
2. Giemsa's stain
3. Wright's stain.

Each of the stain contains acidic stain, basic stain and buffer solution. Generally, methylene blue or toluene are basic stains, and Eosin, Azure-I, Azure-II are the acidic stains in use.

It is advisable to stain a slide soon after preparation of blood smear.

Leishman Stain

Leishman stain is the most common and cheapest of all stain.

Composition

- *Leishman stain powder*: 0.15 g
- *Methyl alcohol*: 100 mL

Leishman stain crystals are grounded in a glass mortar. This powder is first dissolved in few mL of methyl alcohol, and then the remaining quantity of alcohol is added, so that the entire volume becomes 100 mL. Pour the stain in a clean dry bottle, close it well. Do not open it or filter it within 3 weeks. After 3 weeks, it is ready for use.

Blood films are placed in a staining tray. The dry blood film is then covered with stain. The stain should be evenly distributed over the entire slide. After 1 minute add distill water or buffer solution (sodium-potassium phosphate buffer at pH 6.8) to the slide. The distilled water/buffer solution should be carefully mixed with the stain. Keep it as it is for about 7 to 8 minutes. Then wash the slide with distill water to remove excess of stain. Air dry the film and observe under oil immersion objective of microscope.

■ MICROSCOPIC EXAMINATION

First examine stained blood smear under low power objective. Note the background color and distribution of cells.

In an ideal staining smear, three zones can be identified:
1. Thick area or head of smear
2. The central area is body
3. At the end of smear is tail region.

Choose the portion of the smear in the body region, slightly before the tail end.

Observe the slide under oil immersion objective by putting a drop of oil over the slide.

Examine the slide in tail region using OIO (oil immersion objective) and move the slide as shown in **Figure 18.2**.

Count each type of white cell observed. Record the observations either on a piece of paper in a tabular form or on a cell counter. The cell counter has different keys for different types of WBC. Continue the counting till 100 cells are counted. This will give the average number of white cells.

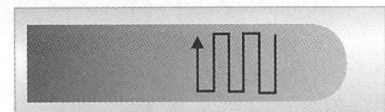

Fig. 18.2: Observation of smear.

Observation

With Leishman stain, the cells are observed as **(Fig. 18.3)**:

- *Neutrophil:* Purple colored nuclei with pink cytoplasm.
- *Eosinophil:* Cytoplasm is faint pink, nucleus is purple and granules are orange red.
- *Basophil:* Granules stain dark blue with purple nucleus.
- *Monocytes:* Pink cytoplasm with purple color nucleus.
- *Lymphocyte:* Dark blue nucleus with light blue cytoplasm.
- *Platelets:* Violet colored granules.
- *Red cells:* Pink color.

Wright Stain

Wright stain is very similar to Leishman stain.

Composition

- *Wright stain powder:* 0.3 g
- *Glycerol:* 3 mL
- *Methyl alcohol:* 97 mL

Left this solution as it is for a week.

Procedure

Cover the slide with stain for 5 to 10 minutes. Take care that the stain does not dry. Now add equal amount of buffer solution/distilled water to the slide. Allow it to react for 2 to 3 minutes. Then wash the slide with water, and air dry it. Now observe under microscope.

Observation

Wright stain gives the same color reaction, as that of Leishman stain.

Giemsa's Stain

This is one of the best stain for malarial and other blood parasite. It is also satisfactory as a routine blood stain.

Composition

- *Giemsa's stain powder:* 0.75 g
- *Glycerin:* 25 mL
- *Methyl alcohol:* 75 mL

Place 75 mL methyl alcohol and 25 mL glycerin in a beaker. Put in a water bath and add 0.75 g of dry Giemsa's power. Warm up to 60°C. Stir with a glass rod. Filter the solution. This is a stock solution. For use, mix 1 mL of stock solution of stain with 4 mL of methyl alcohol.

Procedure

Cover the slide with 15 drops of stain for 1 minute. Add 30 drops of distilled water, mix well and allow to stand for 5 minutes. Wash with water, air dry the smear, and observe under OIO.

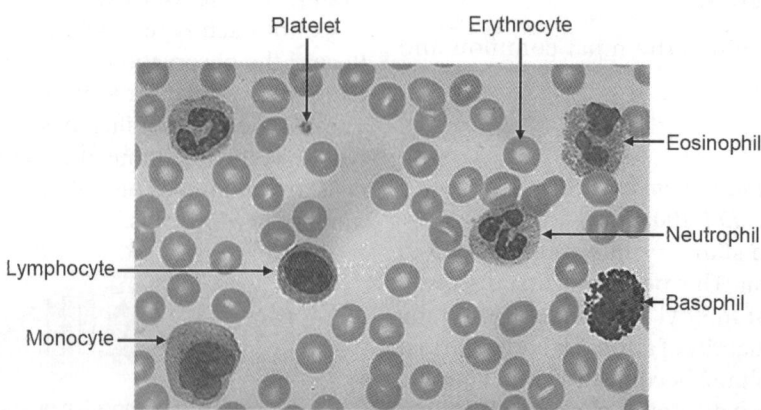

Fig. 18.3: Peripheral blood smear.
(For color version See Color Plate 5)

Observation

- *Nuclei of neutrophil*: Reddish purple color
- *Eosinophilic granules*: Red to orange color
- *Basophilic granules:* Blue color
- *Lymphocyte:* Dark blue nucleus with light blue cytoplasm
- *Platelets:* Violet to purple granules

■ CLINICAL SIGNIFICANCE

The basic use of DLC is to identify changes in distribution of white cells. These changes are related to specific infection, like bacterial, viral, parasitic, leukemic, etc. Different clinical terms are used for the different changes in normal values of the cells.

Normal values

Cells	In %	Per cu mm
Neutrophil	60 to 70	3,000 to 7,000
Lymphocyte	25 to 35	2,000 to 3,000
Monocyte	2 to 6	100 to 600
Eosinophil	1 to 6	50 to 400
Basophil	0 to 0.5	0 to 50

Thus, differential leukocyte count gives us the idea about distribution of different proportions of white cells.

When an infection or inflammatory condition occurs, the body releases white blood cells to help fight the infection. As a part of immune system, different white blood cells perform following functions:
- Basophils secrete chemicals to help fight allergies and infectious agents
- Eosinophils attack parasites and cancer cells and assist with allergic response
- Lymphocytes produce antibodies against bacteria, viruses, and other invaders
- Neutrophils kill bacteria and fungi
- Monocytes help fight bacteria, viruses, and other infections in your body.

Low or high count of each cell is associated with certain pathologic condition.
- *Neutrophils*: These are most abundant cells. They can move freely through the walls of veins and into the tissues of body to immediately attack all antigens.

Having a high percentage of neutrophils in blood is called neutrophilia. This is an indication of an infection. Neutrophilia can point to a number of underlying conditions and factors, including:
  - Infection, most likely bacterial
  - Noninfectious inflammation
  - Injury
  - Surgery
  - Smoking cigarettes or sniffing tobacco
  - High stress level
  - Excessive exercise
  - Steroid use
  - Heart attacks
  - Chronic myeloid leukemia

Neutropenia is the term for low neutrophil levels. Low neutrophil counts are most often associated with medications but they also can be a sign of other factors or illness, including:
  - Some drugs, including those used in chemotherapy
  - Suppressed immune system
  - Bone marrow failure
  - Aplastic anemia
  - Febrile neutropenia, which is a medical emergency
  - Congenital disorders, such as Kostmann syndrome and cyclic neutropenia
  - Hepatitis A, B, or C
  - HIV/AIDS
  - Sepsis
  - Autoimmune diseases, including rheumatoid arthritis
  - Leukemia
  - Myelodysplastic syndromes

- *Lymphocytes:* Most of the lymphocytes move through lymphatic system, but some enters in bloodstream.

A low lymphocyte count, called lymphocytopenia, usually occurs because body is not producing enough lymphocytes, lymphocytes are being destroyed or in case, where lymphocytes are trapped in spleen or lymph nodes.

Lymphocytopenia can point to a number of conditions and diseases. Some, like the flu or mild infections, are not serious for most people. But a low lymphocyte count increases risk of infection.

Other conditions that can cause lymphocytopenia include:
- Undernutrition
- HIV and AIDS
- Influenza
- Autoimmune conditions, such as lupus
- Some cancers, including lymphocytic anemia, lymphoma, and Hodgkin disease
- Steroid use
- Radiation therapy
- Certain drugs, including chemotherapy drugs
- Some inherited disorders, such as Wiskott-Aldrich syndrome and DiGeorge syndrome.

Lymphocytosis or a high lymphocyte count, is in case of an infection. High lymphocyte levels that persist may point to a more serious illness or disease, such as:
- Viral infections, including measles, mumps, and mononucleosis
- Adenovirus
- Hepatitis
- Influenza
- Tuberculosis
- Toxoplasmosis
- Cytomegalovirus
- Brucellosis
- Vasculitis
- Acute and chronic lymphocytic leukemia

For clinical significance of eosinophils, refer Chapter 19.

- *Basophill*: The following conditions can cause basophil level to be high:
  - *Hypothyroidism*: This occurs when thyroid gland does not produce enough thyroid hormone.
  - *Myeloproliferative disorders:* This refers to a group of conditions that cause too many white blood cells, red blood cells, or platelets are produced in your bone marrow. Major types of myeloproliferative disorders include:
    - *Polycythemia rubra vera*: Polycythemia rubra vera (PRV) or polycythemia is a myeloproliferative (Myelo refers to the bone marrow, proliferative describes the rapid growth of blood cells) disorder, which means the bone marrow makes too many blood cells.
    - *Myelofibrosis*: This disorder occurs when fibrous tissues replace blood-producing cells in the bone marrow
    - Thrombocythemia
    - Autoimmune inflammation

The following can cause basophil level to below:
- *Hyperthyroidism*: This happens when your thyroid gland produces too much thyroid hormone.
- *Infections*: Acute hypersensitivity reactions: In this case, body overreacts to a substance in the form of an acute allergic reaction.
- *Symptoms include*: Watery eyes, runny nose, red rash and itchy hives

- *Monocyte*: When monocyte level is high, this condition is known as monocytosis. It is defending the body against infection. Some conditions that can cause an increase in the monocytes in your blood are:
  - Viral infections, such as infectious mononucleosis, mumps, and measles
  - Parasitic infections
  - Chronic inflammatory disease
  - Tuberculosis (TB), a chronic respiratory disease caused by a type of bacteria
  - Chronic myelomonocytic leukemia.

Low levels of monocytes tend to develop as a result of medical conditions that lower overall white blood cell count or treatment for cancer and other serious diseases that suppress the immune system.

Causes of low monocyte count include:
- Chemotherapy and radiation therapy, which can injure bone marrow
- HIV and AIDS, which weaken the body's immune system
- Sepsis, an infection of the bloodstream.

CHAPTER 19

Absolute Eosinophil Count

Learning Objectives
- This test determines total number of eosinophils present in blood. Eosinophils play a significant role in the inflammation related to allergies, eczema and asthma.
- This chapter shares information of direct method as well as indirect method (using formula) of eosinophil count.
- It also discuss role of eosinophils in immune system and clinical significance of absolute eosinophil count.

Keywords
Fuchs-Rosenthal Chamber, Eosinophil diluting fluid, Sahli's pipette, Eosinophilia, Ulcerative colitis, Scarlet fever, Cortisol

INTRODUCTION

Eosinophils are part of immune system. It performs important functions:
i. Eosinophils destroy invading viruses, bacteria, or parasites.
ii. They also have a role in the inflammatory response, especially if an allergy is involved.

An absolute eosinophil count (AEC) is a blood test that measures the number of eosinophils. This test helps to detect allergic diseases, infections, and other medical conditions.

INDIRECT METHOD

Differential count gives the relative count of eosinophil out of total leukocytes. It is possible to get absolute number of eosinophil indirectly by following mathematical formula:

$$\text{Eosinophil/mm}^3 = \frac{\% \text{ of Eosinophil from DLC} \times \text{TLC}}{100}$$

This is an indirect method, which involves two techniques—DLC and TLC.

DIRECT METHOD

It is possible to get direct eosinophil count. The direct method is quick and gives exact value of eosinophil. In this method, the blood is diluted to 1 : 10 with a special diluting fluid. The diluted blood specimen is then charged in the counting chamber and the number of eosinophil are counted usually under 10× or high power (45×). The amount of eosinophil in undiluted blood is then calculated with a formula using the area of chamber, dilution proportion and the depth.

Equipments Required

For absolute eosinophil count, following equipments are required:
1. Blood sample
2. Eosinophil diluting fluid
3. Hemocytometer

Blood Sample

Direct capillary blood or EDTA anticoagulated blood is used for absolute eosinophil count.

Eosinophil Diluting Fluid

It removes other white cells and red cells. It also stains eosinophils with orange red color. Thus, making the microscopic field clear and easy identification.

Composition

- *Eosin 1% (aq) solution*: 5 mL
- *Acetone*: 5 mL
- *Distilled water*: 100 mL

Hemocytometer

For absolute eosinophil count, Fuchs-Rosenthal chamber is commonly used. The chamber has ruled area 16 sq mm and the depth is 0.2 mm, therefore, it occupies more amount of fluid compared with Neubauer counting chamber. Because the number of eosinophil is only 5% of white cells, it will be easier and accurate way to calculate the amount in large volume of fluid.

Procedure

Take 0.45 mL of diluting fluid in a test tube. Transfer 20 microliter of blood in the same test tube with the help of Sahli's pipette. This will give dilution 1 : 10. Take any pipette (RBC, or WBC, or Hb), suck the diluted blood and charge the chamber. Allow it to settle for few minutes. and then observe under microscope.

Fuchs-Rosenthal Chamber

In this chamber, count the cells in entire 16 sq mm area. The depth of chamber is 0.2 mm. Therefore, the formula is:

Eosinophil count =

$$\frac{\text{No. of cell counted} \times \text{Diluting factor}}{\text{Area} \times \text{Depth}}$$

∴ If number of cell counted = N

∴ Eosinophil count $= \dfrac{N \times 10}{16 \times 0.2}$

$= N \times 3.12$

Normal value = 50 to 500 cells per cu mm

The direct method gives absolute number of eosinophil per cu mm of blood.

For example, if total number of cells counted in entire 16 sq mm area = 73

Therefore, N = 73

Eosinophil count = 73 × 3.12 = 227.76
= 228 (round off) cells per cu mm.

■ CLINICAL SIGNIFICANCE

If more than 500 eosinophil cells per microliter of blood, then it indicates disorder known as eosinophilia. Eosinophilia is classified as either mild (500–1,500 eosinophil cells per microliter), moderate (1,500 to 5,000 eosinophil cells per microliter), or severe (greater than 5,000 eosinophil cells per microliter). This can be due to any of the following:

- An infection by parasitic worms
- An autoimmune disease
- Severe allergic reactions
- Eczema
- Asthma
- Seasonal allergies
- Leukemia and certain other cancers
- Ulcerative colitis
- Scarlet fever
- Lupus
- Crohn's disease
- A significant drug reaction
- An organ transplant rejection

An abnormally low eosinophil count can be the result of intoxication from alcohol or excessive production of cortisol, like in Cushing's disease. Cortisol is a hormone naturally produced by the body. Low eosinophil counts may also be due to the time of day. Under normal conditions, eosinophil counts are lowest in the morning and highest in the evening.

Unless alcohol abuse or Cushing's disease is suspected, low levels of eosinophils are not usually of concern unless other white cell counts are also abnormally low. If all white cells counts are low, this can signal a problem with the bone marrow.

CHAPTER 20

Erythrocyte Sedimentation Rate

Learning Objectives
- ESR is relatively simple, inexpensive, non-specific test that has been used for many years to help, detect and monitor inflammation of various infections, cancers and autoimmune diseases.
- This chapter has information about two methods of ESR and factors affecting it. Stepwise diagrammatic representation makes it easy to understand.
- It also discusses possible errors in ESR, its importance and limitations.

Keywords
Westergren method, Wintrobe method, Trisodium citrate, Hemolysis, Toxemia, Polycythemia, Syphilis

■ INTRODUCTION

When an anticoagulated blood is allowed to stand vertically, sedimentation of erythrocyte occurs. The rate at which erythrocytes fall down, is known as erythrocyte sedimentation rate (ESR).

Principle

Anticoagulated blood is taken in a tube and kept undisturbed in vertical position in a rack. This will allow the sedimentation of erythrocytes. After a specific time, generally 1 hour, the level of red cell is noted. The distance traveled by erythrocytes in 1 hour is called as erythrocyte sedimentation rate (ESR).

Methods

There are two different methods of determination of ESR:
1. Westergren method
2. Wintrobe method

■ WESTERGREN METHOD

Requirements

1. Westergren pipette
2. Westergren stand
3. Anticoagulant

Westergren pipette is open at both the ends. It is 30 cm in length and 2.5 mm in diameter. The lower 20 cm are marked with 0 at top and 200 at bottom.

The anticoagulant used in this method is 3.8% trisodium citrate solution. About 0.4 mL of trisodium citrate is added in 2 mL of blood.

Procedure (Fig. 20.1)

Fill the pipette by sucking blood up to 0 mark and fix it vertically in Westergren stand. Read the upper level of RBC column exactly after 1 hour.

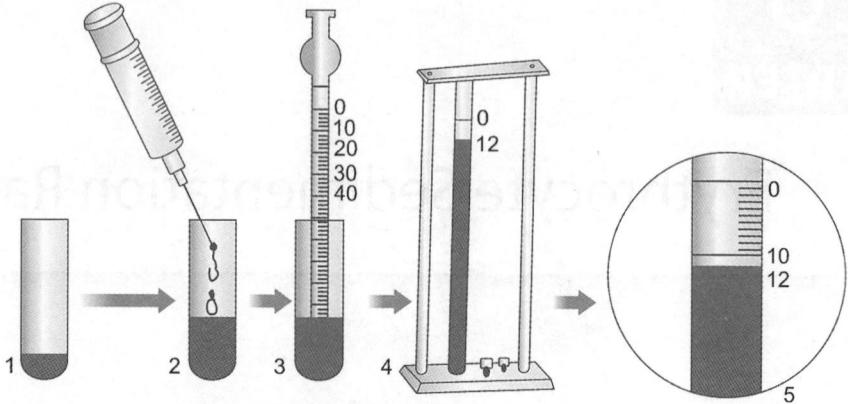

Fig. 20.1: Steps showing Westergren method.
1. Tube with anticoagulant
2. Addition of blood in the tube
3. Filling of Westergren pipette
4. Pipette on stand
5. The ESR level

Normal Values

- *For males*: 3 to 10 mm/hr.
- *For females*: 5 to 15 mm/hr.

■ WINTROBE METHOD

Requirements

1. Wintrobe pipette
2. Anticoagulant
3. Wintrobe stand

Wintrobe tube is open at one side only. The length of Wintrobe tube is 11 cm and the diameter is 2.5 mm. The lower 10 cm are marked. The marking is 0 at top and 100 at bottom for ESR, and it is also used for PCV (packed cell volume).

The anticoagulant used in Wintrobe method is EDTA solution, 0.4 mL of anticoagulant is required for 2 mL of blood.

Procedure (Fig. 20.2)

With the help of long necked Pasteur pipette or a special syringe, fill the Wintrobe tube up to '0' mark. Place the tube in an exactly vertical position in a Wintrobe stand. Read the upper level of RBC column exactly after 1 hour.

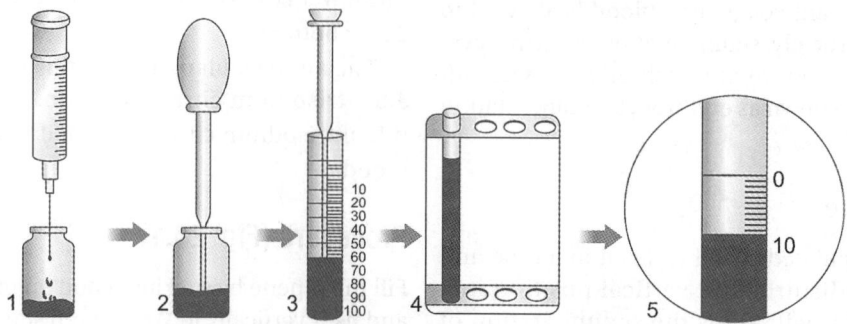

Fig. 20.2: Steps showing Wintrobe method.
1. Addition of blood in anticoagulant
2. Taking blood in Pasteur pipette
3. Filling of pipette
4. Wintrobe tube in stand
5. The ESR level

Normal Values

- *In males*: 0 to 9 mm/hr
- *In females*: 0 to 20 mm/hr

Readings can be taken with a gap of every half hour in both methods.

The Wintrobe method is commonly practiced and more advantageous over Westergren method. This is because of following reasons:

- By Wintrobe method, we can find out PCV in addition to ESR.
- Icteric index, volume of packed leukocytes and platelets can be known.
- Amount of blood required for Wintrobe method is less than that of Westergren method.

■ POSSIBLE ERRORS IN ESR

The value of ESR can be affected by following errors:

- Improper anticoagulant.
- The tube is not exactly vertical in position. Slight inclination may result in great difference in ESR value. Three degrees angle of inclination may raise ESR up to 30%.
- Dirty tube.
- Bubble caused by too vigorous mixing of blood and anticoagulant.
- Hemolysis may modify ESR.
- Blood should be tested within 3 hours of collection. The prolonged storage may modify ESR.
- The stand should not be kept on vibrating surface.
- The reading should be taken exactly after 1 hour.
- The stand should be kept away from window to avoid temperature variations.

■ FACTORS AFFECTING ESR

There are three factors affecting ESR:
1. Plasma
2. RBC
3. Anticoagulant

Plasma

Plasma proteins and other constituents of plasma affect the ESR level. Increased level of fibrinogen and globulin accelerate ESR. Albumin retards ESR. Extreme increase in plasma viscosity slows down ESR. Cholesterol accelerates ESR and lecithin retards ESR.

Red Cell

Change in erythrocyte plasma ratio affects ESR. Anemia is responsible for accelerating ESR. Microcyte sediment slowly. The macrocyte sediment rapidly and normocyte sediment with normal speed. Poikilocytosis retards ESR. Besides these, high sugar, high phospholipids, administration of certain drugs, may affect ESR level.

Anticoagulant

The use of anticoagulant with different proportion and improper anticoagulant may affect ESR value.

Importance and Limitations

ESR is not diagnostic test for any particular disease. A raised ESR suggests progressive increase of disease. Therefore, normalization of ESR indicates the recovery from disease.

The rapid increased ESR is found in any chronic infection like, tuberculosis, lymphatic fever, toxemia, etc.

In pregnancy, after second month, ESR is increased. Myocardial infarction, anemia, syphilis, malignant tumor, menstruation, liver disease, etc. are related with rapid ESR.

The slow ESR is found in:
- Newborn infants
- Polycythemia
- Allergic conditions
- Heart failure, etc.

In this way, ESR is helpful to indicate the relative progress of the disease.

21 CHAPTER

Packed Cell Volume

Learning Objectives
- Packed cell volume is measure of proportion of red blood cells in blood. This test is a part of complete blood cells count.
- This chapter illustrates two methods for detection of packed cell volume. One with large volume of blood cells (macrohematocrit) and other with small amount of blood (microhematocrit)
- Chapter includes information on clinical importance of PCV.

Keywords
Macrohematocrit, Microhematocrit, Wintrobe tube, Card reader, Hemolytic anemia, Lymphoma, Polycythemia vera

■ INTRODUCTION

When anticoagulated blood is centrifuged at a standard speed, erythrocytes, which are heavier than white cells and plasma, will settle down at bottom. This red cells volume is known as hematocrit or packed cell volume (PCV).

Hematocrit or PCV is the volume of red cells expressed as a percentage of whole blood.

Methods

There are two methods, used for the determination of hematocrit:
1. Macrohematocrit
2. Microhematocrit

■ MACROHEMATOCRIT

A large volume of blood is required in this method. Approximately 2 to 4 mL is required.

Principle

Anticoagulated blood is taken in a Wintrobe tube. Fill up to the uppermost mark and then rotate for desired length of time.

The packed cell volume (PCV) of red cells is directly read from the graduated tube as %.

Requirements

- *Blood specimen:* Ethylenediaminetetraacetic acid (EDTA) or double oxalated anticoagulated blood is used in this method. Determine PCV within six hours of blood collection.
- *Wintrobe tube:* It is 110 mm in length and 2.5 mm in diameter. The lower 100 mm are graduated or marked, from 100 at top and 0 (zero) at bottom for PCV.
- Long-necked Pasteur pipette or a special type of syringes is used for filling Wintrobe tube.
- Centrifuge machine with known speed.

Procedure

Mix 0.4 mL of EDTA with 2 mL blood. Fill the Wintrobe tube up to upper most mark with the help of Pasteur pipette or syringe. Fill the another Wintrobe tube to balance first one. If the blood sample is not available, fill the tube with water. Place the Wintrobe tube in opposite side in centrifuge. Turn the centrifuge to slow speed, then slowly increase the speed to 3,000 rpm. Centrifuge for 30 minutes at 3,000 rpm. After 30 minutes switch off the centrifuge and allow it to stop by itself. Take out the Wintrobe tube and read PCV directly with the help of graduation mark given on the tube.

Normal Value

- *In male*: 42 to 50%
- *In female*: 36 to 42%

■ MICROHEMATOCRIT

This method requires small amount of blood, 2 to 3 drops only. The blood can be obtained by finger puncture.

Principle

Anticoagulated blood is centrifuged in a sealed capillary tube, then PCV is determined by a special hematocrit reader.

Requirements

- *Blood specimen:* Blood from finger puncture may be used or EDTA or double oxalate venous blood can also be used.
- *Capillary tube:* Use plain capillary tube for anticoagulated venous blood and use heparinized capillary tube (coated with heparin internally) for blood obtained from finger puncture. The capillary tube is approximately 75 mm in length.
- *Microhematocrit centrifuge:* This is a special type of centrifuge. It has speed about 15,000 rpm. The top of centrifuge is flat with grooves. The centrifuge also has timer, which is usually set for 5 minutes.
- *Hematocrit reader:* There are several types of readers used for reading HCT. The simplest method is use of card reader, which can be made by hand.
- *Clay:* This is used to seal the end of capillary tube.

Procedure

Draw the blood sample into appropriate capillary tube with capillary action. Use plain tube for anticoagulated blood and heparinized tube for plain blood. In case of finger puncture, the blood should flow freely with little pressure. Now wipe off the first drop and then collect the blood specimen. Fill the tube about 3/4th length with blood. Seal the another end of the tube with clay or wax or ultimately by heating. The sealing should be about 2 mm deep. Place two HCT tubes in the groove of centrifuge exactly opposite to each other. It is not necessary that the capillary tube have exact amount of blood level. In case, if there is no filled capillary tube to balance we can use an empty capillary tube. Centrifuge at $13,000 \pm 2,000$ rpm.

Remove capillary tube from centrifuge. It will show three layers. Top layer is of plasma or serum; the middle layer is thin creamy white in color and is known as buffy coat. It is a layer of WBC; the last layer is the column of RBC. Use the HCT reader for finding the value of HCT.

Card Reader (Fig. 21.1)

The reader is used as, hold the tube against scale, so that the bottom of red cell is matched with 0 (zero) line of the card. Move the tube across the card until the uppermost line of plasma is matched to 100% line of card. Check to make sure that bottom of red cell column is still in the line of zero and the tube should be straight and vertical. The line that passes through the top of the column of RBC gives the HCT value.

Clinical Significance

The PCV test measures how much of the blood consists of cells. If the PCV returns a reading of 50%, it means that 50 ml of the cells

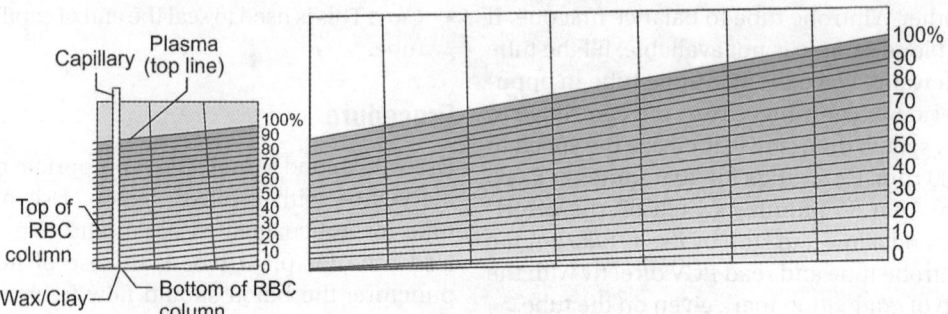

Fig. 21.1: Card reader.

are present in exactly 100 ml of blood. If the RBC number increases, then the total reading of the PCV is also up.

A lower number of the PCV means that the RBC count loss is due to reasons such as blood loss, cell destruction and less bone marrow production. It may be a sign of:
- Bone marrow diseases
- Chronic inflammatory disease
- Deficiencies in nutrients such as iron, folate or vitamin B_{12}
- Internal bleeding
- Hemolytic anemia
- Kidney failure
- Leukemia
- Lymphoma
- Sickle cell anemia

Increased PCV can generally mean that a person is dehydrated and there is a higher number of RBC productions. High hematocrit levels can indicate:
- Congenital heart disease
- Dehydration
- Kidney tumor
- Lung diseases
- Polycythemia vera

22 CHAPTER

Hemoglobin Estimation

Learning Objectives
- Hemoglobin is a protein in red blood cells that carry respiratory gases. It is a part of complete blood count test, used to diagnose or monitor various blood related disorders.
- This chapter points out principle and procedure of different methods of estimation of hemoglobin.
- Chapter includes information on clinical importance of hemoglobin.

Keywords
Sahli's acid hematin method, Colorimetric method of hemoglobin, Specific gravity method, Gasometric method, Hemodilution, polycythemia

■ INTRODUCTION

Hemoglobin is the main constituent of red blood cell (RBC). It carries out the important function of transportation of oxygen (O_2) from lungs to various parts of body, and it also transports back carbon di oxide (CO_2) from body to lungs. Hemoglobin consists of two components—heme and globin.

Heme is combination of iron and protoporphyrin and globin is the protein, formed of amino acid chain.

Normal Red Cell Value

	Red cells	Hb (%)	PCV (%)
Men	5–5.5 million/mm³	13.5–18 g	40–54

(Contd...)

(Contd...)

	Red cells	Hb (%)	PCV (%)
Women	4–4.5 million/mm³	11.5–16.5 g	35–47
Infants	4.0–5.6 million/mm³	13.6–19.6 g	44–62
Children (1 year)	3.6–5.0 million/mm³	11–33 g	36–44
(10–12 years)	4.5–5.2 million/mm³	11.5–14.8 g	37–44

Blood Specimen

Capillary blood can be used directly. If veins blood is used, EDTA or heparin or double oxalate anticoagulants are used.

There are various methods for estimation of Hb.

■ SAHLI'S ACID HEMATIN METHOD (FIG. 22.1)

Principle

Hemoglobin (Hb) is converted to acid hematin by the action of hydrochloric acid (HCl). The acid hematin solution is further diluted until its color matches exactly to that of permanent standard comparable tube. The hemoglobin (Hb) is read directly from the graduated tube.

Procedure

Fill the Hb cylinder up to the lowest mark with 0.1 normal HCl solution. Add 20 µ liter (0.02 mL) blood with the help of Sahli's pipette. Make sure

Section 2: Hematology

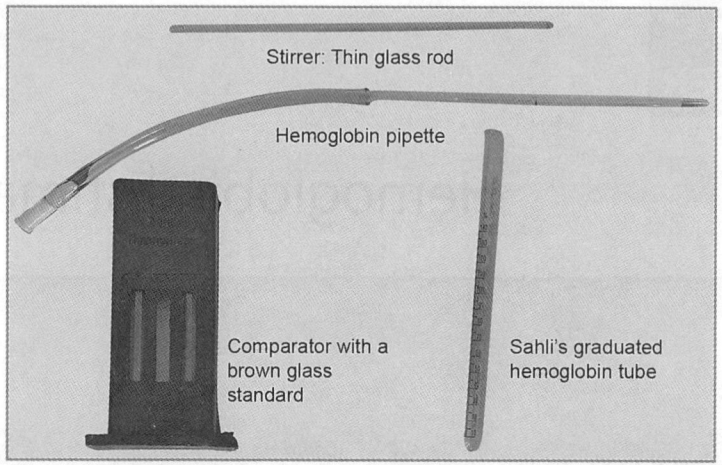

Actual anemia				Suggestive Anemia		Normal	
Men and women blow 70%				Men - 70 to 85% Women - 70 to 80%		Men - Above 85% Women - Above 80%	
30%	40%	50%	60%	70%	80%	90%	100%
4.7 gms.	6.3 gms.	7.8 gms.	9.4 gms.	10.9 gms.	12.5 gms.	14.1 gms.	15.6 gms.

Fig. 22.1: Hemoglobin estimation by Sahli's acid hematin method.
(For color version See Color Plate 5)

that there is no air bubble inside the pipette. Mix the blood with HCl, which is already placed in the cylinder. Take care that there is no blood left to the sides of the cylinder. Rinse the pipette twice in the blood solution. Allow it to react for about 10 minutes till the solution become dark brown in color. Acid hematin is produced in cylinder after combination of Hb and acid. Dilute the solution by adding drop of distill water, until perfect match is obtained with standard, comparable tube. Read the Hb concentration directly from the level of diluted solution. The reading may be in percentage (%) or g/L.

■ COLORIMETRIC METHOD

Colorimetric method of hemoglobin estimation is also known as cyanomethemoglobin method.

Principle

A small quantity of blood is taken and allowed to react with potassium cyanide and potassium fericynide (Drabkin's solution). The chemical reaction gives product of stable color. This product is called as cyanomethemoglobin. The intensity of color is directly proportional to Hb concentration.

Equipment

Colorimeter with green filter (540 nm) Sahli's pipette, test tubes, etc.

Reagent

1. Drabkin's solution
2. Cyanomethemoglobin—standard solution.

Composition

- *Potassium cyanide*: 50 mg
- *Potassium fericyanide*: 200 mg
- *Distill water*: 1000 mL

Store in dark bottle at room temperature.

Standard solution with Hb content of 5 g, 10 g, 15 g is recommended.

Procedure

Take two test tubes and label it as 'B' (Blank) and T (Test solution), add 5 mL of Drabkin's solution in each test tube. Avoid mouth pepetting as Drabkin solution is poison. Stopper the tube with rubber cap, add 0.02 mL of blood specimen into the tube marked with 'T'.

The specimen is taken with the help of Sahli's pipette. Wipe off the tip of the pipette before adding blood into test tube. Mix the content of the tube and wait for 10 minutes with the help of blank and standard solution, find out absorption of test solution in colorimeter at 540 nm. Hb can be calculated as:

Hb concentration =

$$\text{Absorbance of test solution} \times \frac{\text{Conc. of Std}}{\text{Ab. of Std}}$$

■ SPECIFIC GRAVITY METHOD

Principle

When a drop of whole blood is dropped into a copper sulfate solution with a particular specific gravity, the density of drop is directly proportional to the amount of Hb in that drop. If the drop is denser than the specific gravity of solution, the drop is settled down to the bottom. If not, it will float on the top.

Procedure

Copper sulfate solution of specific gravity 1.055 for male and 1.053 for female is taken in two test tubes. The specific gravity corresponds to minimum Hb level. For both the respective sexes 1.055 specific gravity corresponds to 13 g/dL of Hb and specific gravity 1.053 corresponds to 12 g/dL of Hb. A drop of blood is collected by skin puncture and taken into long necked pasteur pipette and then immediately drop the blood into proper copper sulfate solution, observe for 15-20 seconds.

If the person is normal, the drop of blood will settle down and if the person is anemic, the drop will float on the top.

This test does not give the exact amount of Hb. This technique is usually applied in blood blanking for screening the door. It is quick and easy, accurate technique.

■ GASOMETRIC METHOD

In this method, Van Slyke apparatus is used for gasometric determination of Hb. This is indirect method of hemoglobin is estimation, as oxygen carrying capacity of the blood is measured here.

In this method, blood is first of all saturated with oxygen. Then oxygen is taken off and collected, depending upon the amount of oxygen collected, the amount of Hb can be calculated.

For 1 g of Hb-1.34 mL of oxygen is present in blood.

■ CHEMICAL METHOD

In chemical method, Hb is found out by finding the amount of iron present in blood. The amount of iron is directly proportional to the amount of Hb present in blood. Iron content of Hb is 0.347%. It is a complex method.

■ CLINICAL IMPORTANCE

- Decrease in Hb concentration below normal value is sign of anemia.
- The Hb concentration is lower in adult female than in adult male.
- Hb values are low during pregnancy due to hemodilution. Children also have low Hb.
- An increase in Hb concentration can occur due to hemoconcentration, like loss of body fluid, in case of diarrhea, vomiting.
- In case of reduced oxygen supply, like heart disease, ploycythemia, Hb is low.
- Decrease or increase in concentration of Hb should be reported, as it is a sign of disease.

CHAPTER 23

Hemoglobinopathies

Learning Objectives
- A hemoglobinopathy is an inherited blood disorder in which an individual has an abnormal form of hemoglobin. Different disorders of hemoglobin are based on the physical and chemical properties of the different hemoglobin molecules.
- This chapter has detail explanation of structure of hemoglobin and different conditions of disorders of hemoglobin.
- This chapter also guides readers with tests to diagnose hemoglobinopathies.

Keywords
Hemoglobin A, F, A2, Thalassaemia, Variant hemoglobins, Hb EPG, Kleihauer stain, HbH inclusions, Sickling, High Performance Liquid Chromatography (HPLC), Isoelectric Focusing (IEF), Cellulose Acetate Electrophoresis (CAE), DNA tests

A hemoglobinopathy is an inherited blood disorder in which an individual has an abnormal form of hemoglobin.

STRUCTURE OF HEMOGLOBIN

Each red blood cell (RBC) contains about 20 million hemoglobin molecules. A hemoglobin molecule consists of a protein called globin. Globin is composed of four polypeptide chains. Each chain consists of a ring-like non-protein pigment called heme. At the center of each heme ring is an iron ion (Fe^{+2}). Each iron ion combines with one molecule of oxygen. Thus one molecule of hemoglobin can transport four oxygen molecules (**Fig. 23.1**).

Normal hemoglobin types include:
- *Hemoglobin A*: Makes up about 95–98% of Hb found in adults; it contains two alpha and two beta protein chains.
- *Hemoglobin A2*: Makes up about 2–3% of Hb in adults; it has two alpha and two delta protein chains.
- *Hemoglobin F (fetal hemoglobin)*: Makes up to 1–2% of Hb found in adults; it has two alpha and two gamma protein chains. This is the primary hemoglobin produced by the fetus during pregnancy; its production usually falls shortly after birth.

HEMOGLOBINOPATHIES

Hemoglobinopathies are inherited disorders of globin. Hemoglobinopathies occur when changes (mutations) in the genes that code for the globin chains cause alterations in the proteins. There are mainly two kinds of disorders related to hemoglobin.

1. *Thalassaemia syndromes*: When these genetic changes results in reduced production of one of the normal globin chains, it is called the thalassaemia syndromes. These mutations in genes affect the quantity of hemoglobin chain. Thalassaemia syndromes are sub-classified based on the

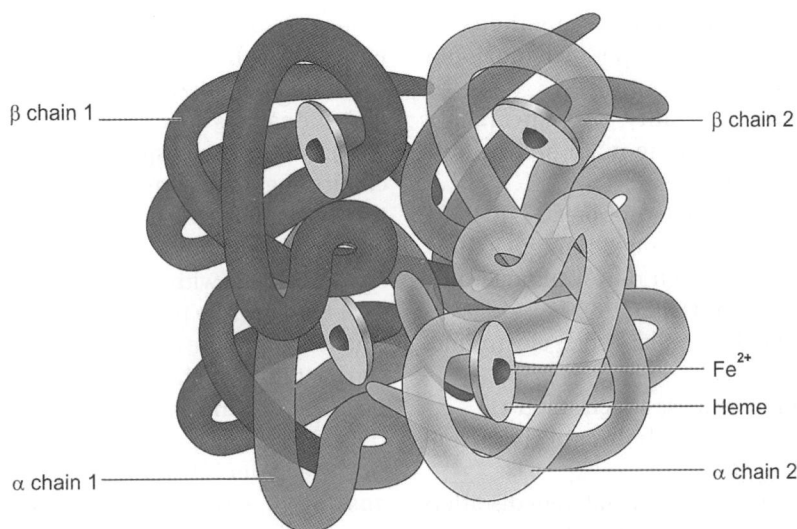

Fig. 23.1: Four polypeptide chains of globin with a ring like heme.
(For color version See Color Plate 6)

gene involved. If mutation is with gene on chromosome 11, it is β thalassaemia and if it is gene on chromosome 16, it is α thalassaemia. α and β thalassaemias are further sub-divided into $α^+$, $β^+$ or $α^o$, $β^o$ depending on whether some (+) or no (o) globin protein is produced as a result of the causative mutation. This is quantitative disorders of globin chain.

2. *Variant hemoglobins:* When these genetic changes results in the production of structurally altered globin chains, it results in formation of variant hemoglobins. These mutations in the globin genes affect quality and structure of hemoglobin. The presence of abnormal hemoglobin within RBCs can alter the appearance (size and shape) and function of the red blood cells. Red blood cells containing hemoglobin variants may not carry oxygen efficiently and may be broken down by the body sooner than usual (a shortened survival), resulting in hemolytic anemia.

Some of the most common hemoglobin variants include:
- Hemoglobin S, the primary hemoglobin in people with sickle cell disease that causes the RBC to become misshapen (sickle), decreasing the cell's survival;
- Hemoglobin C, which can cause a minor amount of hemolytic anemia; and
- Hemoglobin E, which may cause no symptoms or generally mild symptoms.

Many other less common hemoglobin variants include Hb C, Hb E, Hb D-Punjab, Hb O-Arab, Hb G-Philadelphia, and many more, these are usually called after the place in which they were discovered. Most of these do not produce any detectable pathology but are clinically important, while others affect the function and/or stability of the hemoglobin molecule.

The thalassaemia syndromes and some of the Hb variants are inherited as autosomal recessive conditions. Very rarely, β thalassaemia and some Hb variants demonstrates an autosomal dominant inheritance pattern.

DIAGNOSIS

In case of symptoms of unexplained anemia or abnormal results of a complete blood count (CBC), an investigation of a hemoglobin disorder is done. This is to detect or identify hemoglobin abnormality or thalassemia.

Several different laboratory methods are available to evaluate the types of hemoglobin. Some of these include:
- Hemoglobin solubility test—specifically for hemoglobin S, the main hemoglobin in sickle cell disease
- Hemoglobin gel electrophoresis (Hb ELP)
- Hemoglobin isoelectric focusing (Hb IEF)
- Hemoglobin by high performance liquid chromatography (HPLC)
- Hemoglobin by capillary zone electrophoresis
- Hemoglobin by mass spectrometry
- Hemoglobin electrophoresis of globin proteins (Hb EPG)

These methods evaluate different disorders of hemoglobin based on the physical and chemical properties of the different hemoglobin molecules. The relative amounts of any variant hemoglobin detected can aid in a diagnosis. Most of the common hemoglobin variants or thalassemias can be identified using one of these tests or a combination. The results of several different tests are considered. Examples of other laboratory tests that may be performed include:
- CBC, e.g., α/β globin protein ratio is imbalanced in the thalassaemia syndromes. In these conditions, the imbalance is reflected in a low MCV and low MCH.
- Blood smear, e.g., observe a blood film for the presence of sickle cell disease (HbS) or an unstable Hb. Other changes such as stippling and target cells are important clue.

Reticulocyte count, iron studies such as serum iron, TIBC (total iron binding capacity), transferrin (serum iron divided by the total iron-binding capacity) are also important diagnostic tests for hemoglobinopathies.

Genetic testing may be used to detect mutations in the genes that code for the protein chains (alpha and beta globulin) that comprise hemoglobin. This is not a routine test but can be used to confirm whether a person has a mutated gene and whether there is one or two mutated copies (heterozygous or homozygous).

Some specialized tests to detect hemoglobunopathies are discussed in **Table 23.1**.

One of the useful specialized test helpful in confirming thalassemia and whether it is due to α or β globin gene problem is the α/β globin protein ratio. This requires the incubation of red blood cells with a radioactive tracer such as H-leucine. The peaks representing α and β globin proteins are then quantitated to provide an α/β ratio which should equal 1. A ratio > 1 indicates β thalassemia while a ratio <1 is caused by α thalassemia.

Other special hematological tests are possible, particularly when investigating the more uncommon variant hemoglobins. These include tests for oxygen affinity, hemoglobin stability and detection of methemoglobin. Mass spectrometry has been used to characterize various variant hemoglobins. The following techniques can be used in antenatal screening for hemoglobin variants:
- *High performance liquid chromatography (HPLC)*: This can be used for the quantification of hemoglobins S, A2 and F and for the detection, provisional identification and quantification of many variant hemoglobins.
- *Isoelectric focusing (IEF)*: It is satisfactory for the analysis of whole blood samples, hemolysates or dried blood spots. IEF gives good separation of Hb F from Hb A and clinically significant variant haemoglobins (S, C, D-Punjab, E and O-Arab).
- *Cellulose acetate electrophoresis (CAE)*: Hemoglobin electrophoresis at pH 8·4–8·6 using a cellulose acetate membrane is simple, reliable and rapid. It enables the provisional identification of hemoglobins A, F, S/G/D, C/E/O-Arab, H and a number of less common variant hemoglobins.
- *DNA tests*: For detection involving individual cases, DNA based approaches are needed. The DNA laboratory needs to know whether the α or β globin genes or both

TABLE 23.1: Specialized tests to detect hemoglobinopathies.

Test	What does it measure or detect	What does it mean
Hb EPG	Electrophoresis of globin proteins. Different techniques possible from gel or membrane based kits to HPLC. Abnormal bands apart from the usual HbA, HbF and HbA2 peaks can be detected.	(1) Gives some idea of the HbA2 level but more importantly and (2) identifies if there are any variant hemoglobins such as HbE and HbS.
HbA2	Globin electrophoresis and quantitation of the HbA2 peak. Different techniques used from membrane or column based kits to the more universally suited HPLC are in use.	A raised HbA2 is the key parameter indicating the presence of β thalassaemia. A low HbA2 is also important to note as this might indicate δ thalassaemia
HbF	Globin electrophoresis and quantitation with different methods available for the latter.	A slightly raised HbF to 2–3% (normal is <1% in an adult) might indicate heterocellular HPFH or may be silent β thalassaemia. HbF levels 5% and above are more likely to be due to δβ thalassaemia.
Kleihauer	Red blood cells are stained to detect HbF. This test is used to distinguish heterocellular (lower expression of HbF) from pancellular (higher expression of HbF) HPFH (hereditary persistence of fetal hemoglobin).	The Kleihauer stain is useful in fetal blood sampling to confirm that maternal blood has not contaminated a fetal sample (the latter would be homogeneously stained for HbF). Any cells not staining for HbF would represent maternal blood.
HbH inclusions	Red blood cells are stained to detect HbH inclusions (aggregates of β globin protein)	Definitive test to confirm the presence of α thalassaemia (Refer Chapter 25 Heinz Bodies)
Sickle solubility and instability tests	Various tests ranging from biochemical to immunoassay are used to detect HbS and unstable variant hemoglobins.	HbS disease as well as interactions of HbS with β thalassaemia. Efficient and accurate tests for sickling (sickle solubility, Hb EPG) are important components of the hemoglobinopathy workup (Refer Chapter 27 Sickle Cell Anemia)

need to be characterized. DNA technology in hemoglobinopathy testing is based predominantly on PCR (polymerase chain reaction) and Southern blotting.

CHAPTER 24

Red Cell Indices

Learning Objectives
- Red blood cell indices provide information about the hemoglobin content and size of red blood cells. Abnormal values indicate the presence of anemia and which type of anemia it is.
- Three red cell indices, MCV, MCH and MCHC are discussed in this chapter.
- Calculations and clinical significance of these indices are interpreted here.

Keywords
Mean Cell Volume (MCV), Mean Cell Hemoglobin (MCH), Mean Cell Hemoglobin Concentration (MCHC), Macrocytic, Microcytic, Hypochromic, Hyperchromic, Thalassemia

■ INTRODUCTION

Red blood cell is pale red in color because of presence of hemoglobin. It is shaped like a disc, where thinner area in the middle and corners are thick. RBCs are normally all the same color, size, and shape. However, certain conditions can cause variations that impair their ability to function properly. The RBC indices measure the size, shape, and physical characteristics of the RBCs.

There are three different red cell indices calculated from:
1. Hemoglobin concentration
2. Picked-cell volume (PCV)
3. Total red cell count.

The results of these indices are helpful in diagnosis of different types of anemia.

■ MEAN CELL VOLUME

Mean cell volume (MCV) is the average volume of red cell. Because, the size of red cell is very small, it is expressed in femtoliter (Fl).

$$1 \text{ Fl} = 10^{-15} \text{ L}$$

MCV can be calculated as:

$$MCV = \frac{Hct(\%) \times 10}{Total\ RBC\ count\ in\ million}$$

Normal value = 78–94 Fl

Mean cell volume is reduced in microcytic anemia, and raised in macrocytic anemia, in deficiency of vitamin B_{12}, folic acid, etc.

■ MEAN CELL HEMOGLOBIN

Mean cell hemoglobin (MCH) is the average Hb content of red cell. Because the amount is very small, it is expressed in picogram.

$$1 \text{ picogram} = 10^{-12} \text{ g}$$

$$MCH = \frac{Hb(\%) \times 10}{Total\ RBC\ count}$$

Normal value = 27–32 picograms

Mean cell hemoglobin is raised in macrocytic anemia and reduced in hypochromic anemia.

MEAN CELL HEMOGLOBIN CONCENTRATION

Mean cell hemoglobin concentration (MCHC) is the average Hb concentration per unit volume of PCV.

$$\text{MCHC} = \frac{\text{MCH}}{\text{MCV}} \times 100$$

$$= \frac{\text{Hb} \times 10}{\text{TRC}} \div \frac{\text{PCV}(\%) \times 10}{\text{TRC}} \times 100$$

$$= \frac{\text{Hb} \times \cancel{10}}{\cancel{\text{TRC}}} \times \frac{\cancel{\text{TRC}}}{\text{PCV}(\%) \times \cancel{10}} \times 100$$

$$= \frac{\text{Hb}}{\text{PCV}(\%)} \times 100$$

The value is expressed in % or g/L. The normal value is 32–38%. Below 32% is found in iron deficiency or hypochromic anemia. It cannot increase above 38% as the red cells cannot hold higher concentration of hemoglobin.

CLINICAL SIGNIFICANCE

The RBC indices help to determine the cause of anemia.

MCV: The MCV is the most useful value in the RBC indices to help determine the type of anemia.

High MCV: The MCV is higher than normal when red blood cells are larger than normal. This is called macrocytic anemia. Macrocytic anemia can be caused by vitamin B_{12} deficiency, folate deficiency, chemotherapy, pre-leukemias.

Low MCV: The MCV will be lower than normal when red blood cells are too small. This condition is called microcytic anemia. Microcytic anemia may be caused by iron deficiency, which can be caused by poor dietary intake of iron, menstrual bleeding or gastrointestinal bleeding. Rarely it is because of thalassemia, lead poisoning and chronic diseases.

MCH: It represents average hemoglobin content of the cell.

Low MCH: Low value typically indicates the presence of iron deficiency anemia, as iron is important for the production of hemoglobin.

In more rare cases, low MCH can be caused by a genetic condition called thalassemia. In this condition, production of hemoglobin is limited. This means there are not as many red blood cells circulating in bloodstream.

High MCH: This means that there is a larger amount of hemoglobin present per red blood cell.

High MCH value can often be caused by anemia due to a deficiency of B vitamins, particularly B_{12} and folate. Both of these vitamins are required by body in order to make red blood cells.

MCHC: High MCHC means that the relative hemoglobin concentration per red blood cell is high. The red blood cells will take on a brighter color when viewed under the microscope. Individuals with anemia and a corresponding high MCHC are said to be hyperchromic. MCHC can be elevated in diseases such as hereditary spherocytosis, sickle cell disease and homozygous hemoglobin C disease.

Low MCHC means that the relative hemoglobin concentration per red blood cell is low. The red blood cells will take on a lighter color when viewed under the microscope. Individuals with anemia and a corresponding low MCHC are said to be hypochromic. Conditions that can cause low MCHC include the same conditions that cause low MCV, including iron deficiency, chronic diseases, thalassemia and lead poisoning.

CHAPTER 25

Special Blood Cell Tests

Learning Objectives
- There are certain disorders associated with blood cells. This chapter deals with three different special red cell tests.
- Lupus erythematosus, osmotic fragility, and fetal hemoglobin are analyzed in this chapter.
- Test procedure, principle and clinical significance of all three tests are discussed here.

Keywords
Lupus erythematosus, Rotary bead method, Phagocytosis, Buffy coat, Osmotic fragility, Osmosis, Hemolysis, Fetal hemoglobin, Hemoglobinopathy

■ LUPUS ERYTHEMATOSUS

Systemic Lupus Erythematosus (also called lupus or SLE) is a disease in which a person's immune system attacks and injures the body's own organs and tissues. Almost every system of the body can be affected.

The body's immune system is a network of cells and tissues responsible for clearing the body of invading organisms like bacteria, viruses, and fungi. Antibodies are special immune cells that recognize these invaders, and begin a chain of events to destroy them. In an autoimmune disorder like SLE, a person's antibodies begin to identify the body's own tissues as foreign. These antibodies are called "autoantibodies," which reacts with the "self" antigens to form immune complexes. These include antinuclear antibodies (ANA), and anti-DNA antibodies, which are directed against genetic material (DNA). These cells and chemicals of the immune system damage the tissues of the body. The reaction that occurs in tissue is called inflammation. Inflammation includes swelling, redness, increased blood flow, and tissue destruction. It results in breakdown of certain blood cell nuclei in vitro. This degenerated nuclear material attracts phagocytic cells, particularly segmented neutrophils (occasionally monocyte or eosinophil), which engulf this nuclear mass. The resulting phagocyte and inclusion material is termed as lupus erythematosus (LE) cell. The LE cell is a neutrophil that has engulfed the antibody-coated nucleus of another polymorph. Occasionally, a group of polymorphs will collect around an altered nuclear material and will form a rosette.

Types of Lupus

There are three types of lupus: discoid, systemic, and drug-induced.
1. Discoid (cutaneous) lupus is usually limited to the skin. It is identified by a rash that may appear on the face, neck, and scalp. Discoid lupus is diagnosed by examining a biopsy of the rash. Discoid lupus does not generally involve the body's internal or-

gans. Therefore, the ANA test, a blood test used to detect systemic lupus, may be negative in patients with discoid lupus. In approximately 10% of patients, discoid lupus can evolve into the systemic form of the disease, which can affect almost any organ or system of the body.
2. Systemic lupus is usually more severe than discoid lupus and can affect almost any organ or system of the body. For some people, only the skin and joints will be involved. In others, the joints, lungs, kidneys, blood, or other organs and/or tissues may be affected.
3. Drug-induced lupus occurs after the use of certain prescribed drugs. The symptoms of drug-induced lupus are similar to those of systemic lupus. The drugs most commonly connected with drug-induced lupus are hydralazine (used to treat high blood pressure or hypertension), procainamide (used to treat irregular heart rhythms), and isoniazid (a drug used to treat TB).

Cause

The cause(s) of lupus is/are unknown, but there are environmental and genetic factors involved. Some of the environmental factors that may trigger the disease are—infections, antibiotics (especially those in the sulfa and penicillin groups), ultraviolet light, extreme stress, certain drugs, and hormones.

Symptoms

Many SLE patients have fevers, fatigue, muscle pain, weakness, decreased appetite, and weight loss. The spleen and lymph nodes are often swollen and enlarged. Recurrent infections, particularly those caused by bacteria, are common in patients with SLE. The development of other symptoms in SLE varies depending on the organs affected.
- *Joints:* Joint pain and problems, including arthritis, are very common. About 90% of all SLE patients have these types of problems
- *Skin:* A number of skin rashes may occur, including a red butterfly-shaped rash that spreads across the face.
- *Hair loss:* It is common. SLE patients tend to be very easily sunburned (photosensitive).
- *Lungs:* Pleuritis, with fluid accumulating in the lungs. The patient frequently experiences coughing and shortness of breath.
- *Heart and circulatory system:* Pericarditis; inflammation of the heart itself causes myocarditis. These heart problems may result in abnormal heartbeat (arrhythmias), difficulty pumping the blood strongly enough (heart failure).
- *Nervous system:* Headaches, seizures, changes in personality, and confused thinking (psychosis) may occur.
- *Kidneys:* They may become unable to adequately filter the blood, leading to kidney failure.
- *Gastrointestinal system:* Patients may experience nausea, vomiting, diarrhea, and abdominal pain. The lining of the abdomen may become inflamed (peritonitis).
- *Eyes:* The eyes may become red, sore, and dry. It may cause vision problems, and blindness can result from inflammation of the blood vessels (vasculitis) that serve the retina.

Diagnosis

Laboratory tests that are helpful in diagnosing SLE include several tests for a variety of antibodies commonly elevated in SLE patients (including antinuclear antibodies, anti-DNA antibodies, etc.). A blood test called the lupus erythematosus cell preparation (or LE prep) test is also performed. The LE prep is positive in 70–80% of all patients with SLE. SLE patients tend to have low numbers of red blood cells (anemia) and low numbers of certain types of white blood cells. The erythrocyte sedimentation rate (ESR), is quite elevated. Samples of tissue (biopsies) from affected skin and kidneys show characteristics of the disease.

Two methods of demonstrating the LE cell and antinuclear antibodies are the rotary bead method and fluorescent antibody method. The rotary bead method is positive in 75-80 erythematosus. The fluorescent antibody method is positive in 95-100 patients with lupus erythematosus. The rotary bead method is presented in the next paragraph. The fluorescent antibody method requires equipment that limits its use to larger laboratories.

Rotary Bead Method

Principle

Leukocytes are broken down in vitro allowing the abnormal plasma protein to react on the altered nuclear material. Incubation enhances the nuclear deterioration and phagocytosis. Slides are prepared and examined for the peculiar "LE" cell.

Procedure

- 1 mL of patient blood is collected in heparin and transferred to glass tube.
- Four glass beads are added and tube is sealed with tightly fitting rubber cork.
- The preparation is rotated at 33 rpm for 30 minutes and placed at 37°C for 10-15 minutes.
- The contents of tube are transferred to wintrobe tube and centrifuged at 200 rpm for 10 minutes.
- The grayish-white layer that forms above the erythrocyte layer is called the "buffy coat."
- This concentrated layer of leukocytes (with the platelets) can be removed and formed into a smear for staining. This is the buffy coat smear.
- This is air dried, fixed with methanol and stained with Romanowsky stain.

Examination of Blood Film

The films specially their edges and tails are searched for minimum of 10 min (minimum 500 polymorph should be counted) before a negative report is given. The neutrophils show intracytoplasmic inclusion pushing the homogenous degenerated nucleus to the periphery. With Romanowsky stain LE bodies appear as homogeneously stained pale purple colored cellular inclusions (**Fig. 25.1**).

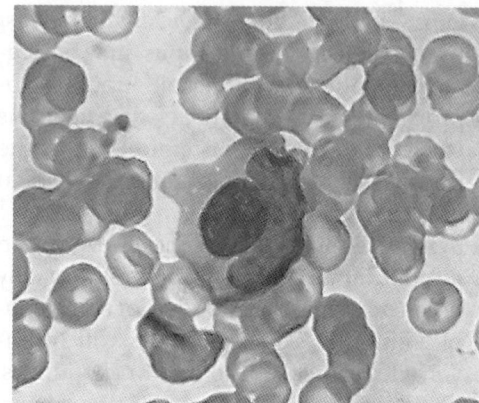

Fig. 25.1: Blood film showing LE bodies.
(For color version See Color Plate 6)

■ OSMOTIC FRAGILITY

Osmosis

Osmosis is the passive movement of water through a semipermeable (which is permeable to water, but impermeable to certain solutes) membrane from a compartment of relatively low osmotic pressure to a compartment of relatively high osmotic pressure, toward equilibrium.

The osmotic pressure responsible for osmosis is generated by these impermeable solutes. The greater is the concentration of impermeable solutes, the greater the osmotic pressure.

Biological membranes are inherently semipermeable. They are permeable to water and other molecules, but they are impermeable to solutes, including all charged molecules (ions). Thus, biological membranes are impermeable to all those inorganic ions found in the extracellular and intracellular fluids, such as Na^+, K^+, Cl^- and Ca^{++}, just to name a few. These ions, contribute to the osmotic pressure of the extracellular and intracellular fluids.

Osmotic pressure is often expressed in relative terms, i.e. by comparing the osmotic pressure of one solution to some standard solution. It also applies to living systems.
- Isotonic solutions are solutions that have an osmotic pressure equal to that of body fluids or to intracellular fluids
- Hypotonic fluids have an osmotic pressure less than that of cellular fluids
- Hypertonic fluids have an osmotic pressure greater than that of cellular fluids.

Osmosis across the Red Blood Cell Plasma Membrane

For red blood cells, a 0.85% NaCl solution is isotonic (iso—equal, tonic—concentration) to plasma. Any NaCl solution that has a NaCl concentration less than 0.85% is considered hypotonic, (hypo—less than, tonic—concentration) and any NaCl solution that has a NaCl concentration greater than 0.85% is considered hypertonic, (hyper—more than, tonic—concentration).
- Inside the body, red cells are bathed in isotonic plasma, in which case water movement into the cell is equal to water movement out of the cell, and there is no net osmosis.
- When red blood cells are taken out of their natural environment and placed in a sufficiently-strong hypertonic fluid (e.g. NaCl solution >0.85% NaCl) there is a net outward osmosis and the cells shrink. This is because the higher osmolarity (salt concentration) outside the cell relative to inside creates osmotic pressure directed towards outside the cell.
- Conversely, when red blood cells are placed in a sufficiently-strong hypotonic fluid (e.g. NaCl solution <0.85% NaCl), there is an uncontrolled net inward osmosis, resulting in the continuous uncontrolled swelling of the cells until the cells break open, a process known as cell lysis. This is because the lower osmolarity (salt concentration) outside the cell relative to inside creates osmotic pressure directed towards inside the cell.

Osmotic Fragility Test

Osmotic fragility is a test to measure red blood cell (RBC) resistance to hemolysis when exposed to a series of increasingly dilute saline solutions. The sooner hemolysis occurs, the greater the osmotic fragility of the cells.

This test is performed to detect thalassemia, hereditary spherocytosis and anemias like autoimmune hemoltytic anemia.

Hereditary spherocytosis is a common disorder in which red blood cells are defective because of their round, ball-like (spherical) shape. These cells are more fragile than normal. Spherical cells are said to have increased osmotic fragility because they are less likely to expand and break open in salter water than normal red blood cells (which are indented or curved inward on both sides). Hemolytic anemia also have increased hemolytic fragility.

Thalassemia is an inherited condition that affects the portion of blood (hemoglobin) that carries oxygen. Thalassemic RBCs are microcytic and hypochromic. Cells that are flatter than normal are more likely to expand, and thus have decreased osmotic fragility. Most of these red blood cells are less fragile than normal and tend to shrink. Sickle cell anemia also have decreased osmotic fragility.

Principle

Small volumes of blood are mixed with a large excess of buffered saline solutions of varying concentration. The fraction of red cells lysed at each saline concentration is determined colorimetrically. The test is normally carried out at room temperature (15-25°C). The resistance which erythrocytes offer to the hemolytic actions of hypotonic saline is used as an index of the osmotic fragility of RBC's.

Specimen

Five mL whole blood (sodium heparin tube or lithium heparin tube) hemolyzed sample should be rejected.

Procedure

- Place the 14 test tubes on the wooden rack labeled serially from 1.00% to 0.00%. Fill the tubes up to three-fourth with sodium chloride solutions of corresponding serial strengths (Table 25.1).
- Add 50 microns of whole blood to every tube. Let the tubes at RT for 30 minutes.
- Mix well by using the vortex.
- Centrifuge for 5 minutes at 2500 rpm.
- Carefully transfer supernatants to cuvettes.
- Set the optical density 0 using supernatant in test tube no. 1, which represents blank, or 0% hemolysis. Test tube no. 14 represents 100% hemolysis.
- Estimate the amount of lysis in each using a spectrometer at a wavelength setting of 540 nm or a photoelectric colorimeter provided with a yellow–green (e.g. Ilford 625) filter.

- Calculate the % of hemolysis for each tube by using:
% of hemolysis = Absorbance of tube/absorbance of 14th tube × 100

The results of the test may be then graphed, with the percent hemolysis plotted on the ordinate (vertical axis) and the sodium chloride concentration on horizontal axis as shown in **Figure 25.2**.

Observation

In tubes with solutions of higher concentration, blood settles down with a clear, colorless supernatant. As the concentration decreases gradually, the supernatant starts getting a reddish tinge. The strength of the sodium chloride solution in which the reddish tinge is first seen indicates the begginning of hemolysis (most fragile RBCs are lysed). The solution in which hemolysis is complete (all RBCs are lysed) is uniformly red, clear and transparent without any sediment. In all the solutions of lower concentration the same picture is seen. Osmotic fragility is expressed as the range of saline concentrations in which, beginning and completion of hemolysis occurs.

Normal Results (at 20°C and pH 7.4)

Table 25.2 shows normal test result of osmotic fragility test.

TABLE 25.1: Procedures for osmotic fragility test.

Test tube	1%Nacl (mL)	Distill water (mL)	Final conc. (%)
1	10.0	0.0	1.00
2	8.5	1.5	0.85
3	7.5	2.5	0.75
4	6.5	3.5	0.65
5	6.0	4.0	0.60
6	5.5	4.5	0.55
7	5.0	5.0	0.50
8	4.5	5.5	0.45
9	4.0	6.0	0.40
10	3.5	6.5	0.35
11	3.0	7.0	0.30
12	2.0	8.0	0.20
13	1.0	9.0	0.10
14	0.0	10.0	0.00

■ FETAL HEMOGLOBIN

Hemoglobin is the oxygen-carrying protein in red blood cells. It is also the pigment that gives red blood cells their color. Red blood cells deliver hemoglobin throughout the body, ensuring that all body tissues have the oxygen they need for life and proper function. Hemoglobin consists primarily of iron-bearing proteins called heme groups and moiety globin protein, which together give hemoglobin its ability to carry oxygen. The heme groups are molecular chains of different types and actually create six different hemoglobins that vary in their amino acid composition and also

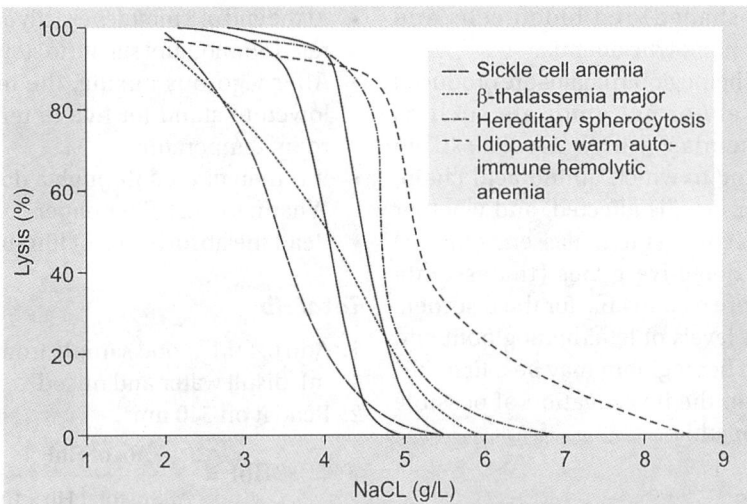

Fig. 25.2: Osmotic fragility curves of patients suffering from the following: sickle cell anemia, β-thalassemia major, hereditary spherocytosis, and "idiopathic" warm autoimmune hemolytic anemia. The normal range is indicated by the unbroken lines.

TABLE 25.2: Test result at 20°C and pH 7.4.	
Hemolysis	Fresh blood (g/l NaCl)
Initial lysis	5.0
Complete lysis	3.0
MCF (50% lysis)	4.0–4.45

(MCF: median corpuscular fragility)

in the genes that control them. Among the six types of hemoglobin, HbA is the normal adult hemoglobin, and HbF is the major fetal hemoglobin.

During fetal development, fetal hemoglobin composes about 90 percent of total hemoglobin. At birth, the newborn's blood is composed of about 70% fetal hemoglobin. As the infant's bone marrow begins to produce new red cells, fetal hemoglobin begins to decrease rapidly. Normally, only 2% or less of total hemoglobin is found as fetal hemoglobin after six months and throughout childhood; in adulthood, only traces (0.5% or less) are found in total hemoglobin.

Clinical Significance

In some diseases associated with abnormal hemoglobin production (hemoglobinopathy), fetal hemoglobin may persist in larger amounts. For example, HbF can be found in higher levels in sickle cell anemia and other hereditary anemias. It has also been reported to be elevated in some other conditions, such as leukemia, pregnancy, diabetes, thyroid disease, and sometimes as a side effect of anticonvulsant therapy. It may also reappear in adults when the bone marrow is overactive, as in disorders such as pernicious anemia, multiple myeloma, and invasive (metastatic) cancer affecting bone marrow. When HbF is elevated after age four, the cause is typically investigated. (Persistence of fetal hemoglobin in inherited hemolytic anemias can be associated with less severe disease symptoms).

Defects in hemoglobin production may be either genetic or acquired. The genetic defects are subdivided into errors of heme production (porphyria) and those of globin production, known collectively as the hemoglobinopathies. There are two categories of hemoglobinopathy:
1. Abnormal globin chains give rise to abnormal hemoglobin molecules—like that of in sickle cell anemia, the inherited condition characterized by curved

(sickle-shaped) red blood cells and chronic hemolytic anemia.
2. Normal hemoglobin chains are produced but in abnormal amounts such as thalassemias, which are classified according to which amino acid chain, alpha or beta, is affected, and whether one defective gene (thalassemia minor) or two defective genes (thalassemia major) are responsible for the disorder.

Testing for levels of fetal hemoglobin and other types of hemoglobin may be a first, important step in the investigation of possible hemoglobinopathies.

Test Sample

Hemolysate is prepared from whole blood (EDTA, citrated or heparinized).

Principle

A red blood cell hemolysate is prepared to lyse the red blood cell and free the hemoglobin.

These tests utilize the characteristics of Hb F to resist denaturation in an alkaline solution. The hemolysate is added to cyanmethemoglobin reagent and then exposed to an alkaline reagent, sodium hydroxide, for specified period. During this time normal Hb is destroyed, but the fetal Hb remains intact.

Ammonium sulfate is added to stop the denaturation process and to precipitate the denatured hemoglobin. The solution is filtered, measured spectrophotometerically, cyanmethemoglobin solution to determine the percent of hemoglobin.

Procedure

- Prepare hemolysate (R1) by add 0.5 mL blood to 9.5 mL Drabkin's solution then mixed.
- Transfer 2.8 mL from R1 to new tube and add 200 µL NaOH (2N) mixed and incubation 2 minutes at RT.
- At the end of 2 minutes exactly add 2 mL saturated ammonium sulfate to stop the reaction.
- After vigorous mixing, the mixture is allowed to stand for five to ten minutes at room temperature.
- It is then filtered through a double layer of Whatman no. 6 filter paper.
- Read the absorbance of filtrate at 540 nm.

Total Hb

1. Add 0.4 mL blood sample from (R1) to 6.75 mL distill water and mixed
2. Read it on 540 nm

$$\% \text{ HbF} = \frac{\text{Abs of HbF}}{\text{ABS of total Hb} \times 10} \times 100$$

Normal amount:
- One day newborn = $77 \pm 7.3\%$ HbF
- 3 weeks = 70.0 ± 7.3 % HbF
- 6–9 weeks = $52.9 \pm 11.0\%$ HbF
- 3–4 months = $23.2 \pm 16.0\%$ HbF
- 6 months = $4.7 \pm 2.2\%$ HbF
- 8–11 month = $1.6 \pm 1.0\%$ HbF
- Adult = <2.0% HbF.

Increased HbF seen in:
- Hereditary causes
  - Homozygous beta thalassemia (20–100 HbF).
  - Heterozygous beta thalassemia (up to 5% HbF).
  - Hereditary persistence of HbF (homozygous 100% and in heterozygous is 15–35%)
  - Sickle cell anemia (10–30% HbF).
- Acquired causes (up to 10% HbF)
  - Pernicious anemia, refractory normoblastic anemia, pure red aplasia, aplastic anemia, sideroblastic anemia.
  - Pregnancy and molar pregnancy.
  - Juvenile chronic myeloid leukemia.
  - Hyperthyroidism.
  - Erythroleukemia.
  - Chronic renal diseases.
  - Leakage of fetal RBC into maternal circulation fetomaternal hemorrhage (FMH).
  - Thalassemia major (shows HbF 40–90%.)

The continuous production of HbF leads to severe anemia and death.

HEINZ BODIES

Introduction

Heinz bodies are formed by damage and denaturing to the hemoglobin component of red blood cells. This is most commonly done by oxidative stress, but also possibly by genetic abnormalities in hemoglobin. Heinz bodies can be seen as an inclusion body within the cytoplasm of the red blood cells.

Typically, during oxidative damage to hemoglobin, an electron is transferred from the hemoglobin to oxygen, resulting in the formation of a reactive oxygen species (ROS). This ROS can lead to severe damage within the cells, and can even cause lysis of the entire cell.

The ROS denatures portions of the hemoglobin, causing precipitate to produce Heinz bodies. As this is not a normal process, Heinz bodies become an antigenic agent. Macrophages in the spleen detect this antigen and remove the damaged portions of the cell, its damaged membrane and the Heinz body (denatured hemoglobin). As a result, a portion of a red blood cell is phagocytosed due to the presence of Heinz bodies. These morphological abnormalities of red blood cells are called degmacytes or "bite cells".

Clinical Significance

Heinz bodies are present in peripheral blood smear, in one or more of following cases:
- G6PD (glucose-6-phosphate dehydrogenase) deficiency is the most important and most common cause of production of Heinz bodies, and consequently degmacytes.
- NADPH deficiency
- Alpha thalassemia
- Chronic liver disease
- *Hyposplenism and splenectomy*: The spleen helps with clearing the blood and thus removing Heinz bodies from circulation. With a damaged spleen, more of these Heinz bodies remain in circulation and are visible in a blood slide.
- Alpha thalassemia

Specimen: EDTA anticoagulated or double oxalate method.

Heinz bodies can be seen in unstained or stained preparations.

Principle

Unstained Preparations

Heinz bodies may be seen as refractile objects in dry, unstained films, if the illumination is reduced by lowering the microscope condenser. One or more may be present in a single cell. These are usually close to the cell membrane and may cause a protrusion of the membrane; in wet preparations, they may move around within the cells in a slow Brownian movement.

The degradation product of an unstable hemoglobin (e.g. hemoglobin Köln) exhibits green fluorescence when excited by blue light at 370 nm in a fluorescence microscope.

Stained Preparations

Heinz bodies are seen in wet preparation when stained with supravital staining. Red cells allows stain to enter inside, when they are in functional condition.

Reagents and Requirements

Test tubes, glass slides, cover slips, microscope, Pasteur pipettes, normal saline (Nacl 0.85 g/dl) and methyl violet.

Procedure

- Dissolve approximately 0.5 g of methyl violet in 100 mL normal saline and filter.
- Add 1 volume of blood (in EDTA anticoagulant) to 4 volumes of the methyl violet solution and allow the suspension to stand for about 10 min at room temperature.

- Mix and take a drop on a glass slide and cover with cover slip. Examine under high power objective (40X).
- Then prepare films and allow them to dry or view the suspension of cells between slide and coverslip. Examine blood smear under oil immersion objective (100x).

Observation

Heinz bodies stain an intense purple color, which is not taken up by the remainder of the RBC. They vary in size from approximately 1–3 µm. Percentage of Heinz bodies can be calculated by counting 100 red cells **(Fig. 25.3)**.

Heinz bodies also stain with other basic dyes. Brilliant green stains them well. If permanent preparations are required, fix the vitally stained films by exposure to formalin vapors for 5–10 min. Then counter stain the fixed films with 1 g/l eosin or neutral red, after thoroughly washing in water. Do not fix with methanol, as Heinz bodies are decolorized by it.

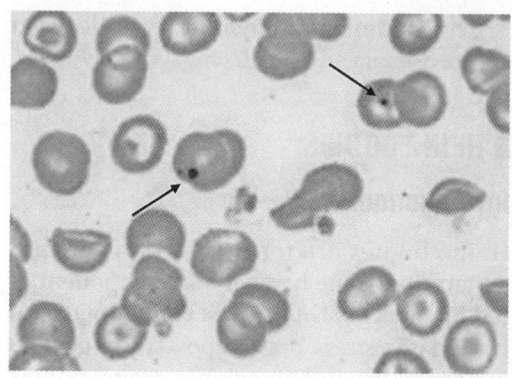

Fig. 25.3: Heinz bodies.
(For color version See Color Plate 6)

CHAPTER 26

Reticulocyte Count

Learning Objectives
- A reticulocyte count is a blood test that measures how fast red blood cells called reticulocytes are made by the bone marrow and released into the blood.
- This chapter throws light on principle, procedure, calculation and importance of reticulocyte count.

Keywords
Romanowsky stain, RNA, Erythropoiesis, Reticulocytosis, Aplastic anemia

INTRODUCTION

Reticulocytes are immature red cells, originated from bone marrow. Reticulocytes stay in circulation for about 24 hours and mature into erythrocytes. Reticulocytes have RNA and cytoplasmic remains, which pick up supravital stain. Reticulocyte cannot take Romanowsky stain because it contains methyl alcohol, which destroys RNA.

PRINCIPLE

Blood is mixed with stain. The stain is allowed to penetrate the cells in living condition. The RNA in the cell is stained as dark blue network inside the cells. The blood smear is made with a drop of blood and stained. Since, direct count is not possible, relative count is taken out of red blood cells. Reticulocytes are expressed as percentage of RBCs.

Requirement

- *Blood specimen:* EDTA anticoagulated or heparinized blood is used. The test should be performed within 2–3 hours of blood collection.
- Clean grease free slide.
- Test tube.
- Microscope.
- Stain—most commonly, brilliant cresyl blue stain is used.

Composition

- *Brilliant cresyl blue*: 1.0 g
- *Sodium citrate*: 0.4 g
- *Sodium chloride solution (0.85%)*: 100 mL

Filter the stain and store in a plastic container. It should be stored in refrigerator at 2–8°C.

Methylene blue can also be used for staining.

PROCEDURE

Filter a small amount of stain. In a test tube, add two drops of blood and two drops of stain by using separate Pasteur pipettes, mix it thoroughly. Cover the tube with rubber

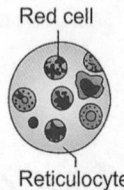

Fig. 26.1: The reticulocyte.

cap and keep it as it for 15–20 minutes. Take a drop of mixed solution of blood and stain on a clean grease free slide. Prepare a smear of this mixture by using spreader slide. Air dry the smear. First observe the smear under low power objective (10×) and locate tail portion of the smear where red cells are evenly distributed. Now, under oil immersion objective count both, red cells as well as reticulocytes. Reticulocytes are observed as fine deep violet cell having network of RNA. The red cells stain pale blue. Observe for about 15 field and count both the cells **(Fig. 26.1)**.

Calculation

The % reticulocyte can be calculated as:

$$\text{Reticulocyte count (\%)} = \frac{\text{No. of reticulocyte counted}}{\text{No. of RBC counted}} \times 100$$

Normal value
- In adults: 0.2–2% of RBC
- In infants: 2–6% of RBC

■ CLINICAL SIGNIFICANCE

The number of reticulocyte in peripheral blood is a reflection of red cell activity (erythropoiesis). Increase in their number indicates increased activity of bone marrow. This is known as reticulocytosis. High reticulocyte levels could be a sign of acute bleeding/chronic blood loss, hemolytic anemia erythroblastosis fetalis (hemolytic disease in a newborn), and kidney disease.

Decreased count of reticulocyte indicates bone marrow suppression, as observed in case of aplastic anemia.

Low reticulocyte levels could also indicate—iron deficiency anemia, folic acid deficiency, vitamin B_{12} deficiency, bone marrow failure caused by drug toxicity, infection or cancer, cirrhosis and as side-effects from radiation therapy.

Reticulocyte hemoglobin content is a good marker of iron function, since it does not change with acute conditions. However, it correlates well with MCV and MCH, and therefore does not appear to provide significant independent diagnostic advantage over MCV.

CHAPTER 27

Sickle Cells Preparation

Learning Objectives
- Sickle cell disease is a group of disorders that have atypical hemoglobin molecules called hemoglobin S, which can distort red blood cells into a sickle or crescent-shape.
- This chapter discusses principle and procedure to analyze presence of sickle cells in blood.
- It also points out difference between sickle cell disease and sickle cell trait.

Keywords
HbS, HbA, Sodium metabisulfite, Sickle cell trait, Normocytic RBC, Normochromic RBC, Sickle cell anemia

■ INTRODUCTION

Sickle cells are abnormal red cells, which are typically narrow, crescent (half-moon-shape) with defective membrane. They contain abnormal Hb (HbS) which is inherited. Hb is insoluble when oxygen tension is lower. This makes the red cell susceptible for sickling. The sickle cells tend to clump together and can not freely flow in circulation. This may block the blood vessel. The area of that organs which is deprived of blood supply due to blockage by these sickle cells damage the tissue or organs.

Importance

Sickle cell anemia is due to homozygous inheritance of abnormal Hb (Hb SS). In heterozygous condition (Hb SA), the disease is milder with no symptoms. This condition is called as sickle cell trait. Sickle cell disease is more severe than sickle cell trait. This disease is not common in India. It occurs mainly in Negro race of Africa. The red cell contains 90–100% Hb S. This disease is usually fatal by the age of 30.

Laboratory Findings

The sickle cells are rarely seen in patient of sickle cell anemia with peripheral blood smear. The other laboratory findings includes normocytic RBC, normochromic RBC, increased reticulocytes, increased platelets, decrease in osmotic fragility of red cell.

■ SICKLE CELL TRAIT

It is found in approximately 10% of American Negroes. The patient is heterozygous containing Hb SA. The red cells of patient contain 20–40% of Hb S and 60–80% of Hb A. The patient lives normal life with no clinical symptoms. The laboratory findings are normocytic, normochromic RBCs **(Fig. 27.1A)**.

The morphology of red cell is seen as normal in peripheral blood smear but these cells sickle under reduced oxygen supply. The degree of sickling however, depends on the concentration of Hb S in the cell. These cells are easily hemolyzed because of their abnormal shape, and results in chronic hemolytic anemia.

Laboratory diagnosis of sickle cell anemia is based on sickling of red cells under deoxygenated condition.

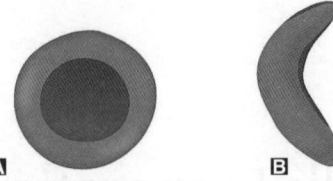

Figs. 27.1A and B: (A) Normal red blood cell (which is shaped a bit like a doughnut); (B) A sickle-shaped red blood cell of sickle cell disease.

Blood Specimen

Ethylenediaminetetraacetic acid (EDTA) anticoagulated venous blood or heparinized blood or capillary blood without anticoagulant can be used.

▮ PRINCIPLE

Whole blood is mixed with sodium metabisulfite ($Na_2S_2O_5$). It is strong reducing agent that deoxygenates Hb. If the cell contains HbS, they become sickle-shaped. This is because, when Hb S becomes deoxygenated, it tends to change them into the sickle shape.

Sickle cells in the circulation increase the blood's viscosity, which will slow the circulation, thereby increasing the time of exposure to a hypoxic condition, particularly in the small vasculature of the spleen. Repeated sickling of the RBCs ultimately damages the membrane permanently.

Requirement

Two percent sodium metabisulfite, dropper, Pasteur pipette, petroleum jelly, slide, etc.

▮ PROCEDURE

The first method, place a small drop of blood in the center of the glass slide. Add equal drop of $Na_2S_2O_5$ with the help of Pasteur pipette, mix it carefully with applicator sticks. Place coverslip. Make sure that no air bubble is present. Using syringe and 19-gauge needle, carefully seal the rims of coverslip with petroleum jelly. This sealing helps avoid entry of oxygen inside the coverslip from the atmosphere, wait for 15 minutes. Examine under 40X or high power objective.

The sickling is visible immediately in case of sickle cell diseased person **(Fig. 27.1B)**. In case of positive results of sickle cell trait sickling is seen within 1 hour so the slide should be kept under observation up to 2 hours and then re-examined after 24 hours.

If still red cells are unchanged, it is reported as negative. In case of positive results, the red cells becomes sickle-shaped, often with spikes. In some cases, red cells like holly leaf are seen in sickle cell trait.

This test does not distinguish between sickle cell anemia and sickle cell trait.

Sickle cell trait	Sickle cell disease
Is not a disease	Can cause mild to severe symptoms
Medical treatment usually not needed	Ongoing medical follow-up needed
Cannot change to disease	Is present at birth and can never be outgrown
There is enough hemoglobin A for normal red blood cell function	There is little or no hemoglobin A. When red blood cells carrying hemoglobin S release their oxygen to the tissue, they change from round to sickle shaped
The normal round red blood cells flow easily through small blood vessels	The sickle shape of the red blood cells gives "sickle cell" disease its name. The hard, sticky sickle red blood cells have trouble moving through small blood vessels. Sometimes they clog up these blood vessels and blood can not bring oxygen to the tissues. This can cause pain and/or damage to these areas

The second method is that put a drop of blood on the slide and seals it with paraffin. Leave the slide for some time and keep on observing the slide for the presence of a sickle cell.

The third method, add dithionite to the blood. HbS will precipitate. A negative test indicates that the patient has no or very little <10% HbS.

Hemoglobin electrophoresis is latest method by which presence of HbS is confirmed.

CHAPTER 28

Morphology of Normal and Abnormal RBCs

Learning Objectives
- Normal RBC's are biconcave in shape with a central pale area, and any deviation in size, shape, volume, structure or color represents an abnormal cell. Such abnormalities are detected by viewing the blood-smear images through a microscope.
- This chapter illustrates all types of abnormalities associated with red cells with proper diagrams.
- It also throws light on clinical importance of different abnormal RBCs.

Keywords
Hypochromic, Hyperchromic, Anisochromic, Polychromic, Microcytic, Macrocytic, Anisocytic, Poikilocytosis, Stomatocytosis, Elliptocyte, Spherocyte, Sickle cells, Target cells, Ovalocytes, Acanthocytes, Echinocytes, Dacryocytes, Schistocytes, Degmacytes, Heinz bodies, Howell-Jolly body

Clinical Significance

Abnormal morphology of RBC must be reported along with peripheral blood smear. This is helpful in the diagnosis of various types of anemia and other diseases like malaria, thalassemia, etc.

Following types of abnormalities are seen with RBC.

■ COLOR REACTION

Hypochromic RBC

Hypochromic RBCs have increased central paler area. It is associated with iron deficiency that decreases Hb concentration. Presence of hypochromic RBCs is called as hypochromatism **(Fig. 28.1)**.

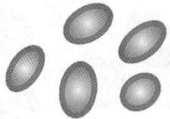

Fig. 28.1: Hypochromic RBC.

■ NORMAL MORPHOLOGY

Normally, RBCs are biconcave, disc-like with diameter 7.2 µ. These are uniformly stained and also known as normochromic (normal color). Mature erythrocytes contain central paler area, and edges are quite thick, containing Hb. Normal RBCs are non-nucleated. The normal morphology of RBC is termed as normocytic (normal cells).

Hyperchromic RBC

Hyperchromic RBCs have decreased central pale area. It is associated with increased iron concentration and Hb concentration. These RBC shows extensive staining than normal RBC. The presence of hyperchromic RBC is known as hyperchromatism **(Fig. 28.2)**.

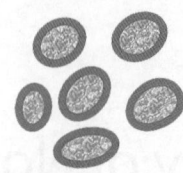

Fig. 28.2: Hyperchromic RBC.

Anisochromic RBC

Anisochromic RBCs have variable intensities, i.e., it has unequal Hb concentration. These RBCs are seen in iron deficiency anemia. Presence of such RBC is known as anisochromatism (**Fig. 28.3**).

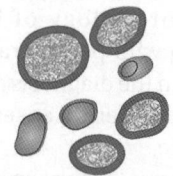

Fig. 28.3: Anisochromic RBC.

Polychromic RBC

Polychromic RBCs are gray colored. It may be slightly larger in size. It is often associated with increased reticulocyte count. Presence of polychromic RBC is known as polychromatism (**Fig. 28.4**).

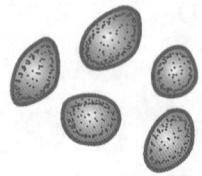

Fig. 28.4: Polychromic RBC.

■ SIZE VARIATIONS

Microcytic RBC

Microcytic RBCs are smaller RBCs, having diameter less than 6 µ. These are present in thalassemia, iron deficiency anemia, or it may be hereditary. Presence of microcytic RBC is known as microcytosis (**Fig. 28.5**).

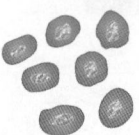

Fig. 28.5: Microcytic RBC.

Macrocytic RBC

The macrocytic RBCs are larger RBCs, having diameter 7.8 µ. It is associated with megaloblastic anemia. The presence of macrocytic RBC is known as macrocytosis (**Fig. 28.6**).

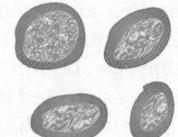

Fig. 28.6: Macrocytic RBC.

Anisocytic RBC

Anisocytic RBCs are variable in their size. It can be seen in various types of leukemia and iron deficiency anemia. Presence of anisocytic RBC is known as anisocytosis (**Fig. 28.7**).

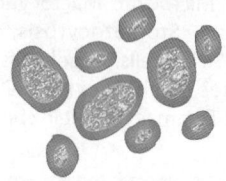

Fig. 28.7: Anisocytic RBC.

■ SHAPE VARIATION

Poikilocytosis

Poikilocytic RBCs have variation in their shape. Defective bone marrow production causes poikilocytic RBCs are of following different types.

Stomatocytosis

These RBCs have stomata like shape, i.e. central paler area is elongated silt like. This is often associated with alcoholism, hepatic disease or it may be hereditary (**Fig. 28.8**).

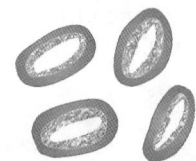

Fig. 28.8: Stomatocytic RBC.

Elliptocyte

These RBCs are elliptical, cigar shaped. Low count of elliptical RBC may be considered as normal. It is associated with various anemia, thalassemia or it may be hereditary elliptocytosis (**Fig. 28.9**).

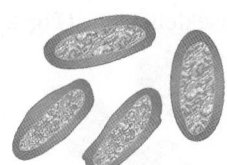

Fig. 28.9: Elliptocytic RBC.

Spherocyte

These are spherical RBC without any central paler area. These are usually slightly smaller in size. Spherocytes can be seen in hemolytic anemia, renal diseases. The presence of spherocyte is known as spherocytosis (**Fig. 28.10**).

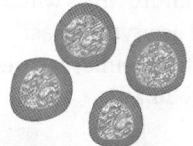

Fig. 28.10: Spherocytic RBC.

Sickle Cells

These are half-moon-shaped cells, which often have pointed ends. Normal RBC tends to be sickle-shaped due to abnormal Hb. The disease is also known as sickle cell anemia (**Fig. 28.11**).

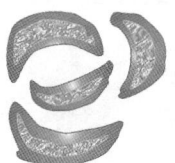

Fig. 28.11: Sickle cells.

Target Cells

Target cells are red blood cells that have the appearance of a shooting target with a bullseye. In optical microscopy, these cells appear to have a dark center (a central, hemoglobinized area) surrounded by a white ring (an area of relative pallor), followed by dark outer (peripheral), second ring containing a band of hemoglobin. Such RBCs are found in hepatitis, thalassemia, etc. (**Fig. 28.12**).

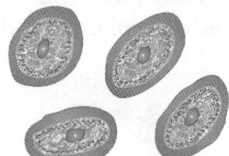

Fig. 28.12: Target cells.

Ovalocytes

These RBCs are oval in shape. The lower count of ovalocytes may be considered to be normal. However, the higher count is associated with various anemias (**Fig. 28.13**).

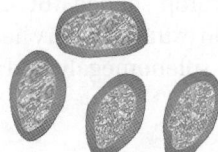

Fig. 28.13: Ovalocytes.

Acanthocytes

These RBCs are irregular-shaped, with throne like projections on their outer edges. Their presence is called as acanthocytosis. Such types of RBCs can be seen in hepatic and renal disorder **(Fig. 28.14)**.

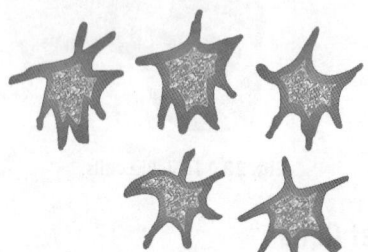

Fig. 28.14: Acanthocytes.

Echinocytes

These are also known as burr cells. These are rounded red cells with evenly spaced cytoplasmic projections on their outer edge. These are found in case of uremia, liver disease, pyruvate kinase deficiency, oxidative or colloid osmotic stress in already dysmorphic erythrocytes (e.g., spherocytes) **(Fig. 28.15)**.

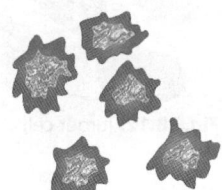

Fig. 28.15: Echinocytes.

Dacryocytes

These are also known as teardrop erythrocytes. These are teardrop-shaped RBCs. Dacryocytes are observed in extramedullary hematopoiesis, mylofibrosis, splenomegaly and thalassemia **(Fig. 28.16)**.

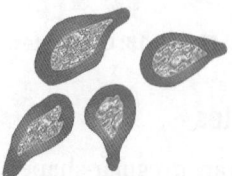

Fig. 28.16: Dacryocytes.

OTHER CONDITIONS

Schistocytes

These are also known as fragmentocytes. These are fragmented RBCs. These are found in case of hemolytic anemia, in case of mechanical damage like presence of artificial cardiac valves **(Fig. 28.17)**.

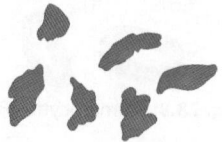

Fig. 28.17: Schistocytes.

Degmacytes

These are also known as bite cells. It appears like one or more semicircular portions removed ("bitten off") from the cell margin. These are found in case of glucose-6-phosphate dehydrogenase deficiency **(Fig. 28.18)**.

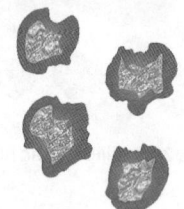

Fig. 28.18: Degmacytes.

ABNORMALITIES IN NORMAL CONTENT OF RBC

Nucleated RBC

These are immature RBCs with nucleus. These are also called as erythroblast. These are seen in megaloblastic anemia, severe bleeding, and leukemia **(Fig. 28.19)**.

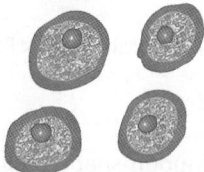

Fig. 28.19: Nucleated RBC.

Heinz Bodies

These are mature cells with deposit of iron which stains dark blue. Heinz bodies are indicative of oxidative injury to the erythrocyte. They are clumps of irreversibly denatured hemoglobin attached to the erythrocyte cell membrane. Heinz bodies can be seen as an inclusion body within the cytoplasm of the Red Blood Cells **(Fig. 28.20)**.

Howell-Jolly Body

In these RBC contains round purple stained nuclear fragment. Normally, these are present in immature RBCs. These can be seen in RBCs with various types of anemia **(Fig. 28.21)**.

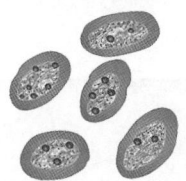

Fig. 28.21: RBCs with Howell-Jolly body.

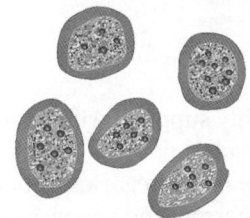

Fig. 28.20: RBCs with Heinz bodies.

RBC Normal and Abnormal Morphology

(For color version See Color Plate 7)

CHAPTER 29

Bone Marrow

Learning Objectives
- The bone marrow produces the cellular elements of the blood. Bone marrow examination is used in the diagnosis of a number of conditions, including leukemia, multiple myeloma, anemia, and pancytopenia.
- This chapter explains structure and function of bone marrow, sample collection by biopsy, preparation of bone marrow film and staining, observation of bone marrow with respect to expected pathologic condition.
- This chapter also points out method for diagnosis of sideroblasts. Percent distribution of normal cellular components of bone marrow is given in a tabular form.
- A sample report is attached to give an idea of different tests results.

Keywords
Red bone marrow, Yellow bone marrow, Microtrephine biopsy, Surgical biopsy, Romanowsky stain, M/E ratio (myeloid/erythroid ratio), Flow cytometry, Fluorescence in situ hybridization (FISH), Sideroblasts Prussian blue (Perls') reaction, Normal distribution of cells and cell maturation stages, Sample report

Bone marrow is the soft, flexible connective tissue within bone cavities. It is a component of the lymphatic system. Bone marrow functions primarily to produce blood cells and to store fat. Bone marrow is highly vascular, meaning that it is richly supplied with a large number of blood vessels.

There are two categories of bone marrow tissue: red marrow and yellow marrow. From birth to early adolescence, the majority of our bone marrow is red marrow. As we grow and mature, increasing amounts of red marrow are replaced by yellow marrow. Adults have on average about 2.6 kg of bone marrow, with about half of it being red (**Fig. 29.1**).

■ STRUCTURE AND FUNCTION

1. *Red bone marrow*: It is also known as myeloid tissue. Red bone marrow consists of a delicate, highly vascular fibrous tissue containing hematopoietic (Blood-forming) stem cells. Stem cells are immature cells

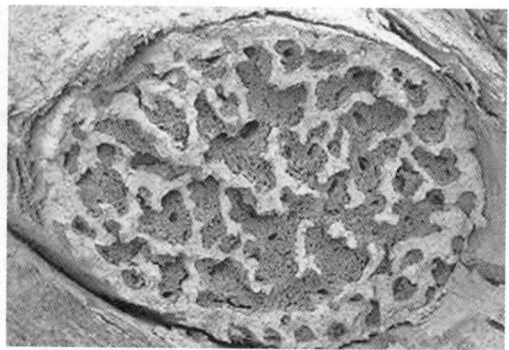

Fig. 29.1: Connective tissue of red and yellow bone marrow.
(For color version See Color Plate 8)

that can turn into a number of different types of cell. These include all red blood cells, platelets and around 60–70% of lymphocytes. Other lymphocytes begin life in the red bone marrow and become fully formed in the lymphatic tissues. The different types of hematopoietic stem cells vary in their regenerative capacity and potency. Some are multipotent, oligopotent or unipotent as determined by how many types of cell they can create.

The process of development of different blood cells from these pluripotent stem cells is known as hematopoiesis. It is these stem cells that are needed in bone marrow transplant.

Together with the liver and spleen, red bone marrow also plays a role in getting rid of old red blood cells.

Red marrow is found mainly in the flat bones such as hip bone, breast bone, skull, ribs, vertebrae and shoulder blades, and in the cancellous ("spongy") material at the proximal ends of the long bones like femur and humerus.

2. *Yellow bone marrow:* Yellow bone marrow contains mesenchymal stem cells, also known as marrow stromal cells. The color of yellow marrow is due to the much higher number of fat cells. These produce fat, cartilage, and bone. It helps to provide sustenance and maintain the correct environment for the bone to function. However, under particular conditions, such as severe blood loss or fever, the yellow marrow may revert to red marrow.

Yellow marrow tends to be located in the central cavities of long bones, and is generally surrounded by a layer of red marrow with long trabeculae (beam-like structures) within a sponge-like reticular framework.

Clinical Significance

A number of diseases pose a threat to bone marrow as it prevent bone marrow from turning stem cells into essential cells. Leukemia, Hodgkin's disease, and other lymphoma cancers are known to damage the marrow's productive ability and destroy stem cells.

A bone marrow examination can help diagnose: Leukemia, multiple myeloma, Gaucher disease, unusual cases of anemia and other hematological diseases.

■ SAMPLE COLLECTION

Before deciding to examine the bone marrow, one should observe something abnormal in peripheral blood smear. Bone marrow can be obtained for examination by bone marrow biopsy and bone marrow aspiration.

Needle aspiration: It is done to remove mainly fluid part by suction. It is a simple, safe and relatively painless method and performed by using a special designed needle, such as Salah or Klema. It is generally aspirated from the posterior iliac crests while the patient is under either regional or general anesthesia.

The disadvantage of this technique is some marrow cells may be destroyed.

Biopsy: Biopsies are samples of tissue that are removed for closer examination. Bone marrow biopsy can be obtained by the following two methods: 1. Microtrephine biopsy and 2. Surgical biopsy.

1. *Microtrephine bsiopsy:* Occasionally, in a very obese patient, it is necessary to use a trephine biopsy needle, which is generally longer than an aspiration needle. This method is not very simple but can be performed in out patient department (OPD) by using needles such as Jasshidi's-Swaim or Islam. The method does not give more than 0.3 mL of fluid at a time.
2. *Surgical biopsy:* This method is carried out under aseptic condition in operation theater. The disadvantages of this method are: (a) It is difficult to repeat and (b) It is not advised in patients with leukemia and bleeding disorders.

Site of Biopsy

- Sternum
- Iliac crest
- Anterior and posterior iliac spine
- Upper end of tibia in children below 2 years.

PREPARATION OF BONE MARROW FILM

Bone marrow smears should be prepared immediately following aspiration. Smears prepared from EDTA samples should be made as soon as possible to reduce storage effect. To prepare smears, the aspirate should be expelled into a small plastic or siliconized glass dish, and a Pasteur pipette used to draw up particles, which are placed on glass slides and then smeared. Alternatively, a drop of aspirate can be placed on each glass slide and the excess blood drained off the slide by tipping the slide, or aspirated with a Pasteur pipette or plastic syringe, before making the smear.

Two types of smears are made:
1. Smears are made with a glass spreader with bevelled edges so that the width of the spreader is narrower than the width of the specimen slide. The spreader is placed in front of the drop of aspirate at an angle of approximately 300 and pulled back to make contact with the drop, to enable the drop to spread along the line of contact with the slide. The spreader is then pushed forward in a smooth action, in contact with the slide.
2. To make a squash slide, a drop of bone marrow containing particles is placed in the middle of one slide, and a second slide is placed on top of the first. The weight of the second slide on the first is sufficient to squash the marrow particles; no downward force should be applied. The slides are drawn apart away from each other, in the direction of the long axis of the slide.

A minimum of six smears and two particle squash ('crush') slide preparations should be made.

STAINING OF BONE MARROW ASPIRATE SLIDES

Two air-dried smears and one squash slide should be fixed with fresh acetone-free absolute methanol and stained with a Romanowsky stain, such as Giemsa stain. Wright's and Wright-Giemsa stains, when performed properly, give sharp and clear nuclear, cytoplasmic, and granule detail.

A methanol-fixed smear and a squash slide should be stained with Prussian Blue (Perls' reaction) and counterstained with Safranin-O or Kernecht Red (nuclear fast red). All bone marrow smears should be cover-slipped using a mounting medium that hardens and dries rapidly. Mounting media may contain toxic organic compounds such as toluene or xylene therefore, as a precautions, it is recommended that this should be performed in a chemical fume hood. Additional slides may be used for cytochemistry (e.g. myeloperoxidase or nonspecific esterases), IHC, FISH, or archived as unfixed, unstained smears, as required.

Observation

Normally, cellularity of bone marrow varies with age. It is more in infants and less in adults. In the bone marrow examination, first of all observe the erythropoietic cells and then look for maturity of leukopoietic cells. The cells appear as dark blue masses and fats as round vacuoles. Normal aspiration contains about 40% of fat cells and 60% of marrow cells. **Table 29.1** for normal distribution of cells and cell maturation stages in aspirates. The cells are evaluated according to number, type, maturity, appearance, etc., and compared to those in the blood using results from a complete blood count (CBC) and blood smear. The bone marrow smear or squash preparation should first be viewed under low power magnification (100 X) to determine the number and cellularity of particles, the number of megakaryocytes, and to scan for clumps of abnormal cells of low incidence.

TABLE 29.1: Normal distribution of cells and cell maturation stages in aspirates or imprints

Cell or cell maturation stage	Distribution	Cell or cell maturation stage	Distribution
Myeloblasts	0–3%	Pronormoblasts/rubriblasts	0–1%
Promyelocytes	1–5%	Basophilic normoblasts/prorubricytes	1–4%
Myelocytes	6–17%	Polychromatophilic normoblasts/rubricytes	10–20%
Metamyelocytes	3–20%	Orthochromic normoblasts/metarubricytes	6–10%
Neutrophilic bands	9–32%	Lymphocytes	5–18%
Segmented neutrophils	7–30%	Plasma cells	0–1%
Eosinophils and eosinophilic precursors	0–3%	Monocytes	0–1%
Basophils and mast cells	0–1%	Histiocytes	0–1%
Megakaryocytes	2–10 visible per low-power field	Myeloid-to-erythroid ratio	1.5:1–3.3:1

Areas of well-spread marrow cells are selected for assessment at higher magnification (i.e. 200X, 400X, 600X, 1000X) for morphological assessment of cells, including cytological detail, parasites or cell inclusions.

Observe for:
- The M/E ratio (myeloid/erythroid ratio)—this calculation compares the number of myeloid cells (WBC precursors) to erythroid cells (RBC precursors).
- Differential count —determines whether cells in each lineage (WBC, RBC, platelet-producing cells) show orderly and complete maturation, and whether the cells are present in normal proportion to one another. The differential count should comprise blast cells, promyelocytes, myelocytes, metamyelocytes, band forms, segmented neutrophils, eosinophils, basophils, mast cells, promonocytes and monocytes, lymphocytes, plasma cells and erythroblasts. The differential count should not include megakaryocytes, macrophages, osteoblasts, osteoclasts, stromal cells, smudged cells or non-hemopoietic cells such as metastatic tumor cells. Lymphoid aggregates, if present, should not be included in the differential count, but their presence should be commented upon. At least 500 cells should be counted in at least two smears when a precise percentage of an abnormal cell type is required for diagnosis and disease.
- Presence of any abnormal cells, such as leukemic or tumor cells.
- Observe for parasites and bacteria.
- Cellularity—the volume of cells is compared to the volume of other components of the bone marrow, such as fat (and whether cellularity is normal for age, increased, or decreased).
- Whether the different cell lineages (myeloid, erythroid and megakaryocytic) are present in adequate numbers. Example: Marrow smear from a patient with hemolytic anemia—erythroid hyperplasia reveals greatly increased numbers of maturing erythroid progenitors (normoblasts).
- If there are any abnormal infiltrates in the marrow (cancer, infection) as well as any changes to the bone marrow stroma (e.g. fibrosis) or bone itself (osteoporosis).

Depending on what condition(s) a healthcare practitioner suspects or is investigating, a number of other tests may be performed on the marrow sample.

A few examples include

In the case of leukemia, tests to determine the type of leukemia may be done. These include determination of antigenic markers for example, immunophenotyping by flow cytometry is done to provide information on the type of leukemia present, including prognostic or therapeutic markers.

Flow cytometry is a laboratory method used to detect, identify, and count specific cells. This method can also identify particular components within cells. This information is based on physical characteristics and/or markers called antigens on the cell surface or within cells that are unique to that cell type.

Flow cytometry involves several steps:
- A sample of cells is suspended in a fluid.
- Prior to testing and depending on the cells being analyzed, the sample may be treated with special dyes to further define cell subtypes.
- The sample containing the cells passes through an instrument called a flow cytometer.
- In the instrument, the fluid in which the cells are suspended passes through very narrow channels so that the cells are organized in a single file as they pass the detector(s). This is accomplished at a high rate of speed (hundreds to thousands of cells per second.)
- The flow cytometer contains one or more lasers and a series of photo detectors that are able to identify certain characteristics unique to various cell types. The single-cell suspension creates unique light-scattering events that occur when each cell passes through the laser light. These initial events are characteristic of the size and shape of the cell, as well as the intensity of the signal that is generated by the specific dyes, thus creating patterns that reflect cell type.
- The signals from the detectors are amplified and sent to a computer. They are converted to digital read-outs displayed on a computer screen or in a printout.
- The data are usually displayed as graphs.

- A chromosome analysis and/or FISH may be ordered to detect chromosomal abnormalities in the case of leukemia, myelodysplasia, lymphoma, or myeloma. Fluorescence in Situ Hybridization (FISH) is a technique used to search DNA of a cell, for the presence or absence of specific genes or portions of genes. Many different types of cancer are associated with known genetic abnormalities. Over a lifetime, cells can make mistakes when they divide and grow. Mutations in the DNA that are associated with cancer may accumulate in these cells. In this method, a single-stranded fluorescent-labeled nucleic acid sequence (probe) complementary to a target genomic sequence is hybridized to detect the presence or absence of a given abnormality. FISH is a method of choice for diagnosis, prognosis, and chemotherapy treatment response in hematopoietic neoplasms (leukemia, lymphomas, multiple myeloma, and myelodysplasia) and solid tumors.
- Special stains may also be used to evaluate iron storage in the marrow and to determine whether an abnormal erythroid (RBC) precursor with iron particles surrounding its nucleus (so-called ring sideroblasts) is present. Presence of iron in bone marrow smear is detected by Perl's staining method.

IMPORTANCE OF DETECTION OF SIDEROBLAST

Presence of iron in bone marrow smear is an important tool to detect: Iron deficiency anemia, where iron stores are completely depleted and in Sideroblastic anemia. It is a form of anemia in which the bone marrow produces ringed sideroblasts rather than healthy red blood cells (erythrocytes). In sideroblastic anemia, the body has iron available but cannot incorporate it into hemoglobin.

Principle

Prussian blue (Perls') reaction is a method for staining non-hem iron in normoblasts (siderocytes), macrophages (hemosiderin), and other cells containing particulate iron. The method allows assessment of both the amount of iron in reticuloendothelial stores and availability of iron to developing erythroblasts.

The granules of non-hem iron are formed of a water-insoluble complex of ferric iron, lipid, protein and carbohydrate. These granules (containing ferric iron) react with potassium ferrocyanide [$K_4Fe(CN)_6$] to form a blue compound ferriferrocynanide), Prussian blue reaction.

Materials

- 2% Potassium ferrocyanide $K_4Fe(CN)_6$.$3H_2O$
- 2N HCl
- 1% aqueous safranin (counterstain)
- Air dried bone marrow smear

Method

- Choose a suitable sample as a positive control and the stain together with a test sample.
- Label the slides as control and patient name/registration number (R/N) accordingly.
- Fix the slides in absolute methanol for 10–20 minutes. Leave it to dry.
- Prepare the working solution by adding 30 mL potassium ferrocyanide and 30 mL HCl in a Coplin jar (v/v potassium ferrocyanide: HCl = 1:1).
- Submerge the fixed and dried slides into the Coplin jar containing the working solution.
- Leave it at room temperature or incubate in a water bath at 50°C for 20 minutes.
- Wash the slides in running tap water for 3–5 minutes.
- Rinse thoroughly in distilled water, and then counterstain with safranin similar to steps 4–6.
- Dry and cover the slides with coverslips with Depex.

Observation: Ring sideroblasts are erythroblasts with iron-loaded mitochondria around the nucleus in the form of a ring. It appears as a blue ring surrounding red nucleus

- Molecular tests may be performed on a sample of bone marrow to help establish a diagnosis. Examples include:
  - T-cell receptor gene rearrangement
  - B-cell immunoglobulin gene rearrangement
  - JAK2 mutation
- Bone marrow may be cultured to look for viral, bacterial, or fungal infections that can cause a "fever of unknown origin." Certain bacteria and fungi can also be detected by special stains.

A peripheral blood specimen is collected for a complete blood count no more than 24 hours before the bone marrow is collected, and the results of the CBC are reported with the bone marrow examination results.

SAMPLE REPORT

Bone Marrow Pathology Report

PATIENT INFORMATION:
LAST NAME, FIRST NAME
GENDER
AGE: DOB:
Patient ID/MRN:
Account #:

PHYSICIAN INFORMATION:
LAST NAME, FIRST NAME
NAME OF HOSPITAL/MEDICAL CENTER
ADDRESS OF MEDICAL CENTER
CITY, STATE
Tel: XXX-XXX-XXX

FINAL DIAGNOSIS:

BIOPSY SITE; BIOPSY:
- ACUTE MYELOID LEUKEMIA WITH t(8;21)(q22;q22.1); *RUNX1-RUNX1T1*, SEE COMMENT

COMMENT:
Peripheral blood film: Leukopenia, few blasts, myelocytes, neutrophils. Relative lymphocytosis. RBCs normochromic, macrocytes, mild anisocytosis, Rare teardrop cells. Normal platelet morphology.
Bone marrow aspirate: Few spicules, blasts 65% with large nuclei with fine chromatin and needle shaped Auer rods. Moderate basophilic cytoplasm with salmon-colored graules. Few mature myeloid precursors. Erythroid precursors markedly decreased, with rare binucleate rubricytes. Few eosinophil precursors noted, Dysmorphic megakaryocytes with increased nuclear lobulation.
Bone marrow imprint: Significantly increased blasts. Few mature myeloid precursors, erythroid precursors markedly decreased.
Bone marrow biopsy: Hypercellular for age: estimated at 80% cellular. Most cells are blasts, few mature myeloid precursors. Erythroid and megakaryocytic precursors markedly reduced.
Iron stain: Stainable iron in macrophages. Sideroblasts and rare ringed sideroblasts.
Flow cytometry: Analysis of the bone marrow aspirate smear demonstrates an abnormal myeloid blast population. Blasts express CD34, CD15, HLA-DR, CD33, CD19 and CD56, No phenotypic abnormalities in the lymphocytes.

Differential Counts

Date	PB	Marrow	Marrow Range (percent)				
Blast, unclassified	4	65	0–2	Normal lymphocytes	50	2	3–24
Myeloblasts			3–5	Reactive lymphocytes			
Promyelocytes			1–8	Lymphoblasts			
Myelocytes		14	5–21	Prolymphocytes			
Metamyelocytes			6–22	Monocytes		3	0–3
Band neutrophils			6–22	Plasma cells			0–2
Segmented neutrophils	40	4	9–27	Rubriblasts			0–4
Eosinophils	3	7		Prorubricytes			1–6
Basophils				Rubricytes			5–25
Other				Metarubricytes			1–21
Other				Erythroid		8	10–30
WBC 2,300	PLT 89,000	MPV 8	HGB 8.1	HCT 23	MCHC	110	

Cytogenetics

ABNORMAL MALE KARYOTYPE: 45,XY,t(8;21)(q22;q22),-Y[20]

Association: This cytogenetics report renders the disease to be classified as "AML with recurrent genetic abnormalities" per the WHO classification 2016. There is also loss of the Y chromosome which is an incidental finding and of no clinical consequence in older male patients.

Prognosis: Good prognosis to chemotherapy and a high complete remission rate

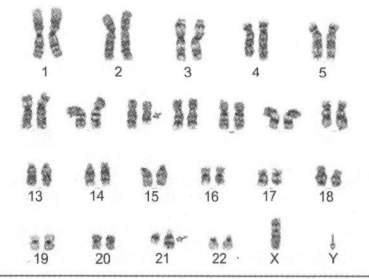

CHAPTER 30

Blood Coagulation

Learning Objectives
- Blood coagulation is an important process that prevents excessive bleeding when a blood vessel is injured.
- This chapter has explanation of a complex chemical process of coagulation, which involves XII factors.
- Mechanisms of coagulation, its three stages are illustrated in flowchart.

Keywords
Hemostasis, Coagulation factors, Thromboplastin, Thrombin, Prothrombin, Fibrin clot

INTRODUCTION

Bleeding occur when a blood vessel is injured. It stops by a process called as hemostasis.

Hemostasis is a complex process that involves three major steps including coagulation.

Coagulation is brought by twelve coagulation factors.

The coagulation factors are numbered in the order of their discovery. There are 13 numerals but only 12 factors. Factor VI later turned out to be the activated form of V. Hence, VI is not now in active use.

COAGULATION FACTORS

The circulating plasma and tissue surrounding the blood vessel contain twelve coagulation factors. These coagulation factors are various organic compounds, proteins, co-enzymes and inorganic element—calcium (Ca). Under normal condition, in circulation these coagulation factors are present in an inactive form. Whenever there is injury, these are converted to active form.

The twelve blood coagulation factors are mentioned here.

Factors	Name of factor
I	Fibrinogen
II	Prothrombin
III	Tissue extract/tissue thromboplastin
IV	Calcium
V	Proaccelerin/liable factor
VI	Combined with factor V
VII	Proconvertin/stable factor
VIII	Antihemophilic factor A/antihemophilic factor (AHF)
IX	Antihemophilic factor B/plasma thromboplastin component (PTC) (Christmas factor)
X	Stuart factor/power factor
XI	Plasma thromboplastin antecedent/antihemophilic (Factor C)
XII	Contact factor/Hageman factor
XIII	Fibrin stabilizing factors (Laki-L or/and Factor)

Platelets are not included in the list of coagulation factors, because platelets release several factors that help in clotting process. In addition, thromboplastin and thrombin are not included in the list, because these are intermediates of coagulation process, and not present normally in the body unless bleeding occurs.

Normal fresh plasma contains all factors listed above, except factor IV (calcium), which is removed by anticoagulant. Thus, absence of calcium (factor IV) prevents clotting of blood.

■ MECHANISM OF COAGULATION

The mechanism of blood coagulation is necessary and significant to understand routine coagulation tests. Any of the deficiency of coagulation factors disturbs coagulation process.

Stage 1

The tissue extract or tissue thromboplastin (III) enters the blood vessel through the site of injury and combines with factor VII and Ca^{++} (IV). This is known as extrinsic system as the reaction is going on out of the blood vessel. The extrinsic system then joins with the intrinsic system, i.e., the blood vessel. The factors that participate in intrinsic system are all present in the blood circulation. The factors are—XII, XI, IX, and VIII.

Now, the extrinsic and intrinsic system joins together and follows a common path. These react with factors X, V and Ca^{++} to produce plasma thromboplastin.

The end product of Stage 1 is plasma thromboplastin, which enters in Stage 2.

Any defect in intrinsic system of Stage 1 is recognized by activated partial thromboplastin time (APTT).

Stage 2

In Stage 2, prothrombin (factor II) is activated by plasma thromboplastin, which is the end product of Stage 1. This results in the formation of active thrombin. Any defect in Stage 2, i.e. deficiency of factor II, will be recognized by prolonged prothrombin time (PT).

Stage 3

In the final stage of coagulation process, inactive fibrinogen is activated by the end product

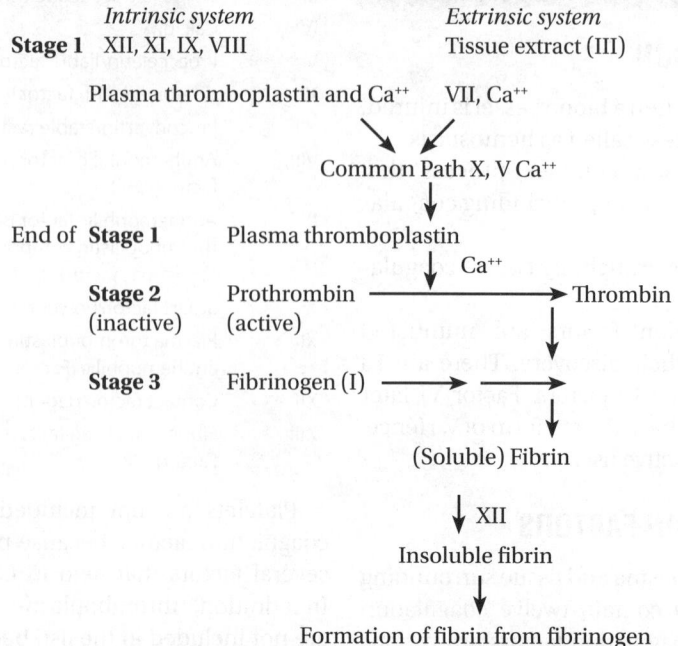

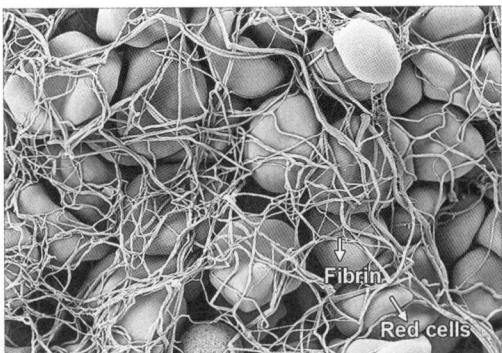

Fig. 30.1: Red blood cell entangled in fibrin to form blood clot.
(For color version See Color Plate 8)

of Stage 2, i.e. thrombin. The fibrinogen is first converted in soluble fibrin. Soluble fibrin polymerizes with the help of factor XIII to form insoluble fibrin clot **(Fig. 30.1)**.

In this way, for the formation of blood clot, twelve coagulation factors work in coordination with one another.

Significance of Blood Clotting

A blood clot is formed to stop bleeding, such as at the site of cut. But clots should not form when blood is moving through the body; when clots form inside blood vessels or when blood has a tendency to clot too much, serious health problems can occur.

■ HEMOSTASIS

Hemostasis is a complex and highly regulated physiological process that maintains a balance between the liquid state of blood within the vasculature and the induction of blood clot formation following injury.

It involves multisystem interactions between components of the vessel wall, blood cells (mainly platelets), and plasma proteins.

The following events are involved in the hemostatic process:
- *Vasoconstriction*: When the blood vessel ruptures, the wall of the vessel immediately contracts to reduce blood flow and thereby prevent blood loss.
- *Platelet activation*: Platelets adhere to the vessel injuries via von Willebrand factor and aggregate with fibrinogen to form platelet plugs (primary hemostasis).
- *Blood coagulation*: Clot formation occurs as a result of coagulation that is mediated by blood-clotting factors.
- *Fibrinolysis*: The blood clot is dissolved when healing is complete, thereby assuring long-term vascular patency.

Disturbances of Blood Coagulation

The human hemostatic system is dependent on a delicate equilibrium between procoagulant and anticoagulant factors that interact with each other to ensure effective hemostasis at the sites of vascular injury. The procoagulant forces include platelet adhesion, aggregation, and fibrin clot formation, while the anticoagulant forces include the natural inhibitors of coagulation and fibrinolysis.

Any disruption in the balance between clot formation and clot dissolution can result in either thrombosis (due to hypercoagulation) or hemorrhage (due to hypocoagulation).

Factors Responsible for Thrombosis/Hypercoagulation

Many factors can cause thrombosis, which is excessive blood clotting including certain diseases and conditions, genetic mutations and medicines. These causes fall into two categories: acquired and genetic.
1. *Acquired* means that excessive blood clotting was triggered by another disease or condition. Smoking, overweight and obesity, pregnancy, use of birth control pills or hormone replacement therapy, cancer, prolonged bed rest, or car or plane trips are a few examples.
2. *The genetic, or inherited*, source of excessive blood clotting is less common

and is usually due to genetic defects. These defects usually occur in the proteins needed for blood clotting and can also occur with the substances that delay or dissolve blood clots.

Effect of Blood Clot

Blood clots can form in, or travel to the blood vessels in the brain, heart, kidneys, lungs, and limbs. A clot in the veins deep in the limb is called deep vein thrombosis (DVT). DVT usually affects the deep veins of the legs. It can cause pain, swelling, redness, or increased warmth in the affected limb. If a blood clot in a deep vein breaks off and travels through the bloodstream to the lungs and blocks blood flow, it is called a pulmonary embolism (PE). Other complications of blood clots include stroke (if it blocks blood supply to brain), heart attack (if it blocks blood supply to heart), and kidney problems like kidney failure (if it blocks blood supply to kidney). Blood clots can cause miscarriages, stillbirths, and other pregnancy-related problems, such as preeclampsia, which is high blood pressure that occurs during pregnancy.

Factors Responsible for Hemorrhage/Hypocoagulation

A deficiency in clotting factors or a disorder that affects platelet production or one of the many steps in the entire process can disrupt clotting. This severely complicates blood loss from injury, childbirth, surgery, and specific diseases or conditions in which bleeding can occur.

Coagulation disorders arise from different causes and involve different complications. Some common coagulation disorders are:
- Hemophilia or hemophilia A (factor VIII deficiency) is genetic disorder is carried by females but most often affects male offspring. It is characterized by spontaneous musculoskeletal bleeding.
- Christmas disease or hemophilia B (factor IX deficiency) is less common than hemophilia A with similar symptoms. Factor IX is produced in the liver and is dependent on interaction with vitamin K in order to function properly. Deficiency in the vitamin can affect the clotting factor's performance as well as deficiency in the factor itself.
- Disseminated intravascular coagulation, also known as consumption coagulopathy, is a clinical emergency that occurs as a result of other diseases and conditions. This condition accelerates clotting, which ironically can result in hemorrhage when the clotting factors are exhausted.
- Thrombocytopenia, the most common cause of coagulation disorder, is characterized by reduced numbers of circulating platelets in the blood.
- Von Willebrand's disease, a hereditary disorder with prolonged bleeding time, is due to a clotting factor deficiency and impaired platelet function. It is the most common inherited coagulation disorder.
- Hypoprothrombinemia is a congenital deficiency of clotting factors that can lead to hemorrhage.

Other coagulation disorders include factor XI deficiency (hemophilia C), and factor VII deficiency. It is also called serum prothrombin conversion accelerator (SPCA) deficiency.

CHAPTER 31

Hemorrhagic Disorders

Learning Objectives
- Hemorrhagic disorders are a group of disorders that share the inability to form a proper blood clot. They are characterized by extended bleeding after injury, surgery, trauma or menstruation.
- Bleeding time, whole blood coagulation time, clot retraction, prothrombin time, platelet count, tourniquet test, activated partial thromboplastin time (APTT) and purpura are used as screening tests of hemorrhagic disorders.
- In this chapter, principle, procedure and clinical importance of all these tests are explained in detail.

Keywords
Inherited and acquired hemorrhagic disorders, Dukes and Ivy's method for bleeding time, Wright and Lee-White method for whole blood coagulation, Fibrinogenemia, Clot retraction, Prothrombin time, Hemolytic disease of new born, Thrombocytopenia, Tourniquet test, Activated partial thromboplastin time (APTT), Hemophilia A, Thromboplastin, Purpura

■ INTRODUCTION

The hemorrhagic disorders are a group of disorders of widely differing etiology, which have in common an abnormal tendency to bleed. This abnormal tendency to bleed is due to a defect in mechanism of blood coagulation.

There are three major components of normal blood coagulation mechanism:
1. Vascular
2. Platelet
3. Coagulation factors.

These act together in coordination to arrest bleeding. A breakdown in the normal coagulation mechanism results in abnormal tendency to bleeding and may result from the defect in any one of these three components. Bleeding is especially liable to occur when one or more than one component is defective.

The various hemorrhagic disorders can result in uncontrolled hemorrhaging into joints, muscles and deep tissues with formation of hematomas. The laboratory investigations are carried out for patients who have a history of spontaneous bleeding after trauma or surgery or patients who have to undergo a major surgery.

The hemorrhagic disorders are either inherited or acquired.

Inherited Hemorrhagic Disorders

These are transmitted as sex-linked disorders and mainly observed among males, while females act as carriers. These disorders are mainly due to deficiencies of factors VIII and IX. Other inherited disorders of coagulation include factor XI deficiency which is transmitted as autosomal disorder and occur with equal frequency in males and females.

Acquired Hemorrhagic Disorders

The most common cause of acquired bleeding disorder includes:
- Thrombocytopenias due to many reasons such as infections, malignant, drug induced immune and non-immune
- Deficiency of vitamin K
- Liver failure
- Therapy of heparin and coumarin group of drugs.

Screening Tests of Hemorrhagic Disorders

These are non-specific tests designed to assess overall coagulation mechanism and are useful for the screening of patients who may have a bleeding disorders. Although, these tests are simple, they lack sensitivity and it does not necessarily mean that a patient has a normal coagulation mechanism if the results of the tests are all normal. The following screening tests are recommended:
- Bleeding time
- Whole blood coagulation time
- Clot retraction
- Prothrombin time
- Platelet count
- Tourniquet test
- Purpura.

Besides these, the routine hemorrhagic disorder tests include—plasma recalcification time, partial thromboplastin time, activated partial thromboplastin time, thrombin sulfate test and fibrinogen determination are used to screen hemorrhagic disorders.

■ BLEEDING TIME

The duration of bleeding from a standard punctured wound of the skin is the bleeding time. It is the measure of function of platelet as well as integrity of the blood vessel wall.

Principle

A standard cut is made in the skin of patient and the length of time required to cease (to stop) the blood is noted. There are two methods for detecting the bleeding time:
1. Dukes method
2. Ivy's method

Dukes Method

It requires sterile needle, filter paper, stop watch, spirit/alcohol.

Procedure

Clean the ear lobe or fingertip with spirit by using a cotton swab. For ear lobe, a glass slide is placed behind the ear lobe to hold it firmly in place. This provides a firm site for incision. Puncture the ear lobe deeply, about 1 mm by using sterile lancet/needle. Start the stopwatch. The blood should flow freely without pressing the ear lobe. Now remove the glass slide from ear lobe after pricking. The blood is allowed to drop on filter paper. The paper should be moved so that each drop will fall on fresh area. The bleeding of wound should be allowed without pressing. When bleeding slows, the wound is touched gently with a fresh area of filter paper at 30 seconds interval. When blood stains disappear from the filter paper, stop the watch and note the time (**Fig. 31.1**).

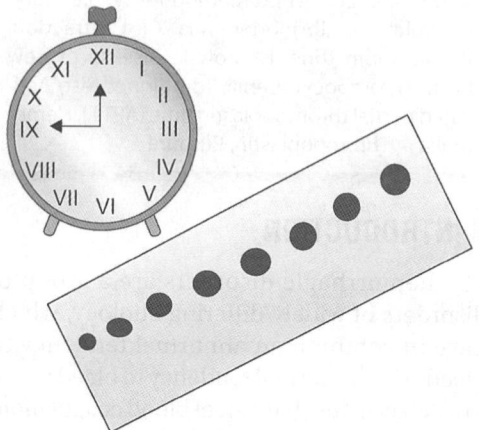

Fig. 31.1: Blood drops on filter paper.

Precautions

- In case of children heel should be used.
- In suspected cases of bleeding disorder, puncture the fingertip.
- The area to be punctured should not be congested.
- The size and depth of wound should be standard.
- If bleeding continues for more than 15 minutes, it should be stopped by placing dry sterilized cotton and applying little pressure on the wound.

Normal value: 1–5 minutes

Ivy's Method

Ivy's method requires sphygmomanometer cuff, which is applied on the patient's arm above the elbow. The puncture site is above the forearm. As soon as bleeding starts, touch the filter paper and start the stopwatch. When the blood drop on filter paper disappears, record the time.

Normal value: 5–11 minutes

Clinical Importance

Prolonged bleeding time (BT) is generally found in thrombocytopenia (platelets below 50,000) in case of Von Willebrand disease, the BT is high. It is also high in case of severe liver disease, leukemia, aplastic anemia, etc.

BT can also be calculated by:

$$BT = \frac{30.5 \times \text{Platelet count}/mm^3}{3{,}850}$$

■ WHOLE BLOOD COAGULATION TIME

The time required for blood to clot out of the blood vessel at 37°C, is known as clotting time. There are two different methods to determine clotting time:
1. Capillary/Wright method
2. Vein puncture/Lee-White method

Principle

Whole blood when removed from vascular system and exposed to foreign surface will form a solid clot. In Wright method, the blood is collected in capillary tube by finger puncture and in Lee-White method the blood is collected from vein in a test tube.

Capillary/Wright Method

By using spirit, disinfect the tip of finger of patient and make about 1 mm deep cut with sterile lancet. Start the stopwatch, wipe-off the first drop of blood, and collect blood in capillary tube up to 2/3rd of its length. After every 30 seconds break off about 1 cm of capillary to find out whether fibrin string/thread has formed. When fibrin string appears, stop the stopwatch and note the time.

The capillary method for clotting time can be advantageously combined with bleeding time test **(Fig. 31.2)**.

Vein Puncture/Lee-White Method

Collect about 2 mL of blood in a syringe and dispense into a clean test tube. Start the stopwatch as soon as the first drop of blood is observed. Plug the tube with cotton and keep them into the water bath at 37°C. After every 30 seconds by tilting the tube find out whether the blood is clotted. When the blood has clotted, stop the watch and note the time.

Blood collected in a test tube should be above 1 mL. As less blood gives shortened clotting time. The water bath temperature should be 37°C ± 0.5°C. The venous puncture should be without trauma.

Vigorous agitation of tube is avoided to prevent air bubble in the tube.

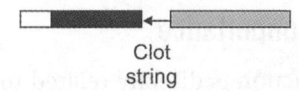
Clot string

Fig. 31.2: Wright method of clotting time.

Normal value (for both methods): 5–10 minutes.

Clinical Importance

Severe deficiencies of any of the coagulation factor indicate prolongation of clotting time.

Prolonged clotting time is noted in afibrinogenemia and hyperheparinemia.

Lee-White method is more reliable than Wright method. Therefore Wright method should be used only when venous blood cannot be obtained.

■ CLOT RETRACTION

A clot forms as the end product of blood coagulation. The clot under normal condition undergoes contraction, where serum is expressed from clot, and a clot becomes denser. This is called as clot retraction. Normal clot retraction starts within 30 seconds after the blood has clotted and is about 50% at the end of 1 hour.

Requirement

Clean dry plane glass graduated centrifuge tube, water bath at 37°C, equipment for collecting the blood, timer, etc.

Procedure

Take 5 mL blood by venous puncture, and transfer it to centrifuge tube. Incubate it at 37°C in vertical position. Record the degree of retraction after 1, 2 and 4 hours. If contraction is not apparent at the end of 1 hour loose the clot gently from the wall of the test tube. The degree and rate of retraction should be noted. Also note the discoloration of serum. Measure the amount of serum expressed by the clot.

Normal value: After 1 hour of blood collection, the clot should express 50% of serum.

Clinical Importance

Clot retraction is directly related to platelet count therefore, it is decreased in thrombocytopenia but normal in hemophilia.

It is requested in case of suspected hemorrhagic disorders.

Precaution should be taken at the time of removal of clot so that serum should not be hemolyzed. Generally, clot is removed by using a hooked long needle. If the clot is small and serum is more, then, patient may have low hematocrit. Patients with polycythemia also have poor clot retraction. Fragile clot represents low fibrinogen values.

■ PROTHROMBIN TIME

Prothrombin time (PT) is the time required for clotting of citrate or oxalate plasma in a glass tube, after the addition of calcium and tissue thromboplastin.

Principle

Stage 1 is crossed by the addition of tissue thromboplastin. The time it takes for plasma to clot after addition of thromboplastin and calcium is a measure of substances in the Stages 2 and 3.

Out of these factors, the most important is prothrombin. Prothrombin time should be performed soon after blood is collected and plasma is obtained, i.e., within half an hour of blood collection.

Procedure

Take 4.5 mL of patient's blood in a clean test tube with 0.5 mL of oxalate or citrate anticoagulant. Mix well and centrifuge at 2000 to 3000 rpm for 10 minutes to get plasma. In other test-tube take 0.1 mL of thromboplastin suspension and 0.15 mL calcium chloride ($CaCl_2$) suspension.

Mix the tube, keeps both the tube at 37°C in water both. After 1 minute contents of second tube are mixed with 0.1 mL of plasma from the first tube, as soon as the contents are added, start the stopwatch and observe for plasma clot. If clot is observed, stop the stopwatch and note the time. This is the prothrombin time.

Normal value: 14 ± 2 seconds.

Clinical Significance

The most common causes of prothrombin time prolongation are liver disorder, vitamin K deficiency, hemolytic disease of newborn (HDN), etc.

■ PLATELET COUNT

Determination of platelet count is requested in the investigation of bleeding disorders. There are two methods by which we can get total platelet count. These are:
1. Direct method
2. Indirect method

Direct Method

In this method, the blood is diluted with platelet diluting fluid and the cells are counted over a specified area under proper magnification.

Requirement

Microscope, improved Neubauer chamber, RBC pipette, platelet diluting fluid.

Composition

- Procaine hydrochloride: 3.0 g
- Sodium chloride: 10 g
- Distilled water: 100 mL

Blood Specimen

Ethylenediaminetetraacetic acid (EDTA) anticoagulated blood or capillary blood also can be used.

Procedure

Mix the blood specimen carefully by using RBC pipette. Draw blood up to 0.5 mark. Wipe off the excess blood from out side of pipette. The diluting fluid is drawn upto 101 mark. This gives the blood dilution 1:200. Mix the contents in the bulb thoroughly. After 5 to 7 minutes discard the first drop, and by using the second drop, charge the chamber. After charging keep the chamber undisturbed for 10 to 15 minutes. This will allow the settling down of cells. Count the cells in the central square of Neubers chamber, i.e., in all 25 squares.

Calculations

$$\text{No. of platelets/cu mm} = \frac{\text{No. of platelets counted} \times \text{Dilution}}{\text{Volume of fluid}}$$

Where,

$$\begin{aligned}
\text{Dilution} &= 200 \\
\text{Volume of fluid} &= \text{Area} \times \text{depth} \\
&= 1 \times 0.1 \\
&= 0.1 \text{ cu mm} \\
&= \frac{\text{No. of platelets} \times 200}{0.1}
\end{aligned}$$

$\therefore$ Platelets/cu mm = No. of platelets $\times$ 2000

Indirect Method

Regents: Dissolve 14 g of magnesium sulfate in distilled water and make up 100 mL.

Procedure

Clean the fingertip and place a drop of 14% aqueous solution of magnesium sulfate on the skin. Puncture through this drop with little pressure and allow the blood to flow into the sulfate solution. When the proportion is about 1 of blood to 5 of magnesium sulfate, mix thoroughly and make a thin smear. Clean the finger and make a RBC count. Stain the smear with Leishman's 'Blood Stain'. Cut a small square in a circular piece of paper and place it in the ocular of the microscope to reduce the size of the field. Count the number of RBCs and the platelets in the field. Count 1000 RBCs. The number of platelets counted to 1000 RBCs is multiplied by the number of thousands of RBCs as determined by RBC count.

Calculation

$$\text{Platelets/cu mm} = \text{No. of platelets} \times \frac{\text{RBC's}}{1000}$$

Normal value: 1.5 to 4 lakh/cu mm.

Clinical Significance

Increased platelet count is often associated with polycythemia vera, following splenectomy and in chronic myelogenous leukemia. This is called as thrombocytosis. Thrombocytopenia, i.e. decreased platelet count is often associated with prolonged bleeding and poor clot retraction, aplastic anemia, megaloblastic anemia, hypersplenism, acute leukemia and in immune thrombocytopenia.

TOURNIQUET TEST

A tourniquet test is also known as a Rumpel-Leede capillary-fragility test or simply a capillary fragility test. It is a clinical diagnostic method to determine a patient's hemorrhagic tendency. It assesses fragility of capillary walls and is used to identify thrombocytopenia.

Principle

A blood pressure cuff is inflated sufficiently to occlude venous return. It is kept in place for a set time. The impact on skin integrity or on capillary walls is subsequently assessed.

Procedure

To do the tourniquet test, a square with an area of 2.5×2.5 cm should be drawn on the forearm and then the following steps are done:
1. Assess the patient's systolic and diastolic blood pressure with the sphygmomanometer
2. Calculate mean value of it, e.g., if systolic blood pressure is 100 mmHg and diastolic is 70 mmHg, it means $(100 + 70) \div 2 = 85$ mmHg
3. Re-inflate the sphygmomanometer cuff to the mean value
4. Wait for 5 minutes with the cuff inflated at the same pressure
5. Deflate and remove the cuff after 5 minutes
6. Let the blood circulate for at least 2 minutes
7. Finally, the amount of red spots, called petechiae, should be evaluated inside the square on the skin to know the result of the test.

Clinical Significance

Capillary fragility tests were designed to detect abnormally weakened capillary walls in the skin that would burst more easily when distended, resulting in the appearance of high numbers of petechiae. The diseases associated with capillary fragility were legion, ranging from coagulopathies, thrombocytopenia (platelet count below 10,000), vitamin deficiencies (e.g., scurvy), infectious diseases (e.g., scarlet fever), and endocrine disorders (e.g., hyperthyroidism) to dermatologic disorders (e.g., Osler-Weber-Rendu syndrome).

ACTIVATED PARTIAL THROMBOPLASTIN TIME

Activated partial thromboplastin time (APTT) is used to measure the efficacy of both the intrinsic (the contact activation pathway) and the common coagulation pathways.

Surface activators like, Kaolin or Celite or Ellagic acids are used in APTT. It binds directly to Factor XII [FXII] resulting in surface activation to XIIa. XIIa cleaves (breaks) FXI to XIa. Hence the name activated. The term partial is due to the absence of tissue factor from the reaction mixture. The term 'thromboplastin' in this test refers to the formation of a complex formed from various plasma clotting factors which converts prothrombin to thrombin and the subsequent formation of the fibrin clot.

Specimen

Blood is collected using 3.2% sodium citrate anticoagulant. The proportions are one part sodium citrate (0.5 ml) to nine parts of blood. Plasma should be removed and test is run within 4 hours of blood collection. This is Platelet Poor Plasma (PPP).

Reagent

- *Kaolin reagent (2 g/dL in normal saline)*: It is used as surface activator which cleaves Factors XI to XIa.

- *Phospholipid substitute*: Platelet poor plasma is used in this test. The use of a commercial phospholipid substitute is used to replace platelet phospholipid, e.g. cephalin.
- *Calcium chloride (0.025 M)*: Calcium is removed (by chelation) when blood is collected into sodium citrate (anticoagulant). Therefore recalcification is necessary to allow coagulation to occur.
- Normal plasma to run control.

Principle

Platelet poor plasma is incubated at 37°C then phospholipid (cephalin) and a contact activator (e.g. kaolin, micronized silica or ellagic acid) are added. This leads to the conversion of Factor XI [FXI] to FXIa. At this step calcium is added and the timer is started. The addition of calcium (pre-warmed to 37°C) initiates clotting. The APTT is the time taken from the addition of calcium to the formation of a fibrin clot. Most laboratories use an automated method for the APTT. In this method, clot formation is deemed to have occurred when the optical density of the mixture has exceeded a certain threshold (clot formation makes the mixture more opaque and less light passes through).

Procedure

- Mix equal volumes of phospholipid reagent and kaolin reagent.
- Incubate at 37°C for one minute.
- Add 0.1 mL of plasma in test tube.
- Add 0.2 mL of phospholipid-kaolin mixture.
- Add 0.1 mL of pre-warmed calcium chloride reagent, mix content and start stopwatch.
- After 20 seconds, observe the formation of the clot by tilting the test tube. As soon as clot is formed, note time.
- Repeat the procedure by using normal control plasma.

Normal value: 25 to 40 seconds.

Clinical Significance

Normal PTT times require the presence of the following coagulation factors: I, II, V, VIII, IX, X, XI and XII. Deficiencies in factors VII or XIII will not be detected with the PTT test. Prolonged APTT may indicate—use of heparin-coagulation factor deficiency (e.g. hemophilia A, B)—antiphospholipid antibody especially lupus anticoagulant, which increases propensity to thrombosis.

To distinguish the causes, mixing tests are performed, in which the patient's plasma is mixed initially at a 50 : 50 dilution with normal plasma. If still it is taking more than 40 seconds to clot, the sample is said to contain an "inhibitor", either heparin, antiphospholipid antibodies or coagulation factor specific inhibitors. If it does correct, a factor deficiency is more likely. Deficiencies of factors VIII, IX, XI and XII and rarely von Willebrand factor, may lead to a prolonged APTT, that corrects on mixing studies.

Prolonged APTT is also found in case of vitamin K deficiency, massive blood transfusion leading to a dilutional coagulopathy or DIC (disseminated intravascular coagulation) due to the consumption of clotting factors. In rare cases where FVIII levels are found, APTT is short. The clot is formed within 20 seconds.

■ PURPURA

Purpura is a skin rash resulting from bleeding into skin from small blood vessels, i.e., capillaries. This results in individual purple spots of the rash called as petechiae. Purpura may be either due to defect in capillaries, called as non-thrombocytopenic purpura or due to a deficiency of blood platelets, i.e. thrombocytopenic purpura.

Acute iodopathic thrombocytopenic purpura is a disease of children in which antibodies are produced that destroy the patient's platelets. The child usually recovers without treatment. Schonlein-Henoch purpura is also seen in young children with unknown cause. It is associated with abdominal pain and kidney disturbance.

CHAPTER 32

Hemophilia and Polycythemia

Learning Objectives
- Hemophilia is a group of hereditary genetic disorders that impair the body's ability to control blood clotting or coagulation, which is used to stop bleeding when a blood vessel is broken. This chapter points out types of hemophilia, its inheritance, symptoms and diagnosis.
- Polycythemia is a condition in which there is a net increase in the total circulating erythrocyte (red blood cell). This chapter points out types of polycythemia, its symptoms and diagnosis.

Keywords
Hemophilia A, Hemophilia B, Hemophilia C, Partial Thromboplastin Time (PTT), Relative polycythemia, Absolute polycythemia, Erythropoietin, Myeloproliferative neoplasms, JAK2 (Janus Kinase 2) gene

■ HEMOPHILIA

Hemophilia is the most common hereditary blood coagulation disorder. It slows down the process of coagulation. This is because of deficiency of one of the clotting factor. This deficiency is mostly because of inherited defective gene. Sometimes, it may be because of sudden mutation in gene linked to the particular clotting factor.

In humans, females have two X chromosomes in their cells, while males have X and Y chromosomes in their cells. The gene for hemophilia is carried on the X chromosome. Hemophilia is inherited in an X-linked recessive manner. Females inherit two X chromosomes, one from their mother and one from their father (XX). Males inherit an X chromosome from their mother and a Y chromosome from their father (XY). That means if a son inherits an X chromosome carrying hemophilia from his mother, he will have hemophilia. Fathers cannot pass hemophilia on to their sons (XY—X from mother and Y from father), as they inherit only Y chromosomes to sons.

But because daughters have two X chromosomes, even if they inherit the hemophilia gene from their mother, and a healthy X chromosome from their father they do not have hemophilia. A daughter who inherits an X chromosome that contains the gene for hemophilia is called a carrier. She can pass the gene on to her children

Severity of Disease

Depending upon percentage of clotting factor present, the disease can be:
- *Severe*—factor levels less than 1%. Patient usually bleeds frequently, about once or twice a week, into their muscles or joints. Bleeding is often "spontaneous," i.e., happens suddenly, for no obvious reason.
- *Moderate*—factor levels of 1–5%. Patients' bleeds less frequently, about once a month, and rarely have spontaneous bleeding. They

may bleed for a long time after surgery, a bad injury or dental procedure.
- *Mild*—factor levels of 6–30%. Patient does not bleed often, but when they do, its a result of surgery or major injury.

Signs and Symptoms of Disease

Hemophilia symptoms include excessive bleeding and easy bruising. The bleeding can occur externally or internally. Any wound, cut, bite, or dental injury can lead to excessive external bleeding.

Spontaneous nosebleeds are common. Signs of excessive internal bleeding include blood in the urine or stools, and large, deep bruises. Bleeding can also happen within joints, like knees and elbows, causing them to become swollen, hot to the touch, and painful to move. Internal bleeding in the brain is very harmful. Symptoms of brain bleeding can include headaches, vomiting, lethargy, behavioral changes, clumsiness, vision problems, paralysis, and seizures.

Many women who carry the hemophilia gene also show some symptoms. This can result in heavy menstrual bleeding, easy bruising, and joint bleeds.

Method of Diagnosis

The majority of patients with hemophilia have a known family history of the condition. If there is no known family history of hemophilia, a series of blood tests can identify which factor of the blood clotting mechanism is defective.

A normal platelet count, normal PT (Prothrombin Time), and a prolonged Activated partial thromboplastin time (aPTT) are characteristic of hemophilia A and hemophilia B. Specific tests for the blood clotting factors can then be performed to measure factor VII or factor IX levels and confirm the diagnosis.

Genetic testing to identify and characterize the specific mutations responsible for hemophilia is also available in specialized laboratories.

Since men with the genetic mutation will have hemophilia, a man cannot be a carrier of the disease. A woman who has a son with known hemophilia is termed an obligate carrier, and no testing is needed to establish that she is a carrier of hemophilia.

Women whose carrier status is unknown can be evaluated either by testing for the clotting factors or by methods to characterize the mutation in the DNA. The DNA screening methods are generally the most reliable.

Prenatal diagnosis is also possible with DNA-based tests performed on a sample obtained through amniocentesis or chorionic villus sampling.

Types of Hemophilia

The main clotting factors involved in hemophilia are factors VIII, IX and XI.

Depending upon the type of clotting factor involved, there are three types of hemophilia:
1. *Hemophilia A*: This is also called as classic hemophilia. It is most common type of hemophilia, caused by deficiency of clotting factor VIII. Most of the time, this is a severe disease. This disease as manifested by bleeding into the large joints such as the knees or hips.
2. *Hemophilia B:* This is also known as Christmas disease. It is caused by a deficiency in clotting factor IX. It can be mild, moderate or severe. Inheritance of hemophilia B is same as that
   Hemophilia A and B are inherited by this X-chromosome as discussed earlier.
3. *Hemophilia C:* This is also known as Rosenthal syndrome. It is caused by a deficiency in clotting factor XI. It can be mild, moderate or severe.
   Hemophilia C is also primarily inherited, but it does not follow an X-linked pattern. This is because the mutation that causes it affects a gene found on chromosome 4— an autosomal or non-sex chromosome. Hemophilia C, therefore, affects both genders equally. For the disease to develop, a

defective copy of the gene must be inherited from each parent. Thus, each parent must either have the disease themselves or be carriers of the disease. The reduced level or activity of factor XI results in moderate bleeding symptoms, usually occurring after trauma or surgery. It is a mild form of hemophilia.

■ POLYCYTHEMIA

Polycythemia ('Poly' means many, 'cyte' means cell and 'hemia' is a condition having to do with blood) is also known as erythrocytosis. This condition is indicated by raised hemoglobin, packed-cell volume (PCV) and red cell count. The values are above those normal for age and sex. The polycythemic condition can be classified as:
1. Relative polycythemia
2. Absolute polycythemia.

Relative Polycythemia

It is caused by decrease in plasma (fluid part) of the blood. The number of red cells in the blood is not increased, but the number of cells per unit volume of blood is increased. This is observed in dehydration, due to stress. This type of polycythemia, is mostly found in hardworking hyperactive middle-aged males. The RBCs are normochromic, normocytic. Morphologically, white cells, red cells and platelets are normal. The hemoglobin, PCV and red cell count is elevated. Bone marrow is normal.

Absolute Polycythemia

Absolute polycythemia can be further categorized as:
i. Primary polycythemia
ii. Secondary polycythemia

Primary Polycythemia

It is one of several "myeloproliferative neoplasms" (MPNs), a term used to group a number of blood cancers that share several features, especially the clonal production of blood cells. All clonal diseases are types of cancer that begin with one or more changes to the DNA in a single cell. The abnormal cells that are in the bone marrow or in the blood are a result of that one mutant cell.

This is also known as polycythemia vera. It results from uncontrolled blood cell production, especially red cells, as a result of acquired mutations in an early blood-forming cell. Because this early cell has the capability to form not only red cells, but also white cells and platelets, any combination of these cell lines may be affected. Mutated gene for PV is *JAK2* (Janus Kinase 2) gene.

In this case, blood volume is increased, while there is no change in volume of plasma. Blood pressure is increased with elevated platelet count. RBCs are normocytic normochromic. Occasional nucleated red cells, immature granulocytes and anisocytic RBCs are seen. Increase in red cell count, hemoglobin, PCV is observed. Bone marrow activity is hypercellular.

Secondary Polycythemia

It is caused by an increased level of erythropoietin. Erythropoietin is a hormone produced in the kidneys that regulate red blood cell production. In polycythemia, the body produces too many RBCs due to an increase in erythropoietin. Its tendency of body to make erythropoietin when it detects there is not enough oxygen being delivered to the tissues. Secondary polycythemia is caused when there is not enough oxygen being delivered, or when there is a tumor that results in an increased output of erythropoietin.

Signs and Symptoms of Disease

The signs, symptoms and complications of PV occur because there are too many red cells, and often, too many platelets. Too many red blood cells can make the patient's blood more viscous (thick) so the blood does not flow efficiently. High platelet counts can contribute to the formation of clots (thrombi). Underlying vascular disease, common in older persons with PV, can increase the risk of clotting complications. The clots may cause serious problems, such as stroke, heart attack, deep vein thrombosis (DVT) or pulmonary embolism.

- Headaches, excessive sweating, ringing in the ears, visual disturbances, such as blurred vision or blind spots, and dizziness or vertigo (a more severe feeling of motion) may occur.
- Fatigue is common.
- Itchy skin, called "pruritus"
- A reddened or purplish appearance of the skin, especially on the palms, ear lobes, nose, and cheeks may occur.
- Some patients may experience a burning sensation in the feet.

Method of Diagnosis

CBC (Complete Blood Cell count) shows:
- High red cell count
- High hematocrit concentration
- An elevated white cell count, especially the neutrophil
- An elevated platelet count, which occurs in at least 50% of patients
- An elevated red cell mass
- A low erythropoietin (EPO) assay in the blood
- Patients may also have a bone marrow analysis as part of their testing
- Gene testing involves—to look for the presence of JAK2 mutation in blood cells.

CHAPTER 33

Anemia

Learning Objectives
- Anemia is the most common blood disorder. It is a condition in which body lack enough healthy red blood cells to carry adequate oxygen to body's tissues, resulting in fatigue and weakness.
- There are many forms of anemia, each with its own cause. Types of anemia depend upon morphology of red cells and upon the etiology of disorder are discussed in this chapter.
- Other pathological parameters associated with each type of anemia and Schilling test is mentioned here.

Keywords
Normochromic normocytic anemia, Hypochromic microcytic anemia, Normochromic macrocytic anemia, Normochromic microcytic anemia, Aplastic anemia, Iron deficiency anemia, Pernicious anemia, Hemolytic anemia, Sickle cell anemia, Sideroblastic anemia, Thalassemia, Schilling test, Vitamin B_{12}

Worldwide anemia is the most common red cell disorder. Anemia lead to a decreased amount of hemoglobin concentration, red cell count and PCV value. The anemia is present when Hb concentration falls below in the following:
- Newborn infants: 14 g/dL
- Child 6 months to 4 years: 11 g/dL
- Child 5 to 11 years: 11.5 g/dL
- Child 12 to 14 years: 12.0 g/dL
- Non-pregnant women: 12.0 g/dL
- Pregnant women: 11.0 g/dL
- Men/adult boys: 13.0 g/dL

In tropical and developing countries, anemia is seen in 50% or more of preschool children and in pregnant women, it is moderate or severe. The main causes of anemia includes malnutrition, protein deficiency, folate deficiency, parasitic, bacterial and viral infections, or it may be inherited.

■ CLASSIFICATION

Anemias may be classified in two ways:
1. Based upon morphology of red cell or
2. Upon the etiology, i.e. the cause of anemia.

Based upon Morphological Classification

It is based on mean corpuscular volume (MCV), mean corpuscular hemoglobin (MCH), mean corpuscular hemoglobin concentration (MCHC) and the red cell morphology on a blood smear.

Normochromic Normocytic Anemia

In this type of anemia, RBCs are normal in size and color, but reduced in number. The packed cell volume is reduced. MCH, MCV, and MCHC are normal. Normocytic normochromic anemia may be found in acute blood loss, anemia of chronic disease aplastic anemia.

Hypochromic Microcytic Anemia

The red cells are small and pale. Decrease in total RBC count, low Hb and PCV, reduced MCV, MCH and MCHC; hypochromic microcytic anemia is found in iron deficiency anemia and thalassemia.

Normochromic Macrocytic Anemia

The red cells are larger in size with no central pale portion. RBC are reduced in number with low Hb, elevated MCV and MCH and normal MCHC. Normochromic macrocytic anemia is found in pernicious anemia, anemia of folic acid and vitamin B_{12} deficiency and in some cases of aplastic anemia.

Normochromic Microcytic Anemia

The RBC are small in size with low Hb, reduced MCV, MCH and normal MCHC. This type of anemia is found in some of the anemias of chronic infections **(Fig. 33.1)**.

Etiological Classification

Based upon the cause of anemia, following types of anemia are found.

Aplastic Anemia

It may occur due to congenital defect, i.e., chromosomal abnormalities in RBC or exposure to various physical and chemical reagents like insecticides, streptomycin, ionizing radiation, etc. Usually, RBCs are normal. But, sometimes anisocytosis or poikilocytosis may be seen. Decreased WBC counts decreased platelets, bleeding time is increased, bone marrow is aplastic, rapid ESR, aplastic anemia may terminate as leukemia.

Iron Deficiency Anemia

The normal adult body contains 4000 mg of iron. About 60% of this iron is present in the circulating blood. The remaining is stored in the liver and reticuloendothelial cells of bone marrow. When iron is being utilized by the RBC at a faster rate and the dietary intake of iron is insufficient to keep up with the increased use, the iron stored in the body is used for the synthesis of hemoglobin. When the iron stores become exhausted, iron deficiency anemia results.

Microcytosis, hypochromia and poikilocytosis are associated with iron deficiency anemia. Reticulocyte count is normal, serum iron is decreased. It is commonly seen in early stages of life and during pregnancy.

Pernicious Anemia

This disease is caused by vitamin B_{12} deficiency. Intrinsic factor, which is necessary for the absorption of vitamin B_{12} is not secreted by the gastric mucosa. This type of anemia is generally found in patients above age of 60 years. It is associated with weakness and shortness of breath, abdominal pain, diarrhea, nausea, pale and sore tongue. The laboratory findings are macrocytic normochromic RBC, moderate to marked anisocytosis and poikilocytosis serum bilirubin may be increased.

Hemolytic Anemia

Hemolytic anemias are characterized by a fall in hemoglobin, jaundice, dark urine, increasing reticulocytosis. It may be hereditary or acquired. Red cells are usually normochromic and microcytic. Serum/plasma appears yellow due to increased bilirubin. Hemoglobin and

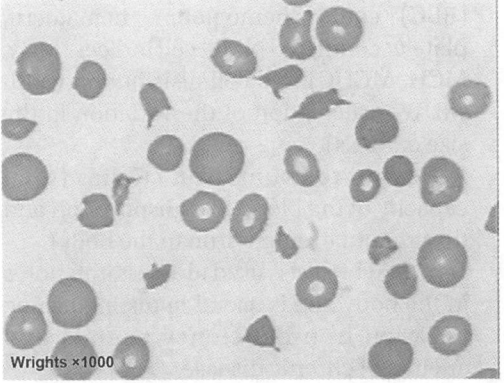

Fig. 33.1: RBCs in normochromic microcytic anemia.
(For color version See Color Plate 8)

hematocrit varies from normal to extremely low levels. Coomb's test is positive.

Sickle Cell Anemia

In this case, the red cells contain 90 to 100% hemoglobin S, and the remaining is Hb F. It is associated with severe abdominal bone and joint pain, enlarged spleen. Sickle cells are found in blood. Reticulocytes and platelets are increased. Osmotic fragility of RBC is decreased.

Sideroblastic Anemias

Sideroblastic anemias may be hereditary or acquired. In case of hereditary sideroblastic anemia, it may be present at birth or during infancy and usually manifests in adolescence. RBCs are hypochromic and microcytic. Increased serum iron level, moderate anisocytosis and poikilocytosis. In case of acquired sideroblastic anemia, normochromic RBCs but very few are hypochromic red cells. It is found in adults above 50 years of age.

■ THALASSEMIA (COOLEY'S ANEMIA)

It is a hereditary blood disease, widespread in Mediterranean countries, Asia and Africa, in which there is abnormality in the protein part of hemoglobin molecule. The affected red cells can not function normally, leading to anemia. Other symptoms include enlargement of the spleen and abnormalities of the bone marrow. Individuals inheriting the disease from both parents are severely affected. This is called as thalassemia major. Those inheriting from single parent are thalassemia minor. These are usually symptom free. Patient with major disease is treated with repeated blood transfusions. The disease can be detected by prenatal diagnosis including amniocentesis.

■ SCHILLING TEST

Schilling test is a test for diagnosing vitamin B_{12} deficiency. In this test, first give 1 mg unlabeled vitamin B_{12} parentally, to the patient. Then give 1 mg labeled vitamin B_{12} orally. It is labeled with ^{57}Co within 24 hours. One-third of absorbed labeled/radioactive vitamin B_{12} is flushed out in urine. Normal excretion is above 10% of oral dose. In anemic patients with vitamin B_{12} deficiency, patients excrete less that 5%. If the test is normal, no further testing is necessary.

If it is abnormal, repeat the said procedure with simultaneous oral administration of intrinsic factor, i.e. vitamin B_{12} binding protein. If excretion increases, it implies lack of intrinsic factor. If it does not, then there is some defect in absorption. The test should be repeated after 48 hours.

Signs and Symptoms of Anemia

Depending upon type and severity, signs and symptoms of anemia include fatigue, weakness, shortness of breath, dizziness, headache, cold hands and feet, pale skin, hair loss, chest pain, irregular heartbeats and difficulties with memory and concentration.

Diagnosis of Anemia

- Complete Blood Count (CBC) is often used as a broad screening test to evaluate overall health. It can be used to diagnose various conditions including anemia, infection, inflammation, bleeding disorder or leukemia. CBC includes the following:
  White blood cells count, Red blood cell (RBC) count, hemoglobin, hematocrit, platelet count, red blood cell indices (MCV, MCH, MCHC), red cell distribution width (RDW—calculation of the variation in the size of RBCs)
- Reticulocyte count, iron studies (total capacity of the blood to transport iron and the amount of stored iron in the body)
- *Ferritin:* This test is used to assess iron stores in the body and is useful in distinguishing between iron deficiency anemia and anemia of chronic disease.
- Vitamin B_{12} and folate
- Erythropoietin (EPO) level.

CHAPTER 34

Leukemia

Learning Objectives
- Leukemia is a cancer of the blood or bone marrow. Bone marrow produces blood cells. Leukemia can develop due to a problem with blood cell production. It usually affects the leukocytes.
- This chapter has brief discussion on different types of leukemia, its characteristics and other pathological conditions associated with it.
- Acute and chronic leukemias are compared here.

Keywords
Acute leukemia, Chronic leukemia, Myelocytic, Lymphoblastic, Metamyelocytes

Leukemia is malignant disorders of white blood cells. Bone marrow is always involved in this disease. The exact cause of leukemia is unknown, but hereditary or viral or exposure to radiation may be suggested. The major symptoms of leukemia include weight loss, fever and increased sweating. Liver, spleen and lymph nodes are enlarged. Basal metabolic rate is also increased.

■ CLASSIFICATION
(On the Basis of Course of Disease)
Based on the course of disease, leukemia is classified as acute and chronic.

Acute Leukemia

Acute leukemia is a sudden onset, generally occurs in children under 14 years of age. It is associated with normocytic, normochromic anemia, with decreased platelet count. Bleeding time is prolonged and white blood cell count may increase up to 1 lakh cells/cu mm. Immature and blast cells are present in peripheral blood smear. Acute leukemia is rapid progressive disease.

Chronic Leukemia

Chronic leukemia is slow progressive disease, anemia may occur at later stages. White cell count is markedly increased and may go up to 9 lakhs/cu mm. Blast cells are seen occasionally.

In between these two, subacute leukemia is also found in some cases. It is quite similar to acute leukemia. But the total leukocyte count may be normal, decreased or increased up to 50,000.

■ CLASSIFICATION
(On the Basis of Cell of Origin)
Leukemias are further classified on the basis of the cell of origin, i.e., whether myelocytic or lymphocytic as:
1. Acute myelocytic leukemia (AML)
2. Acute lymphocytic leukemia (ALL)

3. Chronic myelocytic leukemia (CML)
4. Chronic lymphocytic leukemia (CLL)

Acute Myelocytic Leukemia

Acute myelocytic leukemia (AML) occurs in all age groups, but more common in adults than in children. It is also called as acute granulocytic leukemia (AGL). It is characterized by the presence of large number of myeloblasts in the bone marrow and their appearance in the peripheral blood. Myeloblasts in the peripheral blood may vary from few to as much as 95%. Many variants of AMC have been described depending upon the type of cell predominating in the peripheral blood. These could be myeloblasts, promyelocytes, monoblasts or blasts of both myeloid and erythroid series. In AMC, there is often inflammation of the gums, skin involvement, rectal ulceration, face tumor is observed. It is generally associated with normochromic normocytic anemia. AML is rapidly fatal with most patients dying from hemorrhage or infection due to bone marrow failure.

Acute Lymphoblastic Leukemia

Acute lymphoblastic leukemia (ALL) is more common in children than in adults, that too in males than in females. It is less severe than AMC and in many cases it is cured by intensive and sustained treatment. ALL is the malignancy of the cells of lymphocytic series and it is characterized by the presence of increased number of lymphoblasts in bone marrow as well as in peripheral blood smear. Bone pain, fever, bleeding, purpura, thrombosis, lymphadenopathy and central nervous system involvement is common in ALL. To differentiate between the diagnosis of AML and ALL, several special cytochemical stains and immunological markers can be used **(Fig. 34.1)**.

Chronic Myelocytic Leukemia

Chronic myelocytic leukemia (CML) is also called as chronic granulocytic leukemia

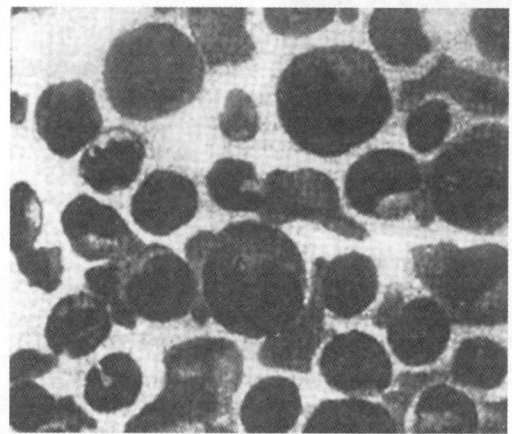

Fig. 34.1: Acute lymphoblastic leukemia.

(CGL). It is common in middle age group. It is characterized by the presence of marked increase in the cells of myelocytic series. The predominant cells are neutrophilic myelocytes and metamyelocytes. Total leukocyte count is generally higher than 50,000/µL to 2000,000/µL. Symptoms due to hypermetabolism are common in chronic myelocytic leukemia. Anemia is normocytic normochromic. Platelet count is usually increased. The abnormal Philadelphia (Ph) chromosome is present in the leukemic cells of more than 95% of patients with CML. CML may develop into AML at later stages.

Chronic Lymphoblastic Leukemia

Chronic lymphoblastic leukemia (CLL) is more often found in older persons (over 60 years) with men affected than women. It is characterized by marked increase of mature lymphocytes (above 15,000 cells/µL). The cell count may go very high and 80 to 90% of the cell look like immature lymphocytes. Prognostically, patients of CLL may live for many years without treatment. Onset of this disease is slow and in early stages asymptomatic. Most patients have weight loss, and develop lymphadenopathy. In later stages of CLL, neutropenia, thrombocytopenia and the loss of normal functioning lymphocytes lead to inadequate immune responses

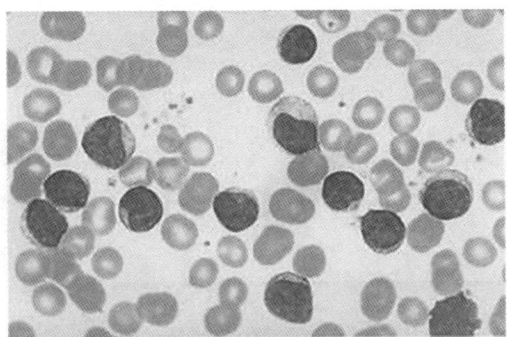

Fig. 34.2: Chronic lymphoblastic leukemia.
(For color version See Color Plate 8)

resulting in various infections. Anemia also develops in last stage **(Fig. 34.2)**.

Comparison of Acute and Chronic Leukemia

Acute	Chronic
Progress rapidly	Progress slowly
Severely ill	Can be asymptomatic
Heals without complication	Complication arises
Common in younger age groups	Common in older age groups
It is prominent	It is mild
Prognosis is predictable	Prognosis is unpredictable
Normal growth factor levels	Lower growth factor levels
Normal level of inflammatory cytokines	Increased level of proinflammatory cytokines
More than 30% blast cells in the bone marrow	Less than 30% blast cells in the bone marrow

Laboratory Diagnosis

There are a number of different tests that can be used to diagnose leukemia:
- Complete Blood Counts determine the numbers of RBCs, WBCs, and platelets. Tissue biopsies can be taken from the bone marrow or lymph nodes to look for evidence of leukemia.
- Flow cytometry examines the DNA of the cancer cells and determines their growth rate.
- *Cytochemistry*: In these types of tests, cells are put on a slide and stained with dyes that react only with some types of leukemia cells. These stains cause color changes that can be seen under a microscope.
- *Cytogenetics*: For this test, the cells are grown in lab dishes until they start dividing. Then the chromosomes are looked at under a microscope to detect any changes.
- *Fluorescent in situ hybridization (FISH)*: This is another way to look at chromosomes and genes. It uses special fluorescent dyes that only attach to specific genes or parts of particular chromosomes. FISH can be used on regular blood or bone marrow samples.
- *Polymerase chain reaction (PCR)*: This is a very sensitive DNA test that can also find certain gene and chromosome changes.

CHAPTER 35

Hemoparasites

Learning Objectives
- The parasites found in the bloodstream of infected people are called as hemoparasite. Four widely spread blood parasites are discussed in this chapter: i. *Plasmodium*, ii. *Leishmania*, iii. *Trypanosoma*, and iv. *Wuchereria bancrofti*.
- Diagrammatic representation of life cycle, pathogenesis and different methods of laboratory diagnosis are described here.
- All latest techniques of diagnosis, such as PCR, rapid diagnostic tests (RDTs), other supportive laboratory investigations are discussed here.

Keywords
Buffy coat, JSB stain, Rapid diagnostic tests (RDTs), PCR, Visceral leishmaniasis, Cutaneous leishmaniasis, Slit skin smear, Montenegro test, ELISA, Novy-MacNeal-Nicolle medium (NNN) medium, Fluorescent antibody test (IFAT), Polycarbonate membrane filtration, Hematoxylin stain, Intradermal test, Saponin method

A parasite is an organism that lives on or in a host organism and gets its food from or at the expense of its host. Most of the parasites are responsible for causing disease in host. The parasites found in the bloodstream of infected people are called as *hemoparasite*. These blood parasites are either protozoa or nematodes. All hemoparasite needed a carrier host, (vector) through which infection is transmitted to humans. Hemoparasites can be transmitted by transfusion of infected blood. Four widely spread blood parasites are discussed here:
1. *Plasmodium*—a protozoan causing malaria
2. *Leishmania*—a protozoan causing kala-azar
3. *Trypanosoma*—a protozoan causing sleeping sickness
4. *Filariasis*—caused by a nematode-*Wuchereria bancrofti*.

■ PLASMODIUM (MALARIA)

Plasmodium is a genus of unicellular eukaryotes that are obligate parasites of vertebrates and insects. The life cycles of *Plasmodium* species involve development in a blood-feeding insect host which then injects parasites into a vertebrate host during a blood meal. The genus *Plasmodium* consists of four species which can infect humans and cause malaria.

The life cycle of malarial parasite is completed in two hosts (**Fig. 35.1**):
1. *Man:* In man it reproduces asexually. Man is a secondary vertebrate host or an intermediate host.
2. *Female Anopheles mosquito:* In mosquito it reproduces sexually. Mosquito is a primary invertebrate host or definitive host.

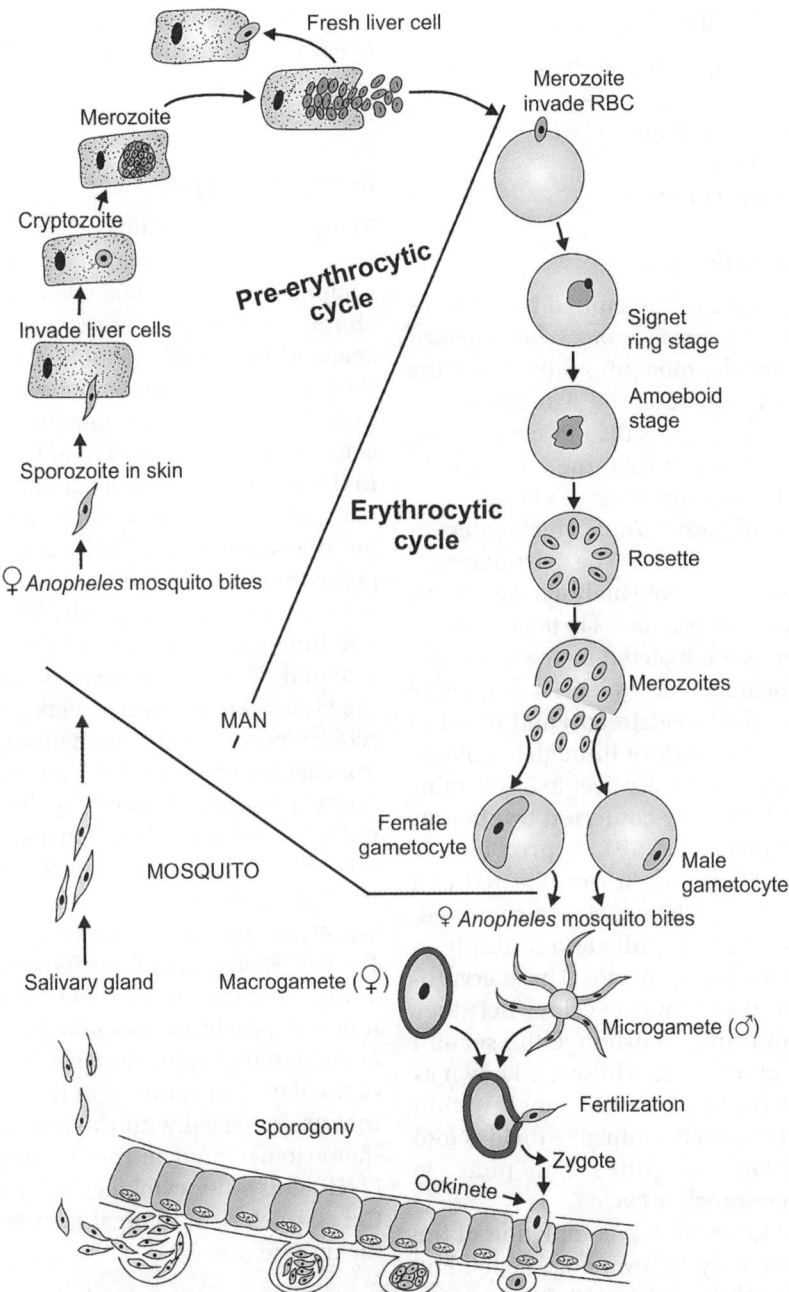

Fig. 35.1: Life cycle of *Plasmodium*.

Life Cycle in Man

In man, life cycle of *Plasmodium* consists of three stages:
1. Pre-erythrocytic cycle
2. Erythrocytic cycle
3. Post-erythrocytic cycle

Pre-erythrocytic Cycle

The *Plasmodium* is transmitted by the bites of female *Anopheles* mosquito. When infected female *Anopheles* mosquito bites a healthy person, first it punctures the skin and inserts an anticoagulant and saliva in man during feeding on blood. At this time, along with saliva, *Plasmodium* enters man's body.

The stage of *Plasmodium* which enters in human body is sporozoite. The sporozoites are long, slender with curved body narrow at both the ends. It contains nucleus in the middle.

Sporozoites are injected by the mosquito into the subcutaneous tissue (less frequently directly into the bloodstream) and travel to the liver either directly or through lymphatic channels. They reach the liver in 30–40 minutes by brisk motility conferred by circumsporozoite protein (CSP). Approximately 8–15 (up to 100) sporozoites are injected, and therefore, only a few hepatocytes are infected. In liver, they grow rapidly and multiply in number to form cryptozoite. These cryptozoites again attack new liver cells, where they grow and multiply to produce the second generation cryptozoite. These are known as merozoites (or metacryptozoites). Within the hepatocyte, each sporozoite divides into 10,000–30,000 merozoites. This phase is called pre-erythrocytic cycle.

The time taken for the completion of the pre-erythrocytic cycle is variable, depending on the infecting species (8–25 days for *P. falciparum*, 8–27 days for *P. vivax*, 9–17 days for *P. ovale*, and 15–30 days for *P. malariae*) and this interval is called as pre-patent period. During this period, man does not show any symptom of malaria fever.

Some of the merozoites again attack new liver cells while the others rupture the liver cell and escape into the blood to infect red blood cells.

Erythrocytic Cycle

The parasite enters in RBC as merozoite. In RBC, it becomes rounded and a contractile vacuole develops inside giving it a ring-like shape. The stage is known as signet ring stage. After this, the vacuole disappears and the parasite becomes amoeba-like in shape. This stage is known as amoeboid stage. This stage feeds on hemoglobin of RBC, increases in size and the nucleus divides into number of daughter nuclei. These nuclei arrange at the periphery of the RBC. Each daughter nucleus gets surrounded by the cytoplasm. This stage is known as rosette stage. The RBC now burst and liberates a number of micromerozoites in blood. These are known as schizonts and the cycle is known as schizogony. Along with schizonts a toxic substance hemozoin (derived from hemoglobin) is also released in the blood. These merozoites released by the lysis of the red blood cell immediately invade uninfected red cells. This repetitive cycle of invasion-multiplication-release-invasion continues. The erythrocytic cycle takes about 48 hours in *P. vivax*, *P. ovale* and *P. falciparum* infections and 72 hours in case of *P. malariae* infection. It occurs synchronously and the merozoites are released at approximately the same time of the day. The contents of the infected cell that are released with the lysis of the RBC (hemozoin) stimulate Tumor Necrosis Factor (TNF) and other cytokines, which results in the characteristic clinical manifestations of the disease.

Post-erythrocytic Cycle

After many erythrocytic cycles some of the micromerozoites changes then into unequal gametes called gametocytes. The larger gamete is female or macrogametocyte and smaller one is male or microgametocyte. This is known as post-erythrocytic cycle. The further development of gametocyte is stopped in man.

Life Cycle in Mosquito

Further development of gametocytes takes place sexually in mosquito. The female *Anopheles* mosquito sucks the blood of malarial patient containing gametocyte and other stages and gets infected. Of these only gametocyte remains active, while the other stages are digested.

In the stomach of mosquito, some changes in gametocytes take place. The nucleus of microgametocyte divides to form six to eight nuclei. These nuclei move towards the periphery and gather some cytoplasm. From each nucleus, flagella like projections arise and each nucleus gets separated. Now the flagellae gets detached from the microgametocyte to form male gamete. On the other side, macrogamete forms a small conical projection on its surface called as cone of fertilization through this area male gamete enters in female gamete and fertilize the egg.

The fertilized egg is called as zygote. It is rounded non-motile. After some time, it becomes active, motile and worm like structure called ookinate. It penetrates the stomach of mosquito and comes outside of stomach. Here, it forms a cyst around itself, called as oocyst. The numbers of oocysts are seen as small rounded structures on the surface of the stomach. The oocyst divides asexually into numerous sporozoites which reach the salivary gland of the mosquito. This phase is called as sporogony. On biting a man, these sporozoites are inoculated into human bloodstream along with saliva. Thus, the life cycle continues.

The sporogony in the mosquito takes about 10-20 days and thereafter the mosquito remains infective for 1-2 months **(Table 35.1)**.

Pathogenicity

Man develops infection by the bite of infected female *Anopheles* mosquito. However, the other modes are:
- Transfusion of blood from patient of malaria (transfusion malaria)
- Transmission to fetus *in utero* through some placental defect (congenital malaria)
- By contaminated syringes particularly in drug addicts.

The incubation period for *P. falciparum* is 12 days, for *P. vivax* and *P. ovale* is 13-17 days, and for *P. malariae* is 28-30 days.

As malarial parasite invades many organs, the pathogenicity can be explained according to the organ affected.

Blood Cells

Red blood cells: Red blood cells are the principal sites of infection in malaria. All the clinical manifestations are primarily due to the involvement of red blood cells.

The growing parasite consumes and degrades the intracellular proteins, mainly hemoglobin. It derives nutrition from the oxyhemoglobin of the red blood cells. The protein material of the erythrocyte is broken down and resynthesized into parasite protein. The waste product of this reaction is hematin, which is liberated in plasma when RBC ruptures. This causes the malarial symptoms to appear. This hematin pigment is filtered out from the blood by reticuloendothelial cells. Hence, the organs rich in reticuloendothelial cells become densely pigmented and assume a color varying from slate gray to black. The transport properties of the red cell membrane are altered, cryptic surface antigens are exposed and new parasite derived proteins are inserted. The red cell becomes more spherical and less deformable. In *P. falciparum* infection, membrane protuberances appear on the red cell surface in the second 24 hours of the asexual cycle. Accretions

Section 2: Hematology

TABLE 35.1: Differentiation of malarial parasites.

	P. falciparum	P. vivax	P. malariae	P. ovale
RBC size	Not enlarged	Enlarged	Not enlarged	Enlarged
RBC shape	Round, sometimes crenated	Round or oval, frequently bizarre	Round	Round or oval, often fimbriated
RBC color	Normal, but may become darker; may have a purple rim	Normal to pale	Normal	Normal
Stippling	Maurer's spots, appear as large red spots, loops and clefts up to 20 or fewer	Schuffner's dots, appear as small red dots, numerous	Ziemann's dots, few tiny dots, rarely detected	Schuffner's dots (James's dots) Numerous small red dots
Pigment	Black or dark brown; in asexual forms as one or two masses; in gametocytes as about 12 rods	Seen as a haze of fine golden brown granules scattered through the cytoplasm	Black or brown coarse granules; scattered	Intermediate between P. vivax and P. malariae
Ring forms (early trophozoites)	Smallest, delicate; sometimes two chromatin dots; multiple rings commonly found	Relatively large; one chromatin dot, sometimes two; often two rings in one cell	Compact; one chromatin dot; single	Compact; one chromatin dot; single
Mature schizonts	Medium size; compact; numerous chromatin masses; coarse pigments; rarely seen in peripheral blood	Large; amoeboid; numerous chromatin masses; fine pigments	Small; compact; few chromatin masses; coarse pigments	Medium size; compact; few chromatin masses; coarse pigments
Gametocyte Microgametocytes	Crescent-shaped, larger and slender; central chromatin	Spherical; compact	Similar to P. vivax, but smaller and less numerous	Like P. vivax, but smaller
Macrogametocytes				

of electron-dense, histidine-rich parasite proteins are found under these 'knobs'. These knobs extrude a strain specific, adhesive variant protein of high molecular weight that mediates red cell attachment to receptors on venular and capillary endothelium, causing cytoadherence. *P. falciparum* infected red cells also adhere to uninfected red cells to form rosettes. Cytoadherence and rosetting are central to the pathogenesis of *P. falciparum* malaria, resulting in the formation of red cell aggregates and intravascular sequestration of red cells in the vital organs like the brain and the heart. This further interferes with the microcirculation and metabolism. Mature forms of *P. falciparum* are rarely seen in the peripheral blood and when found, indicate severe infection. Sequestration does not occur in cases of *P. vivax* and *P. malariae* infections and therefore, all stages of the parasite can be seen in the peripheral blood and complications are very rare.

Anemia is a fairly common problem encountered in malaria and it poses special problems in pregnancy and in children. It can be due to multiple causes. Repeated hemolysis of infected red cells, immune and non-immune hemolysis of non-infected red cells, increased splenic clearance of parasitized as well as non-parasitized red cells, reduction of red cell survival even after disappearance of parasitemia, dyserythropoeisis in the bone marrow, drug induced hemolysis, etc. Anemia depends on the degree of parasitemia, duration of the acute illness and the number of febrile paroxysms. *P. vivax* predominantly invades young red cells and the number of parasites infected rarely exceeds two percent. *P. malariae* develops mostly in mature red cells and the parasitemia is rarely greater than one percent. *P. falciparum* affects red cells of all ages and the parasitemia can be as high as 20 to 30 percent or more.

Anemia of malaria is usually normocytic hypochromic with increase in the number of reticulocytes and polychromatophils. Anemia may be associated with hyperbilirubinemia of the indirect type due to the hemolytic process. Splenomegaly may also be seen.

Leukocyte count is usually low to normal in most cases of malaria. Increased leukocyte count indicates either a severe infection or secondary bacterial infection. Thrombocytopenia is also fairly common in malaria. Erythrocyte Sedimentation Rate (ESR) is usually elevated in malaria up to 30–50 mm in one hour.

Blackwater Fever

In malignant malaria, a large number of the red blood corpuscles are destroyed. Hemoglobin from the blood corpuscles is excreted in the urine, which therefore is dark and almost the color of cola. This is known as blackwater fever.

Clinical Diagnosis and Symptoms

The incubation period for malaria is the time between the mosquito bite and the release of parasites from the liver. This varies, depending on which malaria parasite is causing the disease. In general, it can range from 10 days to a month. The actual attacks of malaria develop when the red blood corpuscles burst, releasing a mass of parasites into the blood. The attacks do not begin until a sufficient number of blood corpuscles have been infected with parasites.

Early symptoms of malaria may be irritable and drowsiness, with poor appetite and trouble sleeping. These symptoms are usually followed by chills, then a fever with rapid breathing. The fever may either gradually increase over 1 to 2 days or may rise very suddenly to 105°F (40.6°C) or above. Then, as fever ends and body temperature quickly returns to normal, the patient has an intense episode of sweating. The same pattern of symptoms—chills, fever, sweating—may repeat at intervals of 2 or 3 days, depending on which particular species of malaria parasite is causing the infection.

Laboratory Diagnosis

Laboratory diagnosis of malarial parasite is performed in following ways:
- Peripheral smear examination.
- Quantitative Buffy Coat (QBC) Test.
- Rapid diagnostic tests (RDTs).
- Other tests for malarial parasite.

Peripheral Smear Examination

For malarial parasite, it is the gold-standard in confirming the diagnosis of malaria. Thick and thin smears prepared from the peripheral blood are used for the purpose.

Preparation of Smear

Thick Smear

The thick smear of correct thickness is the one through which newsprint is barely visible. It is dried for 30 minutes and not fixed with methanol. This allows the red blood cells to be hemolyzed and leukocytes and any malaria parasites present will be the only detectable elements. However, due to the hemolysis and slow drying, the plasmodium morphology can get distorted, making differentiation of species difficult. Thick smears are therefore used to detect infection, and to estimate parasite concentration.

Thin Smear

Air dry the thin smear for 10 minutes. After drying, the thin smear should be fixed in methanol. This can be done by either dipping the thin smear into methanol for 5 seconds or by dabbing the thin smear with a methanol-soaked cotton ball. While fixing the thin smear, all care should be taken to avoid exposure of the thick smear to methanol.

Staining

A number of Romanowsky stains like Field's, Giemsa's, Wright's and Leishman's are suitable for staining the smears. Thick films are ideally stained by the rapid Field's technique or Giemsa's stain for screening of parasites. The sensitivity of a thick blood film is 20 parasites/µl (0.0004%) parasitemia. Thin blood films stained by Giemsa's or Leishman's stain are useful for specification of parasites and for the stippling of infected red cells and have a sensitivity of 200 parasites/µl (0.004%).

Thick Films

The thick film is first dehemoglobinized in water and then stained with Giemsa.

Rapid Giemsa: Prepare a 10 percent Giemsa in buffered water at pH 7.1. Immerse the slide in the stain for 5 minutes. Rinse gently for 1 or 2 seconds in a jar of tap water. Drain, dry and examine.

Standard Giemsa: Prepare a 4 percent Giemsa in buffered solution at pH 7.1. Immerse the slide (at least 12 hours old) in stain for 30 minutes. Rinse with fresh water, drain, dry and examine.

Thin Films

Thin film examination is the gold standard in diagnosis of malarial infection.

Giemsa stain: Fix with 1-2 drops of methanol. Cover the film with 10 percent Giemsa stain and leave for 30 minutes, wash with distilled water, drain, dry and examine.

Leishman's stain: Add 7-8 drops of the stain and leave for 1-2 minutes. Then add 12-15 drops of buffered distilled water, mix thoroughly, leave for 4-8 minutes. Then wash off with clean water, drain, dry and examine.

Jaswant Singh Battacharya (JSB) stain for thick and thin films: This is the standard method used by the laboratories under the National Malaria Eradication Programme in India.

Observation of Blood Films

Thick Blood Film

Infected erythrocytes are counted in relation to a predetermined number of WBCs and an average of 8000/μl is taken as standard. 200 leukocytes are counted in 100 fields (0.25 μl of blood). All parasite species and forms including both sexual and asexual forms are counted together.

If >10 parasites are counted, then the following formulae can be applied:

No. of Parasites/No. of WBCs counted × 8000 = No. of parasites/μl Or if 200 leukocytes are counted.

No. of parasites counted × 40 = No. of parasites/μl. If the parasites are <9, then 500 WBCs should be counted and the formula will be—No. of parasites counted × 16 = No. of parasites/μl.

Thin Blood Film

Determining the percentage of parasitemia will be essential for *P. falciparum*. The number of infected red cells (and not number of parasites) in 1000 RBCs is converted to percentage.

This method estimates the percentage of red blood cells infected with malarial parasites. The smear is scanned carefully, one 'row' at a time. The total number of red cells and the number of parasitized red cells are tabulated separately. If 1,000 red cells are counted, then divide the number of parasitized red cells by 10 to get the percentage (i.e. if 30 out of 1000 cells are parasitized, then the parasitized red cell count is 3%). If lesser red cells are counted, then divide the number parasitized by the total number counted and multiply the result by 100 to obtain a percentage estimate of parasitized red blood cells. If occasional parasites are seen when scanning the smear, but none are identified during the process of counting 300 to 500 red blood cells, a percentage value of less than 1 percent of red blood cells parasitized is assigned. The values of 2 to 3 percent or above that are of clinical concern.

Results in "plus system" are given as:
+   = 1–10 per 100 thick fields
++   = 11–100 per 100 thick fields
+++   = 1–10 per thick field
++++   = >10 per thick field

Advantages of Microscopy

The microscopic method is sensitive. It can detect 5 to 10 parasites per μl of blood if used by skilled technicians. It is informative as the circulating species and stage of the parasite can be seen. It is relatively inexpensive and provides permanent record of the diagnostic findings.

Disadvantages of Microscopy

It is laborious and time-taking. It absolutely depends upon trained technicians, quality staining and microscope.

Quantitative Buffy Coat (QBC) Test

The QBC Test, developed by Becton and Dickenson Inc., is a new method for identifying the malarial parasite in the peripheral blood. It involves staining of the centrifuged and compressed red cell layer with acridine orange and its examination under UV light source. It is fast, easy and claimed to be more sensitive than the traditional thick smear examination.

Method

The QBC tube (**Fig. 35.2**) is a high-precision glass hematocrit tube, pre-coated internally with acridine orange stain and potassium oxalate. It is filled with 55 to 65 microliters of blood from a finger, ear or heel puncture. A clear plastic closure is then attached. A precisely made cylindrical float, designed

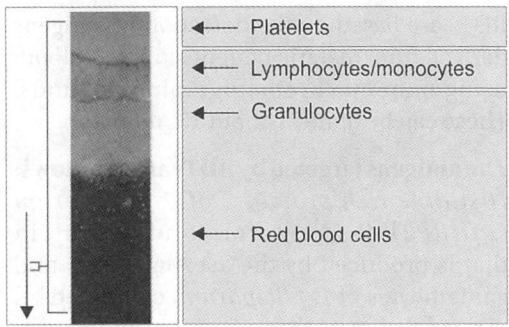

Fig. 35.2: The QBC tube.

to be suspended in the packed red blood cells, is inserted. The tube is centrifuged at 12,000 rpm for 5 minutes. The components of the buffy coat separate according to their densities, forming discrete bands. Because the float occupies 90 percent of the internal lumen of the tube, the leukocyte and the thrombocyte cell band widths and the topmost area of red cells are enlarged to 10 times normal. The QBC tube is placed on the tube holder and examined using a standard white light microscope equipped with the UV microscope adapter, an epi-illuminated microscope objective. Fluorescing parasites are then observed at the red blood cell/white blood cell interface.

The key feature of the method is centrifugation and thereby concentration of the red blood cells in a predictable area of the QBC tube, making detection easy and fast. Red cells containing plasmodium are less dense than normal ones and concentrate just below the leukocytes, at the top of the erythrocyte column. The float forces all the surrounding red cells into the 40 micron space between its outside circumference and the inside of the tube. Since the parasites contain DNA which takes up the acridine orange stain, they appear as bright specks of light among the non-fluorescing red cells. Virtually, all of the parasites found in the 60 microliter of blood can be visualized by rotating the tube under the microscope **(Table 35.2)**.

Rapid Diagnostic Tests (RDTs)

RDTs are based on the detection of antigens derived from malaria patients in lysed blood, using immunochromatographic methods. These can be done in about 15 minutes.

The antigens targeted by RDTs are as follows:

Histidine-rich protein 2 of P. falciparum (PfHRP2): It is a water-soluble protein that is produced by the asexual stages and gametocytes of *P. falciparum*, expressed on the red cell membrane surface, and shown

TABLE 35.2: Comparison between peripheral smear and QBC test for detecting malaria.

Criteria	Peripheral smear	Quantitative Buffy Coat
Method	Cumbersome	Easy
Time	Longer, 60–120 minutes	Faster, 15–30 minutes
Sensitivity	5 parasites/µL in thick film and 200/µL in thin film	Claimed to be more sensitive, at least as good as a thick film
Specificity	Gold standard	False positives, artifacts may be reported as positive by not-so-well-trained technicians
Species identification	Accurate, gold standard	Difficult to impossible
Cost	Inexpensive	Costly equipment and consumables
Acceptability	100%	Not so
Availability	Everywhere	Limited
Other	—	Accidentally can detect filarial worms

to remain in the blood for at least 28 days after the initiation of antimalarial therapy. Several RDTs targeting PfHRP2 have been developed.

Plasmodium aldolase: It is an enzyme of the parasite glycolytic pathway expressed by the blood stages of *P. falciparum* as well as the non-falciparum malaria parasites.

Parasite lactate dehydrogenase (pLDH): It is a soluble glycolytic enzyme produced by the asexual and sexual stages of the live parasites and it is present in and released from the parasite infected erythrocytes.

The Rapid Malaria Tests

The RDTs have been developed in different test formats like the dipstick, strip, card, pad, well, or cassette; and the latter has provided a more satisfactory device for safety and manipulation. The test procedure varies between the test kits.

In general, the blood specimen (2 to 50 µL) is a finger-prick blood specimen, anticoagulated blood, or plasma, and it is mixed with a buffer solution that contains a hemolyzing compound and a specific antibody that is labeled with a visually detectable marker such as colloidal gold. In some kits, labeled antibody is pre-deposited during manufacture and only a lysing/washing buffer is added. If the target antigen is present in the blood, a labeled antigen/antibody complex is formed and it migrates up the test strip to be captured by the pre-deposited capture antibodies specific against the antigens and against the labeled antibody (as a procedural control). A washing buffer is then added to remove the hemoglobin and permit visualization of any colored lines formed by the immobilized antigen-antibody complexes. The pLDH test is formatted to detect a parasitemia of >100 to 200 parasites/µL and some of the PfHRP2 tests are said to detect asexual parasitemia of >40 parasites/µL.

The PfHRP2 test strips have two lines, one for the control and the other for the PfHRP2 antigen. The PfHRP2/PMA test strips and the pLDH test strips have three lines, one for control, and the other two for *P. falciparum* (PfHRP2 or pLDH specific for *P. falciparum*) and non-falciparum antigens (PMA or pan specific pLDH), respectively **(Fig. 35.3)**.

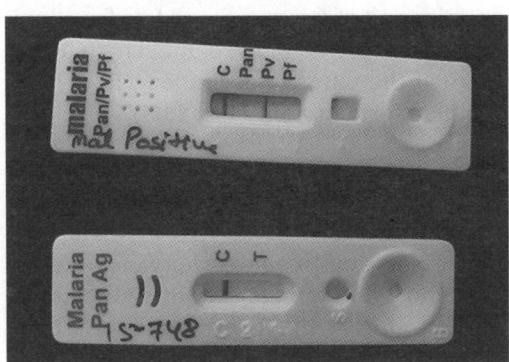

Fig. 35.3: Rapid malaria test.
(Malaria Pan Ag—control; Pv: *Plasmodium vivax*;
Pf: *Plasmodium falciparum*)

Advantages of RDTs

These are easy to perform and interpret. It does not require skilled technician, laboratory equipments and electricity. The RDTs may detect infection even when the parasites are sequestered in deep vascular compartment which are undetectable by microscopic examination of peripheral blood smear.

Disadvantages of RDTs

These are more expensive than microscopy. It cannot differentiate between the species of malaria. It may give false positive result. The RDT may not be able to detect some infections with lower numbers of malaria parasites circulating in the patient's bloodstream. Therefore, all negative RDT's must be followed by microscopy to confirm the result.

Other Tests for Malarial Parasite

Polymerase Chain Reaction (PCR)

Using the non-isotopically labeled probe following PCR amplification, it is possible to detect malaria parasites. PCR have been found to be highly sensitive and specific for detecting all 4 species of malaria, particularly in cases of low level parasitemia and mixed infections.

Detection of Antimalarial Antibodies

Antibodies to the asexual blood stages appear a few days after malarial infection. Malarial antibodies can be detected by immunofluorescence or enzyme immunoassay.

Intraleukocytic Malaria Pigment

Intraleukocytic malaria pigment has been suggested as a measure of disease severity in malaria. The pigment-containing neutrophil count is a simple marker of disease severity in childhood malaria in addition to the parasite count.

Other Investigations

- Moderate elevation in blood urea and creatinine are common. Significant increase is suggestive of renal impairment.
- Hyperbilirubinemia is common in malaria, particularly due to hemolysis.
- Serum albumin levels may be reduced, sometimes markedly.
- Serum aminotransferases, 5'-nucleotidase and lactic dehydrogenase are elevated.
- Prothrombin time and partial thromboplastin time are elevated in 20 percent of patients with cerebral malaria. Some may have features of disseminated intravascular coagulation.
- Urine examination may show albuminuria, microscopic hematuria, hemoglobinuria and red cell casts. With massive intravascular hemolysis, urine may be black in color.

LEISHMANIA (KALA-AZAR)

Habitat

It is an obligate intracellular parasite of reticuloendothelial cells, predominantly of liver, spleen, bone marrow and lymph nodes of man.

Morphology

The parasite exists in two stages:
1. Amastigote stage—occurs in man.
2. Promastigote stage—occurs in gut of sandfly.

Amastigote Stage

In amastigote form the parasites resides in the cells of reticuloendothelial system (macrophages, monocytes, neutrophils, or endothelial cells) of vertebrate hosts. It has non-motile, round or oval body measuring 2–4 µm in length. Cell membrane is delicate and can be demonstrated in fresh specimens only. Nucleus is round or oval situated in the middle of the cell or along the side of the cell wall.

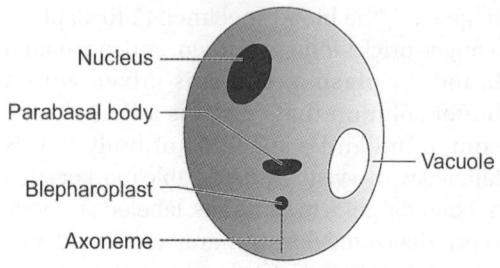

Fig. 35.4: Amastigote.

Kinetoplast consists of parabasal body and blepharoplast which are connected by delicate fibrils. It lies right angle to the nucleus. The axoneme arises from the blepharoplast and extends to the margin of the body. It represents the intracellular portion of the flagellum. Alongside the axoneme lies a clear unstained space known as vacuole **(Fig. 35.4)**.

Promastigote Stage

Promastigotes are found in the digestive tract of insect vector (sandfly) and in the culture media. These are elongated, motile, extracellular stage of the parasite. Fully developed promastigotes measure 15–25 µm in breadth. Nucleus is situated centrally. Kinetoplast lies transversely near the anterior end. In front of the kinetoplast lies a pale staining vacuole. From the blepharoplast arises the axoneme which projects from the anterior end of the parasite as free flagellum. Flagellum may be of the same length as the body of the parasite or longer. There is no undulating membrane **(Fig. 35.5)**.

Life Cycle

L. donovani passes its life cycle in two hosts—man (also dog in some areas) as a vertebrate host and female sandfly of the genus *Phlebotomus* as the invertebrate host. Only about 30 of over 500 species of Phlebotomine sandflies are known to transmit *Leishmania* parasites. These include *P. argentipes* (Indian sub-continent), *P. martini* and *P. orientalis* (in

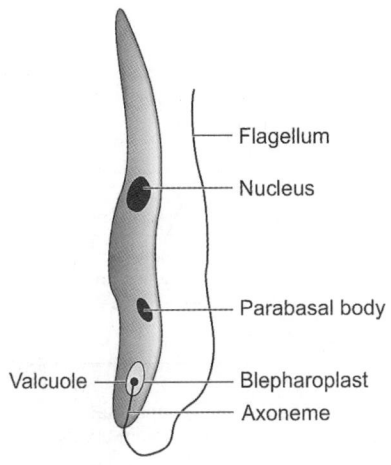

Fig. 35.5: Promastigote.

Africa and Mediterranean Basin), *P. chinensis* and *P. alexandri* (in China).

Infection to man occurs when the infected sandfly bites. The proboscis of sandfly pierces the skin of victim and transfers the promastigotes in the skin along with its saliva. These are engulfed by nearby macrophages and change into amastigotes within the cytoplasm of host cells. Here amastigotes multiply slowly and may remain more or less quiescent for weeks or months. Then the parasitized macrophages are set free into the bloodstream and are carried from the skin to spleen, liver, bone marrow and other centers of reticuloendothelial activity. The amastigotes are now taken up by fixed macrophages such as Kupffer's cells in the liver and multiply by simple binary fission. In the cells of the reticuloendothelial system, the multiplication goes on continuously till the cell becomes packed with the parasites. The host cell is thereby enlarged and eventually ruptures from 50 to 200 or even more amastigotes are found embedded in the cytoplasm of the enlarged host cell. The parasites liberated as a result of rupture into the circulation are again taken up by or invade fresh cells and the cycle is repeated. In this way, the entire reticuloendothelial system becomes progressively infected. In the bloodstream, some of free amastigotes are phagocytosed by the neutrophilic granulocytes and monocytes.

The sandfly vector becomes infected when feeding on the blood of an infected individual or animal reservoir host. The sandflies usually feed up at night when host is asleep. The macrophages are ingested by the fly during the blood meal and the amastigotes are released into the stomach of insect. Almost immediately amastigotes transform into the flagellate promastigote form. The promastigotes then migrate to mid gut of the fly, where they live extracellularly and multiply by binary fission producing enormous number of flagellates. Four to five days after feeding, the promastigotes move forward to the esophagus and salivary glands of the insect. A heavy pharyngeal infection of the sandfly is observed between the 6th and 9th day of infection. At this time, it transfers the promastigotes through the salivary gland, and the cycle is repeated **(Fig. 35.6)**.

The uncommon modes of transmission are through congenital transmission, blood transfusion, and rarely through inoculation of cultures.

Pathogenicity

L. donovani causes visceral leishmaniasis or kala-azar. Incubation period generally varies from 3 to 6 months. The most important immunological feature is a marked suppression of the cell-mediated immunity to leishmanial antigens. In persons with asymptomatic self-resolving infection, T-helper cells predominate, although immune suppression years later can result in disease. An overproduction of both specific immunoglobulins and nonspecific immunoglobulins also occurs. The increase in gamma globulin leads to a reversal of the albumin-globulin ratio commonly seen in this disease. The parasites spread from site of inoculation and multiply in reticuloendothelial cells, especially in the spleen, liver, lymph nodes and bone marrow. The spleen and liver

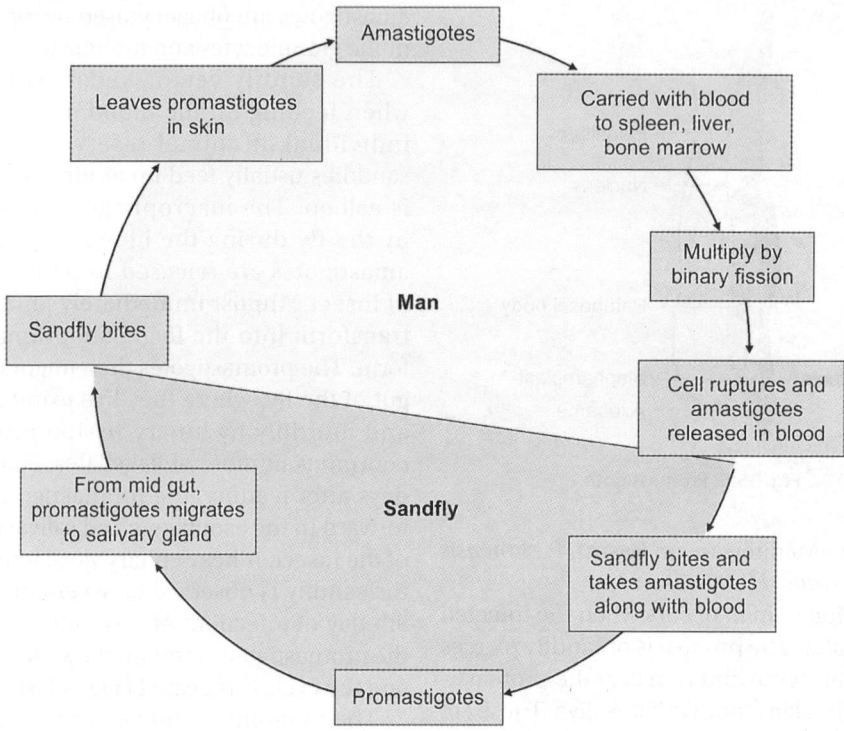

Fig. 35.6: Life cycle of *L. donovani*.

become markedly enlarged and hypersplenism contributes to the anemia. The vascular spaces of spleen are dilated and engorged with blood. In the liver, the Kupffer cells are increased in size and number and infected with amastigote forms of *Leishmania*. Bone marrow turns hyperplastic and parasitized macrophages replace the normal hemopoietic tissue. Lymphoadenopathy is also produced. Human leishmanial infections can result in two main forms of disease, cutaneous leishmaniasis and visceral leishmaniasis (kala-azar). The factors determining the form of disease include *Leishmania* species, geographic location, and immune response of the host.

Clinical Diagnosis and Symptoms

Visceral Leshmaniasis (VL)

The onset of VL is usually insidious with fever, sweating, weakness and weight loss. The most prominent findings are fever, hepatosplenomegaly and anemia. Anemia is normochromic normocytic. The sites mainly affected are the liver, spleen and bone marrow. Enlargement of the liver is due to hyperplasia of Kupffer cells which are packed with amastigotes. The bone marrow is infiltrated with parasitized macrophages. Some organs, notably the kidneys, may show pathological changes secondary to deposition of immune complexes. In advanced cases, ascites and edema can develop. Leucopenia is observed and may contribute to secondary infections. If untreated, deaths are usually due to secondary bacterial infections such as pneumonia, tuberculosis, septicemia or dysentery.

Some people develop post-kala-azar dermal leishmaniasis (PKDL or dermal leishmanoid). It is relatively common consequence of therapeutic cure from visceral leishmaniasis.

It is caused by the reversal of *L. donovani* from viscerotropic to dermatotropic. It generally develops 1-2 years after completion of antimonial treatment for the original disease, when the visceral infection disappears but the skin infection persists. It has occasionally been reported in spontaneously cured patients and in patients with no history of visceral disease. This is probably a sequel to subclinical infection. PKDL has been reported in 10 to 20% of cured cases in India. Patient develops hypopigmented macules anywhere on the body, specially the upper trunk, arms, thighs, forearms, legs, abdomen and neck in that order and erythematous patches (often having butterfly distribution) on nose, cheeks and chin. Later yellowish pink nodules appear mostly on the face. The lesions are soft, painless, granulomatous of varying sizes and unless traumatized, do not ulcerate. If they are more in number, it looks like lepromatous leprosy.

Cutaneous Leishmaniasis

It is characterized by one or more cutaneous lesions on areas where sandflies have fed. Following a bite from an infected sandfly, a small red papule appears at the site of the bite about 2-8 weeks later. The papule increases in size centrifugally. It can be painless or painful. The patient then mounts either a hypersensitive response or an anergic response. In a hypersensitive response, the papule eventually ulcerates, becomes depressed and then eventually heals through scarring. The patient is now immune from subsequent bites. In an allergic response, the nodule grows and spreads over large areas of skin. This resembles leprosy. The skin is dry, thin, and scaly, and hair is lost. As the disease progresses, the skin on the hands, feet, abdomen and face may become darkened, giving the name kala-azar or black fever.

Laboratory Diagnosis

I) Visceral Leishmaniasis

Direct evidence

The parasite can be demonstrated through direct evidence from peripheral blood, bone marrow, or splenic aspirates. The smears are stained in Leishman, Giemsa, or Wright stains and examined under oil immersion microscope. Amastigote forms are seen in plain film, and the promastigote forms in culture.

Fluorescent dyes that stain nucleic acids have been used in the detection of blood parasites. In the *Kawamoto* technique, blood smears on a slide are stained with acridine orange and examined with either a fluorescence microscope or a light microscope.

Staining clinical specimen with acridine orange at low pH (acridine orange acid stain):
- Prepare a smear in a clean grease free slide and allow it to air dry.
- The slide is then fixed with methanol and dried again.
- It is then put in trough with acridine orange staining working solution (i.e 0.01%).
- After 2 minutes of staining, the slides are washed gently with water and dried and then examined in a fluorescent microscope. *Observance*: Leshmania stain orange against a green to yellow background of human cells and debris.

Peripheral blood smear: In the peripheral blood smear, the amastigotes are seen inside the circulating monocytes and neutrophils. However, in view of the small numbers, they often are difficult to locate. The chances of finding *L. donovani* are greatly enhanced by adopting the following methods: (1) thick film, by producing a single straight leukocyte edge when making a peripheral smear, or (2) by centrifuging citrated blood, to get buffy coat which then is smeared, dried, and stained.

Staining of buffy coat smears: Buffy coat films are stained by Leishman stain. An air-dried thin film was made and placed on a staining rack and flooded with Leishman stain. The slide was left for 2 minutes to fix. Two times amount distilled water was added over the flooded stain from a plastic wash bottle for better mixing of the solution. The stain was left for 10 minutes. The stain was washed with running tap water and air-dried again the smear to examine under oil immersion objective.

As a minimum of 1000 fields per slide were examined under oil immersion lens to detect amastigote form of *Leishmania donovani*. Amastigotes appear as round or oval bodies measuring 1-5 µm in length and are found in inside or outside the monocytes and macrophages. In preparations stained by Leishman stain, the cytoplasm appears pale blue, with a relatively large nucleus that stains red.

Culture: Culturing is time consuming and takes about a month. Cultures are made on Novy-MacNeal-Nicolle (NNN) medium. The medium is a rabbit-blood agar having an overlay of Locke solution with added antibiotics. Two mL of blood is taken aseptically from a vein and diluted with 10 mL of citrated saline solution. This is centrifuged and the cellular deposit is inoculated into the water of condensation of Novy-MacNeal-Nicolle medium and incubated at 22°C for 1-4 weeks. At the end of each week, a drop of condensation fluid is examined for promastigote forms. Amastigotes transform to promastigotes in about 24 hours.

Bone marrow aspiration: Bone Marrow is the most common sample collected for diagnosis. Samples are obtained from the sternum or the iliac crest. Although safer than splenic puncture, the parasites are scanty and may give a false-negative test result. Positivity rates ranging from 54 to 86% have been obtained using bone marrow.

Splenic aspiration: When the spleen is enlarged considerably, this is one of the valuable methods for obtaining a positive result. Up to 98% positive results have been obtained using splenic aspiration. Splenic puncture is associated with the risk of uncontrolled hemorrhage and, therefore, should be carried out only when a bone marrow examination is inconclusive. Platelet count and prothrombin time should be checked before the procedure.

Lymph node aspiration or biopsy may be helpful when enlarged lymph nodes are present. In cutaneous disease, tissue can be obtained by a 3-mm punch biopsy, lesion scrapings, or needle aspiration of the non-necrotic edge of the lesion.

Indirect evidence of infection

Detection of hypergammaglobulinemia: The aldehyde and the antimony tests were the initial tests used to diagnose kala-azar.

The aldehyde test is a demonstration of the increase in gamma globulin levels observed in kala-azar. Take approximately 1 ml of blood in a small glass tube and add 1-2 drops of 40% formalin. Formation of milky-white–like opacity and jellification indicates a positive result. The aldehyde test is not positive unless the disease has had at least 3 months duration.

The antimony test also depends on the rise in serum gamma globulin. A positive test is indicated by a white flocculent precipitate seen when a urea stibamine solution comes in contact with serum.

Serology tests: The direct agglutination test, detects the specific immunoglobulin M (IgM) antibody at an early stage. It can be used as a rapid test in primary care settings. VL produces large amounts of specific IgG which can be used for diagnosis. Currently the most used serodiagnostic tests are Indirect immuno Fluorescent Antibody Test (IFAT), Enzyme

Linked Immunosorbent Assay (ELISA) and Direct Agglutination Test (DAT) and the rK39 dipstick tests. These tests indicate the presence of antibodies against Leishmania, therefore confirming the parasite (antigen) is, or was, present in the body.

For patients with a prior history of kala-azar who present with a suspicion of relapse one cannot rely on a serological test for diagnostic confirmation, as specific *anti-Leishmania* antibodies can persist for several years.

Supportive tests: Hematological parameters—blood examination shows a normochromic normocytic anemia, leukopenia, neutropenia, thrombocytopenia, elevated gamma globulins, and a reversal of the albumin-globulin ratio.

Cutaneous Leishmsniasis

Slit skin smear

The margin of the lesion contains amastigotes whereas the center contains debris and dead skin material. This margin of the lesion is aseptically punctured with a hypodermic needle and syringe containing a small amount of saline. The aspirate which is drawn up into the needle is examined microscopically and/or cultured using the method described in visceral leishmaniasis.

Polymerase chain reaction

Gene amplification techniques are sensitive methods useful in diagnosis of cutaneous leishmaniasis particularly when organisms cannot be detected microscopically. It is also very useful for the speciation of *Leishmania* parasites thus the correct treatment can be administered. The PCR-SSCP (Single-stranded conformation polymorphism) technique has been developed for the detection of sequence variation in rRNA genes within the *L. donovani* species. In addition, it can be performed easily and rapidly from clinical samples without prior need of cultivation of the parasite. PCR assay has also been used for post therapeutic follow-up and for detection of relapses among HIV-infected patients using SSU (small subunit) rRNA gene target. The use of fluorogenic real-time PCR using SSU-rRNA gene added with complete automation has made quantification of parasite burden possible. Besides it is a rapid, sensitive and highly specific test.

TRYPANOSOMA (SLEEPING SICKNESS)

Habitat: It inhabits mainly blood and in reticular tissue of lymph node and spleen.

Trypanosoma Brucei Gambiense

Morphology

Trypanosomes are motile, colorless, spindle-shaped bodies with a blunt posterior end and finely pointed anterior end. Body measures about 20×3 μm. The nucleus is large, oval and central in position. Parabasal body and blepharoplast (together called as kinetoplast) are situated at posterior end (**Fig. 35.7**).

A flagellum arises from blepharoplast that covers the body in the form of three to four undulating membrane and continues beyond the anterior end as free flagellum.

During its lifecycle, trypanosome occurs in another two forms—short and stumpy form, which is half in length as compare to fully grown parasite. This form is without flagellum.

Another form is intermediate form. This results as a binary fission of long slender form and changes into short stumpy form.

Life Cycle

T. b. gambiense passes its life cycle in two hosts. The vertebrate hosts are man, and domestic animals and invertebrate host is the tsetse fly of genus *Glossina* (*G. palpalis*, *G. fuscipes* and *G. tachinoides*). Both male and female flies bite man and may serve as vectors (**Fig. 35.8**).

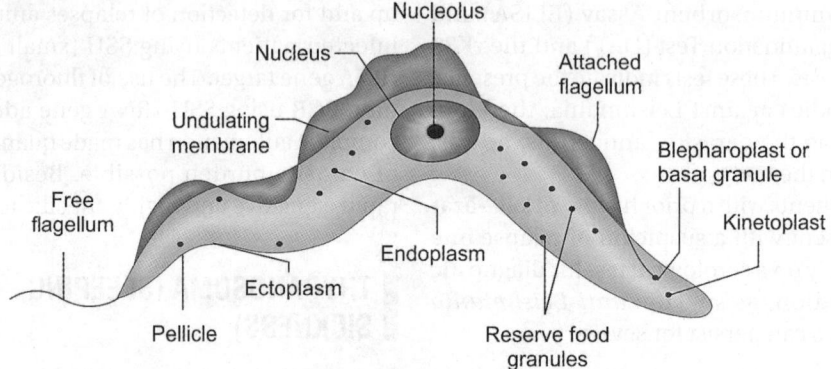

Fig. 35.7: *Trypanosoma brucei gambiense.*

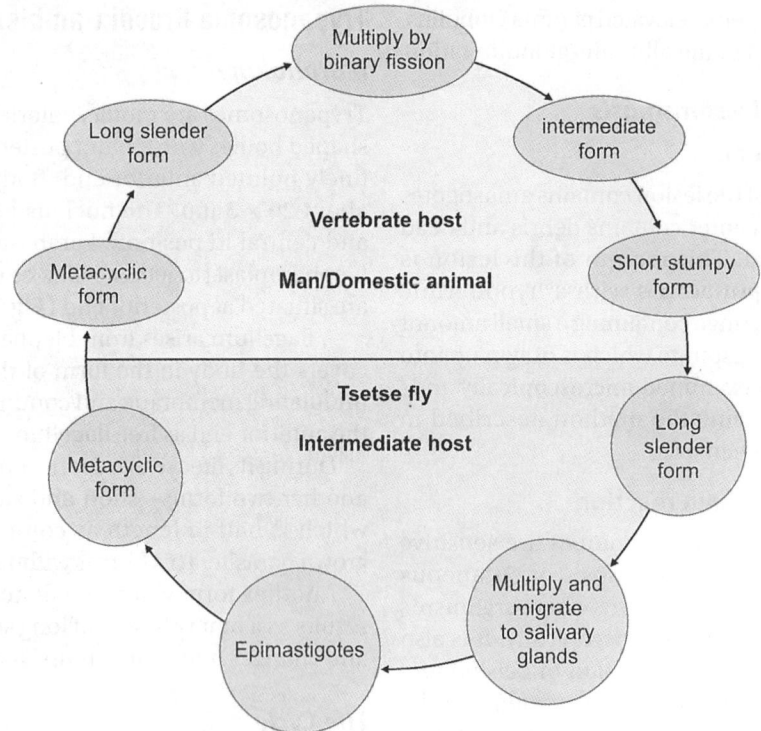

Fig. 35.8: Life cycle of *Trypanosoma*.

Development in man and other vertebrate hosts: The infective metacyclic trypomastigotes are injected into the mammalian host by the bite of infected *Glossina* spp. Trypomastigotes then transform into long slender forms and multiply by binary fission at the site of inoculation. These then transform first into an intermediate stage and then into a non-dividing short stumpy form with no flagellum. Subsequently, the parasites invade the blood stream resulting in parasitemia. These short stumpy forms are taken up by the tsetse fly along with its blood meal.

Development in invertebrate host: When an uninfected tsetse fly bites an infected vertebrate host the development in vector is initiated. In the midgut of the insect, short stumpy forms develop into long slender forms and multiply. These forms then pass to the posterior end of extraperitrophic space (a space between epithelial cells and peritrophic membrane), where they continue to multiply for some days. By the 15th day, they escape to the salivary glands. In the salivary glands, they develop into epimastigotes. The epimastigotes divide repeatedly and then transform into non-dividing metacyclic forms, which are highly motile, short and stumpy. The mature metacyclic forms detach from the salivary gland cells and are infective to the vertebrate host. In fly, the life cycle is completed in about 3–4 weeks.

Pathogenicity

African trypanosomiasis has three symptomatic stages, the last one being the most dangerous eventually leading to death, if left untreated.

Cutaneous: The tsetse fly's mouthpart has tiny serrations on it that saw into skin on its way to suck out blood. A papule may develop at the site of the tsetse fly bite within a few days to 2 weeks. It evolves into a dusky red, painful, indurated nodule that may ulcerate. This typical form is known as trypanosomal chancre.

Hemolymphatic: Several weeks or months later, trypanosomes then multiply in the plasma and interstitial fluid causing an acute to subacute febrile illness. Metacyclic trypomastigotes inoculated by tsetse flies transform into bloodstream trypomastigotes, which multiply by binary fission and spread through the lymphatics and bloodstream after inoculation. Bloodstream trypomastigotes multiply until specific antibodies produced by the host sharply reduce parasite levels. However, subsets of parasites escape immune destruction by a change in their variant surface glycoprotein and start a new multiplication cycle. The cycle of multiplication and lysis repeats.

Central nervous system (CNS): The disease reaches its final stage when the parasites get through the blood-brain barrier entering the brain. The CNS involvement can occur as early as within a month in some cases. This is a meningoencephalitic stage that causes inflammation of the CNS. This can lead to coma and, if left untreated, it may cause death.

Clinical Diagnosis and Symptoms

Each person may have slightly different symptoms. But symptoms tend to happen within 1–4 weeks of infection.

Symptoms in the hemolytic phase are—anemia, cardiac dysfunction, pruritus (itching), fatigue, fever, headache, muscle or joint pain, skin rash, splenomegaly (enlargement of the spleen), swelling of the lymph nodes (most prominently in the back of the neck and in the groin), hands and face, thrombocytopenia (low level of thrombocytes), and weight loss.

After many weeks, the infection may become meningoencephalitis. This is an infection of the brain and the fluid surrounding the brain and the spinal cord. As the illness gets worse, symptoms may include—severe headache, irritability, loss of concentration, progressive confusion, slurred speech, difficulty walking and talking, and worldwide array of behavioral changes ranging from aggressiveness to sleep-like status.

The sleep disturbances that give the disease its name are very characteristic. Typically, the unfortunate patient has an uncontrollable desire to sleep at any time, although, paradoxically, he could suffer insomnia at night. Monitoring the sleep and recording the brain waves of such patients with an electroencephalogram reveal characteristic disruptions of normal, healthy sleep-wake patterns. These changes disappear, if the patient recovers. Otherwise, in the final stages of the illness, the urge to sleep is continuous, and there are seizures, brain swelling, incontinence, coma, and, ultimately, death.

Trypanosoma Rhodesiense

T. rhodesiense differs from *T. gambiense* in following points:
- *T. rhodesiense* is found in east and central Africa.
- Main tsetse vector spp are—*G. morsitans*, *G. pallidipes* and *G. swynnertoni*.
- Reservoir host is mainly animal (e.g. rats).
- The course of disease caused by *T. rhodesiense* is more acute, rarely lasting 9 months before death occurs.
- Lymph node enlargement is not much pronounced.
- *T. rhodesience* are more resistant to treatment in advanced stage.

WUCHERERIA BANCROFTI (FILARIASIS)

Wuchereria bancrofti is a nematode (roundworm) parasite of the family Filarioidea. It is also known as Filariworm, which is the major cause of lymphatic filariasis. It is one of the three parasitic worms, together with *Brugia malayi* and *B. timori*, which infect the lymphatic system to cause lymphatic filariasis.

These filarial worms are spread by a variety of mosquito vector species. *W. bancrofti* is the most prevalent of the three. Adult worms lodge in the lymphatic system and disrupt the immune system. It causes abnormal enlargement of body parts, pain, severe disability, and social stigma.

Wuchereria bancrofti is a parasitic filarial nematode worm spread by a mosquito vector. Adult male and female worms reside in the lymph nodes and lymphatic vessels of man. The microfilariae are found in the blood. Humans are the only known reservoir hosts.

Morphology (Fig. 35.9)

In man, *Wuchereria bancrofti* occurs in two forms—adult worm and microfilaria.

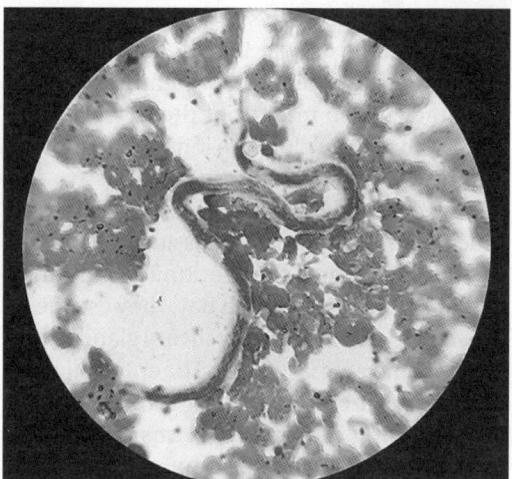

Fig. 35.9: Microfilaria in peripheral blood smear. *(For color version See Color Plate 8)*

Adult Worm

These are long hair like transparent creamy white in color. They are filiform in shape and both ends are tapering. The male measures 2.4 to 4 cm in length and 0.1 mm in thickness its tail end is curved ventrally with numerous pair of papillae and there is one long and one short spicule. The female measures 8 to 10 cm in length and 0.2 to 0.3 mm in thickness. Its tail end is narrow and abruptly pointed. Both male and female worms remain coiled together and it is difficult to separate them. Females are usually more in number than males. The life span of adult worm is 5 to 10 years. The female is viviparous and liberates sheathed embryos (microfilariae) into lymph form where they find way into blood.

Microfilaria

It is transparent, and colorless with blunt head and pointed tail. It measures 245–295 μm in length and 7.5–10 μm in width. It is covered by a hyaline sheath which is much longer (about 359 μm) than the microfilaria. It can move forwards and backwards within the sheath. The somatic cells or nuclei appear as granules in the central axis of the microfilaria. At places, these granules are absent. These

Chapter 35: Hemoparasites

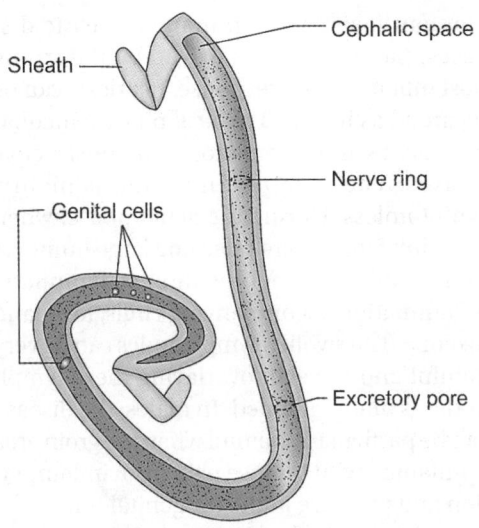

Fig. 35.10: *Microfilaria bancrofti*.

form the landmarks for recognition of various microfilariae. The tail tip is free from nuclei (Fig. 35.10).

The larval forms do not undergo any further development in the human body unless they are taken up by their appropriate intermediate host. The life span of microfilariae in the human body is about 70 days.

Life Cycle

W. bancrofti passes its life cycle in two hosts—man and mosquito (Fig. 35.11).

Life Cycle in Man

The adult worms reside in lymph nodes and lymphatics (usually inguinal, scrotal and abdominal) of man. The lymph provides nutrition to the adult worm. The male fertilizes female and the gravid female gives birth to microfilariae. Through lymphatics they find their way into general circulation. They only appear in the peripheral bloodstream, at a time which coincides with the biting habits with the species of mosquito that predominantly transmits them. They appear during 10 pm to 2 am in the peripheral blood and then rest of the time they remain in pulmonary circulation.

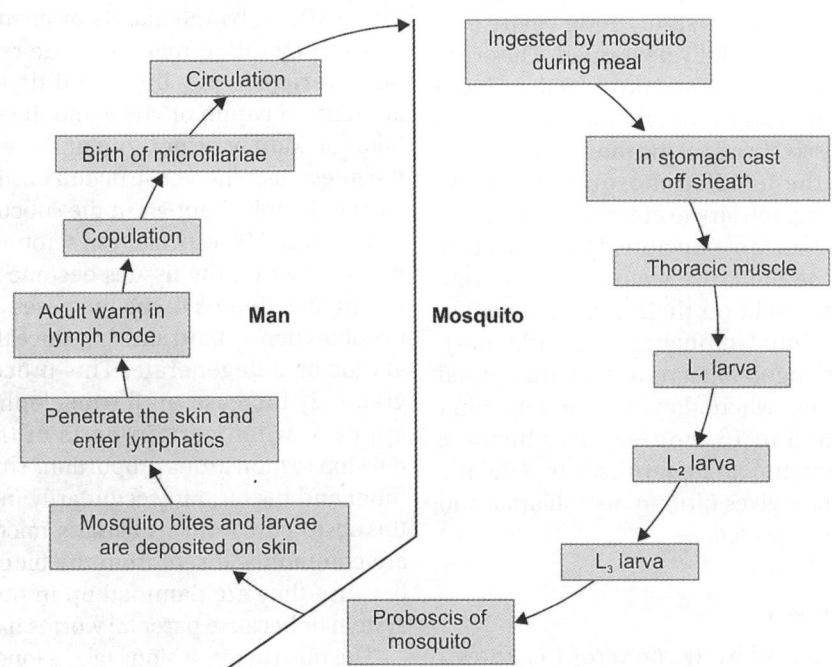

Fig. 35.11: Life cycle of *W. bancrofti*.

Sheathed microfilariae are ingested by the mosquito during its blood meal. In order to infect mosquitoes, there must be about 15 or more microfilariae per drop of blood (20 cu mm). A high concentration of 100 or more per drop is fatal to the mosquitoes.

Life Cycle in Mosquito

A number of species of mosquito belonging to the genus *Culex, Aedes* and *Anopheles*, act as intermediate hosts for *W. bancrofti*. *Culex quinquefasciatus* is responsible for 50% of cases of lymphatic filariasis.

While sucking the blood, the sheathed microfilariae are ingested by the mosquito and reach the stomach of the mosquito. Here, they cast off their sheaths in 2-6 hours penetrate the stomach wall and in the course of 4-17 hours reach thoracic muscles. In next two days, they metamorphose into short, sausage-shaped organisms with a spiky tail. This is first stage larva (L_1). In 3-7 days, they molt once or twice to become second stage larva (L_2) on the 10th or 11th day the metamorphosis become complete. The tail atrophies to a mere stump and the digestive system, body cavity and genital organs are fully developed. These are the third stage larvae and are infective. These larvae then migrate from thoracic muscles to the proboscis sheath of the mosquito.

When the infected mosquito bites the human being the larvae are deposited on the skin near the site of puncture. They then enter through the puncture wound or penetrate through the skin on their own. Thereafter, they enter into lymphatics and settle down usually in inguinal, scrotal and abdominal lymph nodes, where they develop into adult worms. In 5 to 18 months, they become sexually mature. Male fertilizes female, the gravid female gives birth to microfilariae and the cycle is repeated.

Pathogenicity

Disease caused by *W. bancrofti* is known as wuchereriasis or bancroftian filariasis or elephantiasis. As with many parasitic diseases, pathogenesis is driven by the strong host inflammatory response. Filariasis can be regarded as having 3 clinical phases: Incubation, acute or inflammatory, and obstructive phases. The incubation period is mainly symptomless. During the acute phase, when the adult females are releasing large numbers of microfilariae, there is intense lymphatic inflammation accompanying chills, fever and toxemia. The swollen lymph nodes can be very painful and the skin overlaying these lymph nodes is often inflamed. In males, the disease can be particularly painful when the groin area is inflamed with intense pain from inflammation and pressure in the urogenital tract.

At the cellular level, there is inflammatory cell infiltration of the lymph node linings, particularly polymorphs and eosinophils and lymphocytes. Adult worms are frequently killed with abscesses formed around them. In the acute filariasis, symptoms disappear and then reappear frequently.

In the obstructive phase, the effects are varicose lymph or chyle vessels behind places where lymph glands or channels are blocked by inflammatory tissue reactions. Such varicose may burst and divert large amounts of lymph or chyle into the scrotum, bladder, kidney or peritoneum or even into the intestine. When obstruction occurs in the smaller lymph channels in the subcutaneous system and skin, especially in scrotum, limbs, breast or vulva, the tissues become swollen. Eventually, fibrous tissue increases and skin becomes dense, hard and dry, since the sweat glands also degenerate. This process may gradually increase until true elephantiasis appears, when certain parts of the body develop to monstrous proportion. This allows fungi and bacteria to secondarily invade. In this obstructive form of filariasis, microfilariae are commonly absent from the blood either because they are dammed up in the lymph system or because parental worms have died.

The obstructive lesions take a long time to develop may be 20 years.

Clinical Diagnosis and Symptoms

The microfilariae usually produce no symptoms. Filarial symptoms are caused by living or dead adult worms. The sign and symptoms are due to either inflammatory reactions or lymphatic obstruction. Many patients are asymptomatic. Patients may present with fever, chills, aches general malaise, lymphangitis and lymphadenitis. Lymphangitis commonly affects the lower extremities and there may also be genital and breast involvement. An inflammatory reaction occurs in the lymphatic vessels that harbor the adult worms. Edema develops which may resolve after the first few attacks. A late complication resulting in thickening and verrucous changes in the skin known as elephantiasis may occur after recurring lymphangitis. Elephantiasis is the last consequence of the swelling of limbs and scrotum.

Secondary bacterial and fungal infections may occur in patients with long-standing elephantiasis.

Obstruction of the genital organs may result in hydrocoele formation and scrotal lymphedema. Obstruction of the retroperitoneal lymphatics may cause the renal lymphatics to rupture into the urinary tract producing chyluria.

Some patients with filariasis do not exhibit microfilaremia but develop tropical pulmonary eosinophilia which is characterized by peripheral eosinophilia, wheeze and cough. High eosinophilia, high IgE level and high anti-filarial antibody titers are features of this syndrome. This is called as occult filiariasis.

Laboratory Diagnosis

The laboratory diagnosis of wuchereriasis involve following procedures.

Direct Evidence

The direct evidence involve search for microfilariae and adult worms:

Microfilariae

For the direct search of microfilariae, the specimens used are:
- Peripheral blood—the specimen collection time should be selected in accordance with patient's clinical symptoms and travel history. For the species of *W. bancrofti*, in tropics and subtropics, the periodicity is nocturnal. Therefore, the collection time is 12 at midnight. In the Pacific area, the periodicity is diurnal subperiodic, therefore, the collection time preferred is 4 pm.
- In chylous urine.
- In exudates of lymph.
- In the hydrocele fluid.

The detection methods are (i) Polycarbonate membrane filtration and (ii) Saline/Saponin method.

Polycarbonate membrane filtration

This technique is very sensitive, enabling very low parasitemia to be detected. It is now the most widely used technique for separating microfilariae from blood.

Nuclepore polycarbonate membranes, 25 mm diameter, 5 µm pore size, are held in a Millipore Swinnex filter holder, using a rubber gasket to secure the membrane.

Method

- Place the membrane on the holder with a drop of water
- Draw up 10–20 ml of 1:1 saline diluted blood into a 20 mL syringe
- Connect the syringe to the filter and gently push the blood through the filter membrane
- Repeat until all of the blood has been filtered
- Draw up 20 ml of saline into the syringe, flush through the filter, repeat using air
- Unscrew the top of the filter and discard the gasket into chloros; use forceps to transfer the membrane to a slide
- Add a drop of saline to the membrane and cover with a coverslip

- Examine the membrane under the microscope, using a 10X objective. Examine any microfilariae found using a 40X objective to note the presence of a sheath.

Saline/saponin method

Reagent: 1 percent saponin in normal saline.

Method

- Deliver 2 ml of blood (fresh or anti-coagulated) into a centrifuge tube and add 8 ml of 1 percent saponin in saline
- Mix the blood by inversion, and then allow it to stand at room temperature for 15 minutes to allow the blood to hemolyze
- Centrifuge at 2,000 rpm for 15 minutes to deposit the microfilariae
- Discard the supernatant and use the deposit to make a wet preparation
- Examine the slide using the 10X objective. Active microfilariae can be seen and produce a snake-like movement as they disturb the cell suspension
- If it is not easy to inspect the microfilariae due to excess "wriggling", a little 10% formalin can be run under the coverslip to immobilize them
- Confirmation of species can be made by using appropriate staining methods to demonstrate nuclear morphology.

Staining methods for microfilariae

Thick and thin blood films can be examined. However, this is an insensitive method due to the low microfilaremia, and larger volumes of blood need to be examined.

The two methods commonly used are: (i) Supravital staining and (ii) Permanent staining.

Supravital staining

Reagent: 0.75 percent cresyl blue in saline or 1.0% methylene blue in saline.

These reagents can be used to stain live microfilariae by allowing the stain to flow under the coverslip on to a polycarbonate membrane preparation or a centrifuged preparation. The dye will stain the nuclei of the microfilariae and also provide a contrasting background to look for a sheath. It may take several minutes for the dye to penetrate the organisms and the slide should be kept in a moist chamber to prevent the preparation from drying out.

Permanent staining

Permanent stains should show up the nuclei, including the pattern of nuclei in the tail region and stain the sheath if necessary.

The stains of choice are: (1) Hematoxylin (2) Giemsa and (3) Rapid Field's.

Hematoxylin: Delafield's hematoxylin will stain the nuclei and the sheath well and unlike Ehrlich's hematoxylin does not require heating.

Reagents: Delafield's hematoxylin (BDH), 1% acid alcohol mixture, methanol.

Method
- Make thin films, allow to air dry then fix in methanol for 5 minutes
- Stain with Delafield's hematoxylin for 20 minutes
- "Blue" the nuclei by placing the slide in a coplin jar and allow a stream of running water to flow into the jar for 20 minutes
- Decolorize with 1% acid alcohol for 5–10 seconds before "blueing" in tapwater again. Control this process by examination under the microscope until the nuclei are clear and distinct
- Allow the slide to dry before mounting in DPX
- The nuclei should stain blue and the sheath gray.

Giemsa

Reagents: Methanol, Giemsa stain, immersion oil.

Method
- Make a thin film and allow to air dry
- Fix in methanol for 1 minute

- Tip off the methanol and flood the slide with Giemsa stain diluted 1:6 with buffered distilled water pH 6.8. The diluted stain must be freshly prepared each time
- Stain for 20–25 minutes
- Run buffered water on to the slide to float off stain and to prevent deposition of precipitate on to the film. Allow the slide to drain dry
- Examine the film using the oil immersion objective. Nuclei should stain red.

Adult Worm

Adult worm can be seen in:
- Biopsied lymph node
- The calcified worm may be seen on X-ray examination.

Indirect Evidence

- DNA probes can be used for the diagnosis of *W. bancrofti*.

- *Immunological tests:* Filarial antigen may be detected in the patient serum by enzyme immunoassays using monoclonal antibodies against microfilarial larval surface antigens. However, because antigen shedding may be irregular, particularly during times when circulating microfilariae may not be detected, detection of antibody to larval antigens may be more appropriate.

The other test include:

Intradermal test: This is an immediate hypersensitivity reaction. A positive test shows weal over 2 cm after 30 minutes of injection of antigen. However, this test cannot distinguish between past and present reaction.

The blood examination shows 5 to 15% increase in eosinophils.

CHAPTER 36

Analyzers in Hematology

Learning Objectives
- In this machine age, every field is turning in to automatic. Automated hematology analyzers can rapidly analyze whole blood specimens for the complete blood count (CBC). Automated ESR is another test in current trend.
- This chapter introduces readers with a wide range of analyzers based on different principle. Calibration, maintenance, and QC of analyzers are discussed here.
- What to consider while buying analyzer, manual vs automatic analyzers, limitations of analyzers
- Automated ESR

Keywords
Electrical impedance, Flow cytometry, Fluorescent flow cytometry, Software-generated WBC suspect flags, Automated ESR

▌INTRODUCTION

The complete blood count (CBC) and differential leucocyte count (DLC) are the backbone of hematology laboratory evaluation. The CBC and DLC are used to diagnose anemia, to identify acute and chronic illness, bleeding tendencies and white blood cell disorders. During last two decades, blood cell analysis has progressed from the use of labor intensive manual procedures to the use of highly automated instruments. Current trends include attempts to incorporate as many analysis parameters as possible into one instrument platform, in order to minimize the need to run a single sample on multiple instruments. Such instruments are being incorporated into highly automated combined biochemistry/hematology laboratories, where samples are automatically sorted, aliquoted, and brought to the appropriate instrument by robotic track system.

Hematology analyzers are used widely in patient and research settings to count and characterize blood cells for disease detection and monitoring. Basic analyzers return a complete blood count (CBC) with a three-part differential white blood cell (WBC) count. Sophisticated analyzers measure cell morphology and can detect small cell populations to diagnose rare blood conditions. Other parameters of hemogram are calculated in analyzers by means of statistics. Many manufacturers offer integrated slide-making and staining modules that can be added on to the instrument.

▌HEMATOLOGY ANALYZER (CELL COUNTER) TECHNOLOGY

The three main physical technologies used in hematology analyzers are: electrical impedance, flow cytometry, and fluorescent flow cytometry. These are used in combination with chemical reagents that lyses or alter blood cells to extend the measurable parameters. For example, electrical impedance can differentiate red blood cells (RBCs), WBCs, and platelets by volume. Adding a nucleating agent that shrinks lymphocytes more than other WBCs make it possible to differentiate lymphocytes by volume.

Electrical Impedance

The traditional method for counting cells is electrical impedance, also known as the Coulter principle. It is used in almost every hematology analyzer.

Blood cells are suspended in an electrolyte solution (isotone) and made to flow from an outer chamber into an inner chamber through an orifice of 100 of μm diameter. This aperture so narrow that only one cell can pass through at a time. An electrode is placed in each chamber to sense the electric current flowing through the orifice. When a cell (poor conductor of electricity) passes through the orifice, it imparts resistance (impedance) to the electrical. The impedance changes as a cell passes through. The change in impedance is proportional to cell volume, resulting in a cell count and measure of volume. Impedance analysis returns CBCs and three-part WBC differentials (granulocytes, lymphocytes, and monocytes) but cannot distinguish between the similarly sized granular leukocytes—eosinophils, basophils, and neutrophils.

Red cells and white cells are counted separately by diluting the blood in different diluents. The white cell diluent is Drabkin solution, which in addition to the WBC counts, reports Hb concentration. Of all the indices, MCV is actually measured from the average amplitude of voltage pulse in the region of red cell size (6 to 9 μm). Hematocrit value is calculated from MCV and RBC count (MCV × RBC in millions divided by 10). Other indices like MCH and MCHC are calculated in the same way as described earlier (Refer Chapter 24).

Flow Cytometry

Laser flow cytometry is more expensive than impedance analysis, due to the requirement for expensive reagents, but returns detailed information about the morphology of blood cells. It is an excellent method for determining five-part WBC differentials.

In this method, a laser or a tungsten halogen lamp is pointed towards the bloodstream, which passes through a channel that is a so narrow that cells can only pass through one by one. This is achieved through a hydrodynamically focused flow, called sheath flow. When the cell passes through the light beam the light is scattered or reflected into a particular direction, which depends mainly on the size of the cell but also in the shape and the refractive index. A photo detector is placed at the angle at which the light is scattered. The absorbance is measured, and the scattered light is measured at multiple angles to determine the cell's granularity, diameter, and inner complexity. The use of lasers is preferred due to the focused light beam they produce. Calibration of these instruments has to be performed using human blood.

Fluorescent Flow Cytometry

Adding fluorescent reagents extends the use of flow cytometry to measure specific cell populations. Fluorescent dyes reveal the nucleus-plasma ratio of each stained cell. It is useful for the analysis of platelets, nucleated RBCs, and reticulocytes.

Proprietary Technologies

Manufacturers combine these three technologies with innovative uses of reagents, hydrofluidics, and data analysis tools to produce proprietary methods, each of which has strengths in terms of accuracy, speed, or breadth of parameters. Some popularly used analyzers are discussed here.

Siemens: These instruments use peroxidase staining for differential testing. This provides a secondary total WBC that acts as an internal QC check.

The Sysmex: Sodium lauryl sulfate method for hemoglobin analysis is a noncyanide method with very short reaction times. Hemoglobin is determined in a separate channel, minimizing interference from high leukocyte concentrations.

The Abbott: Uses three-color fluorescence combined with patented Multi Angle Polarized Scatter Separation technology to deliver accurate WBC enumeration and identification using four angles of light scatter.

FACTORS TO CONSIDER WHEN BUYING A HEMATOLOGY ANALYZER

Choice of instrument will be driven primarily by the setting of use—patient bedside, consulting room, clinical lab, or research lab. Note that instruments must have regulatory approval for clinical as opposed to research use.

Other considerations include:
- Range of tests
- Time per analysis
- Automation
- Reagent supply
- Sample size and microsampling
- Accuracy, precision, and linearity
- Maintenance, calibration, and QC
- Results analysis and storage
- Footprint.

Range of Tests

Every hematology analyzer returns a CBC and a three- or five-part WBC differential. However, even the simplest analyzer will return multiple parameters. The most basic analyzer from **Sysmex**, the XP-300™ is with some basic parameters: WBC; RBC; HGB; HCT; MCV; MCH; MCHC; PLT; NEUT #,%; LYM #,%; MXD #,%; RDW-SD; RDW-CV; and MPV.

By contrast, the Pentra DX Nexus SPS evolution from **Horiba** measures 50 parameters, some of which are for research parameters only. Consider whether there is a choice of tests to run, or whether every parameter is measured for every sample. Check the cost per run since extensive test menus will incur higher reagent costs.

Time per Analysis

Time per analysis depends on the parameters being measured. The rate limiting step is the reaction time for reagents. A simple CBC can typically be returned in 1 min. More sophisticated analyses can take up to 10 min.

Abbott's CELL-DYN Sapphire provides a reportable CD61 immunoplatelet count in approximately 5 min, and CD3/4 and CD3/8 immuno T-cell count in approximately 7 min.

Automation

High-throughput labs require automation of their hematology workflow and the capability to integrate with other systems. Factors to consider are throughput, autoloader capacity, and whether vials and racks are compatible with other lab equipment.

The **Sysmex** XE-5000 reports 31 whole blood parameters at a rate of 150 samples/hr.

The ADVIA 120 from **Siemens** is a benchtop instrument with a 150-capacity rack-based autosampler, allowing 75 min of walkaway operation.

Pentra DX Nexus SPS evolution from **Horiba** has an autoloader with continuous loading capability. The rack is compatible with most pre- and postanalytical systems.

If barcode tracking is required, check the quality of the imaging technology. Coulter LH 780 analyzers from **Beckman Coulter** are capable of reading most barcode labels, even those with lower print quality.

Many manufacturers offer integrated slide-making and staining modules that can be added on to the instrument.

Check the system's capability for flagging outlying results. Automatic flagging and retesting minimize the requirement for manual review.

Reagent Supply

When choosing an instrument, check how many reagents are required and the costs and safety requirements. Can they be purchased from any supplier, or only the manufacturer?

Erba's ELite 3 measures 20 parameters with only three reagents, which are environmentally friendly and cyanide free. **Beckman Coulter's** DxH 800 and DxH 600 use only five reagents for all analyses, including NRBC and reticulocytes.

Check how often the reagents need to be changed. The ADVIA 120 from **Siemens** carries enough onboard analytical and wash reagents for 1850 CBC/diff tests.

Sample Size and Microsampling

Typical sample size requirements are on the order of 150 μL of whole blood for multiparameter analysis. Many manufacturers offer microsampling, which is particularly helpful for pediatrics. The **Horiba** ABX Micros ES 60 uses 10 μL of whole blood for CBC plus WBC 3-diff.

Accuracy, Precision, and Linearity

Ask to see the manufacturer's data on accuracy, precision, and linearity. The accuracy of volume measurements using impedance can be greater than 1% and depends on the width of the aperture relative to the cell being measured. Some instruments use multiple-sized apertures to improve accuracy for different-sized cells. Temperature also affects accuracy. The **Horiba** Pentra 80 features a preheated analysis chamber to ensure consistent results.

Calibration, Maintenance, and QC

Consider how frequently the instrument must be cleaned and recalibrated. Ask what QC features are included.

IDEXX includes qualiBeads. In its analyzers, qualiBeads are particles with specific characteristics that are used as an internal standard to verify pipetting accuracy and laser performance.

The **Horiba** ABX Pentra manages reagent standardization, validation, and reruns and can also share rules between a central laboratory and satellite laboratories.

Open or Closed Tube Sampling

Closed tube sampling reduces the risk of exposure to blood. Instruments with open or closed sampling options have different stability and calibration requirements depending on the mode of operation.

Results Storage and Analysis

A major differentiator between analyzers is the number of results that can be stored on the system. A small benchtop analyzer might typically save 1000 patient results with histograms. The **Horiba** ABX Pentra DX120 SPS will store 90,000 results plus graphics.

Footprint

Check dimensions and space it needed. Systems vary from small benchtop units to large automated machines. The ABX Micros ES 60 from **Horiba** is a compact benchtop unit that delivers CBC + 3-diff. It has a touchscreen interface and can store 1000 patient results with histograms. It has a footprint of 16.9 in × 14.2 in × 14.2 in and weighs only 14.02 Kg.

The freestanding automated XN-9000 from **Sysmex** is scaleable. The 801 model is 26 ft long × 4 ft deep and can analyze 120 slides/hr and 900 CBCs/hr. If linear floor space is limited, a corner unit can be added.

Consider the ergonomics of operation and the quality of the display screen.

Manual versus Automated Cell Counting

Although peripheral blood smear examination provides information that cannot be obtained

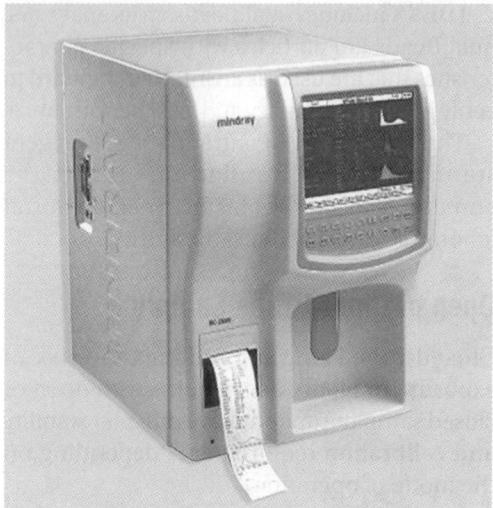

Fig. 36.1: Blood cell counter machine.

from automated cell counting, it has certain limitations and special considerations.

Blood Cell Counter (Fig. 36.1)

Limitations of Manual Cell Counting

- Experience is needed to make technically adequate smears consistently.
- Non-uniform distribution of WBCs over the smear, with larger leukocytes concentrated near the edges and lymphocytes scattered throughout.
- There is a non-uniform distribution of red blood cells as well, with small crowded red blood cells at the thick edge and large flat red blood cells without central pallor at the feathered edge of the smear.
- It is subjective, labor-intensive, and statistically unreliable (only 100-200 cells are counted).
- It is imprecise with reported coefficients of variation (CV) ranging from 30% to 110%.
- *Cell identification errors in manual counting*: This is mostly associated with distinguishing lymphocytes from monocytes, bands from segmented forms and abnormal cells (variant lymphocytes from blasts). The monocytes tend to be underestimated and the lymphocytes tend to be overestimated.

Advantages of the Automated Analyzers

- Cell counting with these instruments is rapid, objective, statistically significant (8000 or more cells are counted), and not subject to the distributional bias of the manual count.
- They are also more efficient and cost effective than the manual method. Some of these cell counters can process 120–150 samples per hour.
- In addition, the precision of the automated differential makes the absolute leukocyte counts reliable and reproducible.

Disadvantages of the Automated Analyzers

- The automated hematology analyzers also may produce cell counts which are falsely increased or decreased.
- Some analyzers, particularly the impedance based counters check only the volume and number of particles and may not be able to correctly distinguish tiny clumps of platelets and nucleated red blood cells. Platelet clumps may be misclassified as leukocytes or erythrocytes, and nucleated red blood cells can be misclassified as leukocytes or, specifically, lymphocytes.
- Furthermore, large or unidentifiable atypical cells, toxic immature neutrophils, and markedly reactive lymphocytes can also be misclassified.

Software-generated WBC Suspect Flags

These 'flags' are warnings generated and displayed by the machine to alert the laboratory personnel that the machine has detected some abnormality in cell population or distribution that needs attention. The machines are preprogrammed by the manufacturers to generate certain flags according to an internal algorithm. Some examples of these flags include, blast flag, atypical flag, flag for discrepancy of the two WBC counts, nucleated RBC (NRBC) flag, flag for immature granulocytes as well as others.

Conclusion

Automation of some of the most commonly requested laboratory tests (the CBC and differential counts) has reduced the number of technologists needed for performance of these tests. As a result, there has also been a dramatic reduction of the numbers of medical technologists and technicians in medical laboratories. While automated blood analyzers count significantly more cells to create a differential count than technicians, they are perhaps still less efficient in detecting abnormal WBCs. Therefore, whenever a hematological malignancy or rare hereditary disorder is suspected in a patient, a microscopic differential count must be performed independently of whether the automated hematology analyzer gives a suspect flag message or not. At present, the automated analyzers are not error-free. With further technological refinements, this situation may well change.

■ AUTOMATION IN ESR

Manual method for ESR is Westergren method. ICSH (International Council for Standardization in Hematology) has recommended this as Gold Standard method. As this method is laborious and time consuming, several modifications of this method are available. These modifications resulted in automation of various steps and reduced test time to as less as 5 minutes to 30 minutes. Erythrocyte sedimentation is measured at 30 minutes or less and extrapolated to 1 hour using a mathematical formula by the instrument. The sedimentation is measured by infrared light, which increases accuracy. Results are automatically printed after the measurement of ESR. Statistical reports are generated with the following features: standard deviation,

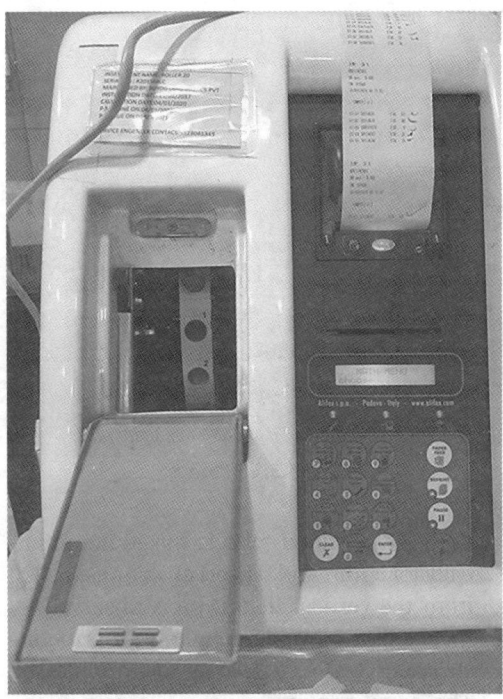

Fig. 36.2: Automated ESR machine.

percent coefficient of variation, mean, and highest and lowest result. Today, there are automated ESR systems that provide faster results and address laboratory safety by minimizing contact with blood samples **(Fig. 36. 2)**.

Steps in two different analyzers are discussed here.

1. The Seditainer system comprises a glass vacuum tube measuring 120 mm × 10.25 mm **(Fig. 36.3)**. The tube contains 1.25 cm^3 of 0.105 M buffered sodium citrate and has a vacuum sufficient to draw 5.0 cm^3 of blood. After the tube is filled to the required level, as marked on the tube, it is inverted 8–10 times to ensure thorough mixing. The tube is then immediately placed in a precalibrated Seditainer rack and left for exactly 1 hour. The tube is filled by vacuum with 1.8 cm^3 of blood and sent immediately to the hematology laboratory. On arrival, the tube is placed in the instrument rack of the measuring

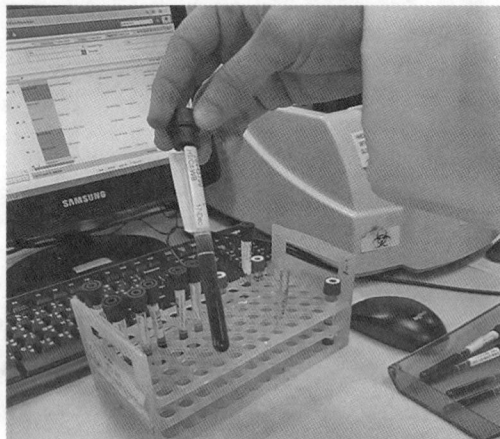

Fig. 36.3: ESR tubes.

device. The blood tube is mixed automatically for 5 min and placed at an angle of 200 from the vertical. The tube is observed by means of a movable camera inside the instrument connected to a microprocessor. The computer records the changes in the height of the red cell column by measuring light transmission differences between sedimented cells and the overlying plasma. After 20 min the system reads the fall of the red cell column and converts it to the equivalent Westergren ESR measurement at 1 hour.

2. RR Mechatronics has developed the Starrsed ST, which is a tube based ESR analyzer with a small footprint. The Starrsed ST, in full operation, produces sample results up to every 30 seconds. After manually applying the sample tube for aspiration, the entire process is fully automated. A built-in barcode reader identifies each sample. The Starrsed ST will then perform an ESR measurement fully unattended.

After presenting a sample tube, the aspiration system is activated. A needle pierces the cap and blood is drawn from the tube. The Starrsed ST has a fully integrated diluting system, which dilutes the blood with the Starrsed citrate diluent in a 4:1 ratio, in full accordance with the Westergren method. The diluted blood sample is then drawn up into one of the 24 Westergren pipettes inside the instrument (for immediate testing, a single sample can be analyzed). The instrument measures the sedimentation for each pipette within 30 or 60 minutes. Most users prefer the 30-minute mode. The built-in printer produces the result that is also sent automatically to the LIMS (Laboratory Information Management System). Simultaneously, the used Westergren pipette is automatically cleaned and prepared to receive a new sample. Additionally, all 24 pipettes receive a fully automated, intensive end-of-day cleaning using Starrsed X-Clean. All waste fluids, i.e., blood, diluent and X-Clean, are collected in a built-in waste container, ready for disposal as stipulated by local regulations.

Controls

Good laboratory practice advises the use of controls to ensure the continued reliability of the test results. RR Mechatronics supports this with Starrsed Control. It is to be used in the ESR analyzer as if it were a real patient sample. Starrsed Control is processed exactly the same way and is fully compliant with the ICSH recommendations and CLSI (The Clinical and Laboratory Standards Institute) procedures. The Starrsed ST recognizes the test tube by its barcode, reads the ESR range, check the expiration date of the control, and analyzes the sample. Starrsed Control gives maximum reliability at minimal effort and costs.

Additional Benefits

- As the Westergren glass tubes are re-usable after each automatic cleaning, there are no additional costs for new pipettes. No disposable plastics of any kind are used.
- As opposed to other test instruments, Starrsed instruments actually identify and report hazy samples so that the lab technician may decide on further testing.
- The Starrsed ST makes use of EDTA sample tubes. The advantage is that EDTA blood

is very stable compared to pre-citrated samples, allowing for accurate ESR test results up to 24 hours after collection. This provides laboratories with even more logistical flexibility.
- Because the Starrsed ST dilutes the blood, which is in agreement with the Westergren method, it compensates for different hematocrit levels. The hematocrit level of the sample therefore will not influence the accuracy of the ESR measured.

Choosing an Automated ESR System

Depending on laboratory's requirements, key considerations for selecting ESR analyzer include capacity, analysis time, throughput, and dimensions.

Section 3

Blood Banking

Blood Banking

CHAPTER 37

Historical Aspect

Learning Objectives
- Present day well equipped Blood Banks have history of around 300 years. This chapter throws light on this long journey which started with the discovery of circulatory system.
- Time line is created in this chapter, which throws light on various milestones of blood banking like Blood grouping, anticoagulant, isolation of blood components, use of plastic bags and apheresis.
- For all significant discoveries, its importance in blood banking and name of inventor included. Discoveries after 2007 are mentioned in last chapter of the section—Recent Advances in Blood Banking.

Keywords
Karl Landsteiner, Cross matching, Alexis Carrel, Glucose citrate solution, Plasmapheresis, Cord stem cell transplant, Coombs test, Somatic nuclear transfer

■ DEFINITION

The blood bank collects, stores, processes and supplies blood or its components for transfusion to patients who need replenishment.

The whole blood and packed red blood cells can be stored for a limited period of time (maximum 42 days). But blood components and derivatives such as platelets, dried or fluid blood plasma, plasma proteins like albumin or globulin or fibrinogen can be stored for much longer period (maximum one year). So today, established blood banks not only store and supply whole blood but also its various fractions too.

■ HISTORY

The modern era blood bank has traveled a long journey which starts from the discovery of circulatory system in 1628.

Discovery of circulatory system and earlier transfusion efforts:

1628	English physician William Harvey discovered the circulation of blood.
1665	The first recorded successful blood transfusion occurred in England: Physician Richard Lower kept dogs alive by transfusion of blood from other dogs.
1667	Jean-Baptiste Denis in France and Richard Lower in England separately report successful transfusions from lambs to humans. Subsequently transfusions failed. Within ten years, transfusing the blood of animals to humans became prohibited by law, delaying transfusion advances for about 150 years.
1795	In Philadelphia, an American physician, Philip Syng Physick, claimed to perform the first human blood transfusion, although he did not publish this information.

1818	James Blundell, a British obstetrician, performed the first successful transfusion of human blood to a patient for the treatment of postpartum hemorrhage. Using the patient's husband as a donor, he extracted approximately four ounces of blood from the husband's arm and, using a syringe, successfully transfused the wife. Between 1825 and 1830, he performs 10 transfusions, five of which prove beneficial to his patients, and published these results. He also devised various instruments for performing transfusions and proposed rational indications.
1829	First exchange transfusion was given in case of Rabies.
1840	At St George's School in London, Samuel Armstrong Lane, aided by consultant Dr Blundell, performed the first successful whole blood transfusion to treat hemophilia.
1867	English surgeon Joseph Lister used antiseptics to control infection during transfusions.
1873-80	US physicians transfused milk (from cows, goats and humans).
1884	Saline infusion replaced milk as a "blood substitute" due to the increased frequency of adverse reactions to milk.

Discovery of Blood Group

1900	Karl Landsteiner, an Austrian physician, discovered the first three human blood groups, A, B and O. The fourth, AB, is added by his colleagues A Decastello and A Sturli in 1902. Landsteiner received the Nobel Prize for Medicine for this discovery in 1930.
1907	Hektoen suggested that the safety of transfusion might be improved by crossmatching blood between donors and patients to exclude incompatible mixtures. Reuben Ottenberg performed the first blood transfusion using blood typing and crossmatching in New York. Ottenberg also observed the Mendelian inheritance of blood groups and recognized the "universal" utility of group O donors.
1908	French surgeon Alexis Carrel devised a way to prevent clotting by sewing the vein of the recipient directly to the artery of the donor. This vein-to-vein or direct method known as anastomosis. The procedure, however, proved unfeasible for blood transfusions, but paved the way for successful organ transplantation, for which Carrel received the Nobel Prize in 1912.
1908	Moreschi described the antiglobulin reaction.
1912	Roger Lee, a visiting physician at the Massachusetts General Hospital, along with Paul Dudley White, developed the Lee-White clotting time. Adding another important discovery to the growing body of knowledge of transfusion medicine, Lee demonstrated that it is safe to give group O blood to patients of any blood group, and that blood from all groups can be given to group AB patients. The terms "universal donor" and "universal recipient" are coined.

Use of Anticoagulant and Refrigerated Storage

1914	Long-term anticoagulants, among them sodium citrate, are developed, allowing longer preservation of blood.

1915	At Mt Sinai Hospital in New York, Richard Lewisohn used sodium citrate as an anticoagulant to transform the transfusion procedure from direct to indirect. In addition, R Weil demonstrated the feasibility of refrigerated storage of such anticoagulated blood. Although, this was a great advance in transfusion medicine, it took 10 years for sodium citrate use to be accepted.
1916	Francis Rous and JR Turner introduced a citrate-glucose solution that permitted storage of blood for several days after collection. Allowing for blood to be stored in containers for later transfusion aids the transition from the vein-to-vein method to direct transfusion. This discovery also allowed for the establishment of the first blood depot by the British during World War I. Oswald Robertson was credited as the creator of the blood depots.
1932	The first blood bank was established in a Leningrad hospital.
1937	Bernard Fantus, director of therapeutics at the Cook County Hospital in Chicago, established the first hospital blood bank. In creating a hospital laboratory that can preserved and store donor blood, Fantus originated the term "blood bank." Within a few years, hospital and community blood banks began to be established across the United States. Some of the earliest are in San Francisco, New York, Miami and Cincinnati.

Discovery of Rh Blood Group System and Isolation of Blood Components

1939-40	The Rh blood group system is discovered by Karl Landsteiner, Alex Wiener, Philip Levine and RE Stetson and was soon recognized as the cause of the majority of transfusion reactions. Identification of the Rh factor took its place next to ABO as one of the most important breakthroughs in the field of blood banking.
1940	Edwin Cohn, a professor of biological chemistry at Harvard Medical School, developed cold ethanol fractionation, the process of breaking down plasma into components and products. Albumin, gamma globulin and fibrinogen are isolated and became available for clinical use.
1943	The introduction by JF Loutit and Patrick L Mollison of acid citrate dextrose (ACD) solution, reduced the volume of anticoagulant, permitted transfusions of greater volumes of blood and permitted long-term storage.
1945	Coombs, Mourant and Race described the use of antihuman globulin (later known as the "Coombs Test") to identify "incomplete" antibodies.
1950	Audrey Smith reported the use of glycerol cryoprotectant for freezing red blood cells.

Use of Plastic Bags and Spreading of Blood Bank

1950	In one of the single most influential technical developments in blood banking, Carl Walter and WP Murphy, Jr, introduced the plastic bag for blood collection. Replacing breakable glass bottles with durable plastic bags allowed for the evolution of a collection system capable of safe and easy preparation of multiple blood components from a single unit of whole blood. Development of the refrigerated centrifuge

	in 1953 further expedite blood component therapy.
Mid-1950s	In response to the heightened demand created by open heart surgery and advanced in trauma care patients, blood use entered its most explosive growth period.
1960	A Solomon and JL Fahey reported the first therapeutic plasmapheresis procedure.
1961	The role of platelet concentrate in reducing mortality from hemorrhage in cancer patients is recognized.
1962	The first antihemophilic factor (AHF) concentrate to treat coagulation disorders in hemophilia patients was developed through fractionation.
1964	Plasmapheresis is introduced as a means of collecting plasma for fractionation.
1967	Rh immune globulin was commercially introduced to prevent Rh disease in the newborns of Rh-negative women.
1969	S Murphy and F Gardner demonstrated the feasibility of storing platelets at room temperature, revolutionized platelet transfusion therapy.
1970s	Blood banks move toward an all-volunteer blood donor system.

Development of Donor Screening Tests and Apheresis

1971	Hepatitis B surface antigen (HBsAg) testing of donated blood began.
1972	Apheresis was used to extract one cellular component, returning the rest of the blood to the donor.
1983	Additive solutions extend the shelf life of red blood cells to 42 days.
1985	The first blood screening test to detect HIV was licensed and quickly implemented by blood banks to protect the blood supply.
1987-2002	A series of more sensitive tests are developed and implemented to screen donated blood for infectious diseases: Two tests that screen for indirect evidence of hepatitis; the Human T-Lymphotropic-Virus-I-antibody (anti-HTLV-I) test; the hepatitis C test; the HIV-1 and HIV-2 antibodies test; the HIV p24 antigen test; and Nucleic acid amplification testing (NAT) that directly detects the genetic material of viruses like HCV and HIV.

The recent development in the field of Blood Banking is Cord Stem Cell Transplant. While most blood stem cell resides in the bone marrow, a small number are present in the blood stream. These multipotent peripheral bloodstream cells (PBSCs) can be just used like bone marrow stem cells to treat leukemia, other cancers and various blood disorders. The multipotent stem cell rich blood is also found in umbilical cord. This cord should be stored after the birth.

2005	Researches at Kingston University in England claim to have discovered a third category stem cell, derived from umbilical cord blood.
2007	In January 2007, Scientists at Wake Forest University led by Dr Anthony Atala report discovery of a new type of stem cell in amniotic fluid. In June 07, Scientist Shoukhrat Mitalipov report the first successful creation of a primate stem cell line through somatic nuclear transfer.

Discoveries and achievements after year 2007 are included in last chapter of this section, Recent Advances in Blood Banking.

CHAPTER 38

Organization and Operation of Blood Bank

Learning Objectives
- Present day multifunctional blood bank has to be properly organized and perfectly operated.
- This chapter discusses objectives and organization of blood bank, requirement of staff and equipments, and day-to-day operations of blood banks.
- This chapter also guides for documentation and record keeping in blood bank.

Keywords
Functions of blood bank, Licensing by FDA, Set-up and space requirement, Requirement of staff and equipments, Processing of donor blood, Component preparation, Pretransfusion tests, Quality control, Record keeping

INTRODUCTION

Blood is the lifeline of human body, supplying oxygen and other nutrition. An adult human body has approximately 5 liters of blood. This circulating liquid plays a vital role in survival of practically all tissues and organs of human body. The blood content is reduced in a disease process, accident and surgery. Blood transfusion plays a vital role in providing support to the treatment procedure. In recent years, blood transfusion services have become an integral part of the health care system.

With the emergence of transfusion medicine department, the definition of blood bank has changed. Today, it is not just a bank to collect and issue blood, it prepares and supplies individual blood component, to the patients as and when the need arises during the course of treatment.

OBJECTIVES OF THE BLOOD BANK

The primary aim of the Blood Bank is to provide quality medical care to patients by dispensing safe and good quality blood and its components for transfusions.
- Proper blood collection facilities.
- By proper donor selection.
- Safe procedures for bleeding donors.
- Promotion of voluntary blood donation and motivation of donors to return for donation.
- Ensuring confidentiality of donor record.
- Providing information to donors.
- Optimal testing, preservation and utilization of blood.
- Providing properly grouped and cross-matched blood.
- Detection of transfusion transmitted infections.
- Providing specially processed blood for patients requiring repeated transfusions.
- Ensuring optimal utilization of blood by preparing blood components.
- Proper preservation of blood.
- Prompt and appropriate disposal of unsafe blood.
- Promptly provide blood, round the clock.

MAIN FUNCTIONS OF THE DEPARTMENT

- *Proper donor selection*: Strictly follow all the norms for donor selection. The donor must be voluntary or friends/relatives of patient without any coercion on them. Promote voluntary blood donor and motivate them to continue the noble task of donating the blood. Professional donors should be identified and rejected permanently since their blood is of poor quality and carry infections of many diseases like HBsAg, HIV, HCV, syphilis, etc.
- *Proper blood collection*: Strictly follow the instructions for procedure of blood collection at each step. Take care that it should be finished in 8–10 minutes.
- *Blood grouping*: All blood units are processed for cell and serum grouping. Serum grouping confirms findings of cell grouping and also detects rare atypical antibodies. Confirmatory testing (Du test) is done on all units which test as Rh negative to rule out weak or partial Rh groups.
- *Detection of transfusion transmitted infections*: HIV, hepatitis B, HCV, syphilis and malaria. Each and every blood unit collected is tested.
- Providing specially processed blood for patients requiring repeated transfusions. For example, saline washed red blood cells.
- Ensuring optimal utilization of blood by preparing blood components. Almost all the blood collected is separated into the various blood components. By doing separation, we can satisfy many recipients from a single donor. Thus, ensuring optimum utilization of blood.
- *Proper preservation of blood*: All blood units are preserved at 2–6 degrees centigrade, in a well-designed walk-in cooler (Cold Room) equipped with a continuous temperature monitor and alarm facility. Plasma and cryoprecipitate are preserved in large freezers maintaining temperature below –30°C, while platelet concentrates are kept on a special rotator for continuous slow agitation which is essential for their proper functioning.
- *Prompt and appropriate disposal of unsafe blood*: All units of blood suspected to harbor infectious agents or be suboptimal for any reason are carefully autoclaved at the blood bank, disposed in biomedical waste and destroyed by incineration at the municipal incinerator.
- *Promptly provide blood, round the clock*: The blood bank crossmatches the blood of donor and recipient and issues blood continuously, all the twenty-four hours, thus making it available during all the emergency hours.

Organization of a Blood Bank

Legal set-up: Human blood is covered under the definition of 'drugs' under section 2 (b) of Drugs and Cosmetics Act. Hence, it is imperative that the blood banks need to be regulated under the Drugs and Cosmetics Act and rules hereunder. The license is granted for operating a blood bank by State Licensing and Central Approving Authorities (FDA—Food and Drug Administration department) after inspection. The processing of whole human blood for components needs separate license. The validity of a license is of five years unless it is suspended or cancelled.

Drugs Controller General of India has formulated a comprehensive legislation to ensure better quality control system on collection, storage, testing and distribution of blood and its components. The set-up of blood bank should be based on these legislations.

Norms to Set-up a Blood Bank

The criteria to set up a blood bank depend on the things like—whether it is attached to hospital, the level of hospital, what kind of patients are expected, and ultimately work load.

Following are the norms that should be followed during set-up of a blood bank:
- *Locations and surroundings*: The blood bank shall be localized at a place which shall be away from open sewage, drain, public lavatory or similar unhygienic surroundings. The wall and floors of the room shall be smooth, washable and such as can be kept clean. The employees should be free from contagious or infectious diseases.
- *Space requirement*: The space requirement again basically depends on the number of units of blood consumed per year. The minimum total area requirement is 100 sq m for whole blood bank operation and additional 50 sq m for preparation of blood components.
- *Blood bank premises design*: In planning, the design of a blood transfusion service, the activities and flow of operation should be considered for adequate utilization of space **(Table 38.1)**.

The functional plan of a blood transfusion service is thus based on the paths taken by

TABLE 38.1: Suggested area requirements for blood banks.

Working hours	Working 24 hours for 7 days		
Categories of hospitals with blood bank	3–7 UOB/Hospital Bed. 1000–6000 UOB consumed per year	8–15 UOB/Hospital Bed. 6000–15000 UOB consumed per year	16 UOB or more per Hospital Bed over 15000 UOB consumed per year
UOB (Units of Blood)	100–800 Bed Hosp. District Hospital Health Service Hospital Corporation Hospital No Super-specialties, Non-teaching	400–1000 Bed Hospital Medical College Specialized Hospital Teaching Hospital	800–1000 Bed Hospital Apex institutes. Metropolitan Medical Colleges Hospital All superspecialties Teaching Hospital, and blood bank
Donor complex (all in square meters)			
1. Reception room	25	25	40
2. Medical examination room		15	25
3. Blood collection room	40	55	100
4. Donor rest room	15	25	30
5. Kitchen/Pantry	5	5	10
6. Apheresis room			40
7. Quarantine storage		30	50
Laboratory area (all in square meters)			
1. Laboratory for routine donor work	25	25	30
2. Laboratory for routine patient and antenatal work		35	50
3. Laboratory for specialized	—	—	50
4. Emergency laboratory	—	—	20
5. Laboratory for transfusion transmitted diseases	20	25	30
6. Wash room, distillation plant, etc.	20	25	30

(Contd...)

(Contd...)

Working hours	Working 24 hours for 7 days		
7. Component basic and coagulation work	—	25	30
8. Component advanced freeze drying	—	—	100
General areas (all in square meters)			
1. Doctors office	15	15 × 3	20 × 1, 15 × 3
2. Donor recruiter, social worker, clerical staff	25	30	50
3. Blood bank office	15	20	25
4. Stores	20	25	35
5. Technicians' common room	15	20	25
6. Toilets	5 × 2	5 × 2	5 × 3
7. Trainee doctors' room			25
8. Library/conference room			30
9. Issue counter	18	20	20
TOTAL	**248 Sq m**	**460 Sq m**	**1000 Sq m**

the donors, the blood unit, blood samples and material.

- *Donor complex*: The donor complex will include:
  – Reception room: For all the activities of reception and to guide donor for further movement.
  – Medical examination room: For detailed history of donor and preliminary testing like Hb, blood pressure, weight, etc.
  – Blood collection room: For collection of donor's blood.
  – Donor rest room/refreshment room: To keep donor in resting position and have some refreshments after donating blood.
  – Kitchen/pantry: To prepare tea, coffee, and other refreshments for donor.
  – Apheresis room: This is required in superspecialties hospitals where apheresis is practiced.
  – Quarantine storage: For initial storage of blood (before testing) it should be in the vicinity of place where donor's blood is collected.

The flow of donors should be uniform and clearly defined to avoid unnecessary traffic in the corridors.

The donor complex should be pleasant and comfortable. Donor educational material can be made available to prospective donors in the reception or waiting room. The donor organizers should be associated with donor complex for donor motivation, recruitment and retention.

- *Laboratory area*:
  – Laboratory for routine work: For blood group (forward and reverse type) and crossmatching.
  – Laboratory for antenatal work: For platelets, HLA and granulocyte serology.
  – Specialized laboratory: Needed in superspecialty hospitals.
  – Emergency laboratory: Needed in superspecialty hospitals when work load is extra like in case of disasters.
  – Laboratory for transfusion transmitted diseases: For hepatitis, HIV, venereal disease research laboratory (VDRL) and malaria.

- Wash room: For washing and cleaning glassware. Distillation plant can be kept here.
- Component work: For separation of blood components.
- Component advanced: In superspecialty hospitals for freezing and drying.
• *General areas*:
  - Storage: To store processed blood
  - Issue counter: To issue the blood as per the need of patient
  - Doctors office
  - Donor recruiter, social worker, clerical staff
  - Blood bank office
  - Technicians common room
  - Toilets
  - Trainee doctors room
  - Library/conference room.

Requirement of Staff

Every blood bank shall have following categories of whole time competent technical staff:
- *Medical officer*: A person adequately trained and experienced in transfusion services should head it, preferably a MD in Transfusion Medicine or Pathology. The person appointed should have the authority to organize, manage, and collaborate and to ensure the fulfilment of safe blood transfusion services.
- *Trained technicians* in all areas of the work of the blood transfusion services along with technical supervisors where blood components are manufactured. He should have a Medical Laboratory Technician (MLT) degree with six months experience in testing blood/its components or diploma in MLT with one year experience.
- *Registered nurses*: Bachelor in Nursing with one year experience in blood banking.
- *Junior doctor*: A degree in medicine with or without experience.
- *Assistant medical officer*: A degree in medicine and having experience in blood bank for at least one year **(Table 38.2)**.

Requirement of Equipments

The blood bank should be equipped with the machines and instrument appropriate to its functions. The quality and quantity of equipment required depends on the number of blood units collected and procured, the techniques used, the infrastructure of the center and the size of the hospital **(Table 38.3)**.

All instruments must be properly maintained and regularly checked for their functioning. The staff must be familiar with the use of all the equipment.

Regular quality monitoring checks on the equipment must be done and recorded.

Uninterrupted power supply should be maintained for all the equipment with efficient back-up system. Intrinsic safety of the equipment and safety of its operation are essential.

Reagent Requirements

All the reagents and kits used in the blood transfusion service must be checked for reactivity, specificity and validity. The oldest reagents should be used first (first in, first out) and there should be a system to check when stocks are low. A regular supply of reagents and kits should be ensured. The antisera must be carefully stored and grossly checked on each day of use for any contamination.

■ OPERATION OF BLOOD BANK

Operation of blood bank is the study of different activities that are going on in a blood bank.
- Processing of donor blood
- Preparation of components
- Pretransfusion test of recipient
- Quality control.

Processing of donor blood: The donor is a voluntary or replacement donor (near relatives and friends of patient). When donor comes to blood bank, first he/she is medically examined by junior doctor, and asked to fill-up a donor form.

Now, predonation tests like BP, Hb, weight and blood group are performed. When donor

TABLE 38.2: Standard for staff in a blood transfusion service.

Working hours		Working 24 hours for 7 days	
Categories of blood bank	5000 donors units processed per year	10,000 donors units processed per year with round the clock service	20,000 donors units processed per year with round the clock service
Blood collection room			
1. Medical officer	1	1	2
2. Assistant officer		1	3
3. Jr Doctors/Residents	2	4	4
4. Nurses	2	3	4
5. Social Worker	1	2	3
6. Attendants	1	2	3
Apheresis room			
1. Nurse	–	1*	3
2. Attendant	–	1*	1
Laboratory			
1. Technician superviser	–	2	4
2. Tech. assistant	2	4	8
3. Technician	5 (+3 for shift works)	11	13
4. Laboratory Assistant	1	2	4
5. Laboratory Attendant	2 + (2 for shift works)	5	6
Donor organizer			
Associated clerical staff	–	1	2
Services staff/clerical staff			
1. Clerk/typist	1	1	1
2. Store keeper	1	1	1
3. Cleaner/sweeper	1	1	2

*If apheresis facilities are available.

is passed in all these criteria of donor selection, the blood is collected in a double, triple, or quadrate bags as per the requirement of blood bank with respect to available stock. After blood is collected, immediately seal the bag and seal the tube at least four places. The two pilot tubes are sent to two laboratories—the one with ethylenediaminetetraacetic acid (EDTA) anticoagulant is send to serology laboratory for blood grouping, where blood grouping (forward and reverse type) is done, along with the check of D^u for negative blood group. The other pilot tube without anticoagulant is sent to laboratory of transfusion transmitted diseases. Here the blood is checked for malaria, VDRL, hepatitis and HIV. Till all these processes of serology and transfusion transmitted diseases are done, the blood collected in bags are kept at initial storage at 2 to 6°C. Once, the results from all these tests are clear, the blood is further processed for component separation. In case, it comes positive for any transfusion transmitted diseases, it should be immediately destroyed. If components are prepared before serology testing and any of the unit show positive result then all components prepared from that unit are also discarded.

Component preparation: For component preparation, take out all the 'tested' bags from initial storage and proceed. From double bags, packed red cells and fresh frozen plasma are prepared. From triple bags, platelets, packed

TABLE 38.3: List of equipments/instruments needed in blood bank.

Donor room	Laboratory	Washing room

▪ Testing kit
  – Disposable lancets
  – $CuSO_4$ containing jars hematocrit weighing
  – Hemoglobinometer or hematocrit
  – Weighing scale
  – Clinical thermometer
  – BP instrument
  – Stethoscope
▪ Bleeding room
  – Donor cot
  – Disposable blood collection bag and set
  – Syringes and needles
  – Shaker
  – Blood bag weighing scale
  – Heat sealer/hand sealer and aluminum clips
  – Artery forceps
  – Khan tubes for collecting blood samples
  – Emergency kit
  – Oxygen cylinder
▪ Apheresis room
Blood cell separators and accessories
▪ General
  – Refreshments
  – Hot plate
  – Coffee thermos
  – Refrigerator
	▪ Blood bank refrigerators or walk in cooler
	▪ Deep freezer (–30°C and lower)
	▪ Incubator 22°C with Rotating shelves
	▪ Incubator 37°C
	▪ Water bath
	▪ Centrifuge
	▪ Automatic cell washer
	▪ Refrigerated centrifuge
	▪ Laminar flow
	▪ Microscope
	▪ Agglutination viewer
	▪ Rh viewing box
	▪ Micropipettes
	▪ ELISA reader
		▪ Autoclave
		▪ Hot air oven
		▪ Distillation plant
		▪ Pipette washer
		▪ Ultrasonic cleaner

*Besides these, glassware, office furniture and other instruments like telephone and computer are also required which are not listed.

red blood cells (RBCs), and fresh frozen plasma (FFP) can be prepared.

The component separation is done at different rotations for different length of times. Before putting the bags into centrifuge, balancing of bags is important. After separation of components the bags are separated, labeled properly and stored at respective storage temperature.

Pretransfusion tests of recipient: In a blood bank, when a person comes in need of blood or its component, he comes along with a sample of patient's blood. This blood is grouped and then crossmatched with the blood of same group in stock. For crossmatching with patient's blood, the blood present in tube of collected bag is used. Crossmatching major and minor both are done to ensure the results. Besides these, the pretransfusion tests also include antibody detection tests. Before issuing blood, all clerical checks are done properly.

Charges of blood and blood products quite vary according to the blood bank. But all the blood banks have adopted replacement policy. Friends or relatives of recipient are encouraged to donate blood to blood bank. This is to cope up with the huge requirement of blood and poor supply of voluntary donors. In case of emergency, person can get the blood by keeping some deposit to blood bank, but to get the deposited money back, he has to donate blood. Blood bank issues the crossmatching report of the blood to the patient together with the blood unit.

Quality control: To prevent any mishap and provide a safe transfusion practice a procedure of continuous monitoring of equipments, reagents and supplies, techniques, products prepared and the personnel must be carried out routinely. This practice of quality control is an assurance for accurate results. The quality control tasks include:

Environment monitoring, testing of the empty bags, documentation review, staff training and supervision, self-inspection and quality audit and equipment calibration.

Cleaning of glassware: Glassware used in blood transfusion laboratory must be cleaned thoroughly. Cell-serum mixture must not be allowed to dry on the glass.

Immediately after completion of any technical procedure, dirty tubes and slides should be placed in a suitable disinfectant. Buckets kept under the work benches containing disinfectants are convenient for this purpose.

Dirty glassware can give rise to erroneous results and/or may cause hemolysis of red cells.

DOCUMENTATION AND RECORD MAINTENANCE

Documentation provides the ability to trace prospectively and retrospectively all steps in all procedures, dating from collection of the blood to monitoring techniques, component preparation, laboratory testing, issue and transfusion of blood.

An effective record system helps to judge the performance of the blood transfusion service to trace any donated unit of blood from its source to the final fate and also helps in legal or investigational purposes.

Record Keeping

The record includes:
- *Donors record*: Blood donor, address and signature of donor with other particulars of age, weight, hemoglobin, blood grouping, blood pressure, medical examination, bag number and patient's details for whom donated (in case of replacement donation), category of donation and deferral records and signature of Medical Officer In-charge.
- *Master record for blood and its components*: It shall indicate bag serial number, date of collection, date of expiry, quantity in mL. ABO/Rh Group, results for testing of HIV I and II antibodies. HCV, malaria, VDRL, hepatitis B surface antigen and irregular antibodies.
- *Issue register*: It shall indicate serial number, date and time of issue, bag serial number, ABO/Rh Group, total quantity, name and address of the recipient, group of recipient, unit/institution, details of crossmatching reports, indication for transfusion.
- *Records of components supplied*: Quality supplied; compatibility report, details of recipient and signature of issuing person.
- Records of bags used with details of manufacturers, batch number and date of supply.
- Register for diagnostic kits and reagents used with details of manufacturers, batch number and date of supply.
- Records of purchase, use and stock in hand of disposable needles, syringes, blood bags should be maintained.

All records must include the date and signature of the laboratory staff performing the test. Records should be retained for at least 5 years and kept confidential. Computers are being widely employed in maintaining the records. With the growing demand for improving the efficiency, accuracy and effectiveness it has become imperative to introduce computers in the blood transfusion service. Blood Bank Management Software is now commercially marketed and provides facility to alter the software as per requirement and demand of blood bank.

Computers can help the functions of a blood bank in:
- Donor identification/registration
- Donor blood collection
- Processing of blood
- Maintenance of records of laboratory testing
- Inventory management
- Issue and labeling of blood.

CHAPTER 39

Immunohematology and Serum Immunoglobulin

Learning Objectives
- Immunohematology is application of immunology to hematology, which is commonly known as blood banking.
- This chapter covers basic introduction of antigens, antibodies and their reactions associated with immunohematology.
- Characteristics, functions and clinical significance of immunoglobulins is also included in this chapter.

Keywords
Antigens, Antibodies, Hemagglutination, Structure of immunoglobulins, Function of immunoglobulins, Characteristics of IgG and IgM antibodies, Clinical significance of IgG, IgM, IgA, IgD, IgE

■ INTRODUCTION

Immunology is defined as the study of resistance (immunity) to disease. Immunohematology is an application of the principles of immunology to the study of the red cell antigens and their corresponding antibodies in blood for resolving the problems of blood transfusion and some complications of pregnancy. Immunohematology is more commonly known as blood banking or transfusion medicine. This is the area of laboratory medicine dealing with preparing blood and blood components for transfusion as well as selection of appropriate compatible components for transfusion.

■ ANTIGENS

Antigens are foreign substances which when introduced into the body can provoke the formation of specific antibodies. Antigens and their specific antibodies react with each other when they come in contact.

In blood banking, red cell antigens are of main importance. White cells, platelets and biological fluids are also known to exhibit antigenic properties. RBC antigens are fixed protein or lipoprotein structures incorporated in the lipid membrane of the RBC. Formations of human RBC antigens are coded by specific nuclear DNA loci and composition known as *genes*. Since RBC antigens are DNA specific, if one is born with an antigen, he has it for life. More than 300 antigens have been discovered on the surface of RBC. Associated inherited variations of allied genes gives rise to the classification of antigens into associated blood groups, i.e. ABO, Rh, Kell, Kidd, Duffy, MNS and others.

Red Cell Antigens

High Frequency Antigens (Public Antigens)
Antigens with a frequency of >99% on human red cells, e.g. Kph, Jsh, Lub, k, vel, Ge, etc.

Low Frequency Antigens (Private Antigens)

Antigens with a frequency of <1% of human red cells, e.g., SW9, Js9, Kpa, etc.

■ ANTIBODIES

Antibodies are produced by circulating lymphocytes and plasma cells (immunocytes) in an individual following antigenic stimulation. The antibodies are immunoglobulins, present in serum and can be demonstrated serologically by reacting with corresponding antigen (immunologic reaction).

The antibodies are mainly of two types—natural antibodies and immune antibodies. The natural antibodies do not penetrate from mother to fetus and thus protects it from incompatible maternal blood.

The natural antibodies can be present naturally in an individual from birth, without any antigenic stimulation. These antibodies are generally of IgM type and with high molecular weight.

Immune antibodies are produced when the red cells carrying corresponding antigens enter into an individual, who normally lacks the antigen (e.g. anti-D). These are usually IgG type antibodies and react best at body temperature. These have low molecular weight. Immune antibodies produced by infectious agents do not interfere normally in blood banking procedure the exceptions are like mycoplasma and some of the bacterial infections.

Antibodies stay in the plasma and form a part of humoral system of the body. Hence, for the identification of the antibody, clotted blood, which yields the serum, is required. Most often the antibodies react specifically with its corresponding antigen that stimulated its production (e.g. D antigen with anti-D). Occasionally however, two antigens have certain chemical groups in common and an antibody made against one of them will react to some degree with the other. This apparent dual specificity is known as cross-reactivity.

Isoantibodies are produced in the same species as the antigen source. Anti-D (anti-Rh) produced by Rh negative individual, after receiving Rh positive cell is an example of isoantibody production. Heteroantibodies however, originate in species other than the source of antigen. The antihuman globulin used in the antihuman globulin reaction (Coomb's reaction) is an example of heteroantibody.

Reactions in Immunohematology

- The red cell antigen involved in the hemagglutination is referred to as agglutinogen.
- The antibody involved in the hemagglutination is referred to as agglutinin.
- The natural antibodies such as anti-A and Anti-B react with corresponding agglutinogens A and B in the saline medium at room temperature.
- The immune antibodies such as anti-D react only in albumin solution with incubation at 37°C.
- The hemagglutination reaction first results in coating of the antibody (adsorption) on the red cells, followed by bridging of the red cells and resulting agglutination.
- Some of the immune antibodies may not produce hemagglutination, but remain adsorbed on the red cells carrying corresponding antigens. This is called sensitization. These cells can be later detected by their reaction with antihuman globulin reagent.
- Visible hemagglutination reactions require proper proportion of antigen and antibody.

Immunoglobulins are glycoprotein molecules that are produced by plasma cells in response to an immunogen and these functions as antibodies.

Basic Structure of Immunoglobulins

- *Heavy and light chains:* The basic immunoglobulin unit consists of two identical polypeptide heavy chains (with high molecular weight: 55,000–75,000 MW) and two identical polypeptide light chains (with low molecular weight: 25,000 MW). Immunoglobulins are named according to structure of heavy chains. These five types of heavy chains are designated as alpha (IgA), delta (IgD), epsilon (IgE), gamma (IgG) and mu (IgM). The light chains are of only two types—kappa and lambda. The two light chains of every immunoglobulin will be identical, either kappa or lambda.

- *Interchain bonding:* The two heavy chains are held together by interchain bonding covalent bonds (disulfide bonds) and by non-covalent bonds. Within each chain there are also interchain disulfide bonds.
- *Variable and constant regions:* Each light chain contains 220 amino acids and each heavy chain has 440 amino acids. The first 110-120 amino acids of both heavy and light chains have a variable sequence and form variable region, which is considered to determine the antibody specificity. The rest of the light and heavy chains represent regions with constant amino acid sequence.
- *Hinge region:* This is the region at which the arm of the antibody molecule forms a Y. It is called the hinge region because there is some flexibility in the molecule at this point. In this region, enzymes or albumins act. The bonds in this region are all covalent bonds.
- *Fragments:* Each molecule of immunoglobulin is divided into three parts—one part of Fc and two parts of Fab pieces. The Fc is a insoluble fraction, which is crystallized in the cold (c for crystallizable) and Fab is a soluble fragment which is having ability of binding (ab for antigen binding).

Production of immunoglobulins: The immunoglobulins make up approximately 20% of total serum proteins. The introduction of red cell antigen into the circulation of an individual (lacking that antigen) may stimulate the production of a corresponding antibody. This may occur as a result of blood transfusion therapy or fetomaternal blood group incompatibility in pregnancy. These are called incomplete or acquired (IgG). Mostly immune antibodies are IgG that reacts best at 37°C and require the use of antihuman globulin serum for detection. Common immune antibodies react with Rh, Kell, Duffy, Kidd and Ss blood group system.

Certain antibodies occur without known antigenic stimulus. These are known as complete or natural antibodies (IgM, IgA). Common naturally occurring antibodies react with the ABO, Hh, Ii, Lewis, MN and P blood group systems.

Classes of Antibodies

- IgG—provides long-term immunity or protection.

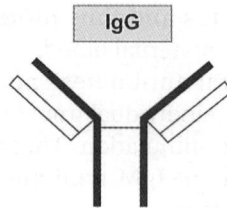

- IgM—first antibody produced in response to an antigenic stimulus.

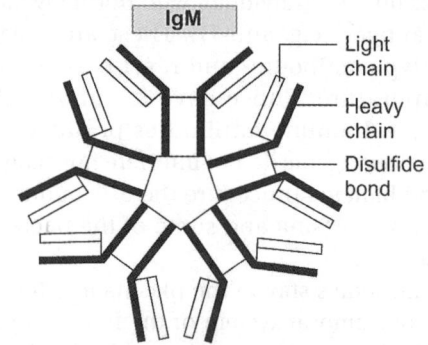

- IgA—found in secretions like tear, saliva, colostrums and mucus. Protects against infections in urinary, GI, and respiratory tracts.
- IgE—involved in allergic reactions.
- IgD—not much known about it. Surface receptor of B lymphocytes.

- Most important classes of antibodies in blood banking are IgM and IgG, and to a certain extent IgA.

Characteristics of IgG and IgM Antibodies

Significance in Blood Banking

Immunoglobulins have a great importance in immunohematology. Approximately one-third of anti-A and anti-B are IgA and two-third are IgM and occasionally IgG.
- IgG can cross placenta, hence plays an important role in HDN. IgM antibodies shows visible agglutination hence plays an important role in blood grouping.
- Clinical significance of red cell antibodies in blood bank depend on whether they can cause in vivo hemolysis, which in turn will cause transfusion reactions or hemolytic disease of the newborn.
- IgG will frequently cause in vivo hemolysis due to antibody coating the red blood cells.
- IgM, with a few important exceptions, usually does not cause in vivo hemolysis. The most important of these exceptions are ABO antibodies.

Size of the Antibodies
- IgG and IgA are relatively small since it is comprised of only one immunoglobulin subunit (monomer).
- IgG is Y-shaped and IgA is T-shaped.
- IgM is relatively large since it is comprised of 5 immunoglobulin subunits (pentamer).

Serum Concentration
- IgG is found in the largest concentration of all immunoglobulins in the plasma.
- IgM is found in relatively small amounts.
- IgA is a second most common serum immunoglobulin (IgG > IgA > IgM).

Complement Activation
- IgG = will do it if conditions are optimal.
- IgM = very good complement activator.
- IgA = does not fix complement unless aggregated.

Placental Transfer
- IgG is small enough to easily cross placenta and is the only immunoglobulin capable of doing so.
- IgM, IgA and the other classes do not cross placenta.

Optimum Temperature of Reactivity
- IgG = 37°C, IgA = 37°C.
- IgM = 4°C (may react at any temperature below 30°C).

Number of Antigen-binding Sites
- IgG has 2 binding sites.
- IgM has 10 binding sites.

GENERAL FUNCTIONS OF IMMUNOGLOBULINS

- *Antigen binding*: Immunoglobulins bind specifically to one or a few closely related antigens. Each immunoglobulin actually binds to a specific antigenic determinant. Antigen binding by antibodies is the primary function of antibodies and can result in protection of the host. The valence of antibody refers to the number of antigenic determinants that an individual antibody molecule can bind. The valency of all antibodies is at least two and in some instances more.
- *Fixation of complement*: This results in lysis of cells and release of biologically active molecules.
- *Binding to various cell types*: Phagocytic cells, lymphocytes, platelets, and basophils have receptors that bind immunoglobulins. This binding can activate the cells to perform some function. Some immunoglobulins also bind to receptors on placental trophoblasts, which results in transfer of the immunoglobulin across the placenta. As a result, the transferred maternal antibodies provide immunity to the fetus and newborn.

Clinical Significance of Immunoglobulins

Immunoglobulin G

Increases in:
- Chronic granulomatous infections
- Hyperimmunization
- Liver disease
- Malnutrition (severe)
- Dysproteinemia
- Disease associated with hypersensitivity granulomas, dermatologic disorders, and IgG myeloma
- Rheumatoid arthritis.

Decreases in:
- Lymphoid aplasia
- Selective IgG, IgA deficiency
- IgA myeloma
- Bence-Jones proteinemia
- Chronic lymphoblastic leukemia.

Immunoglobulin M

Increases (in adults) in:
- Trypanosomiasis
- Actinomycosis
- Malaria
- Infectious mononucleosis
- Lupus erythematosus
- Rheumatoid arthritis.

Note: In the newborn, a level of IgM above 20 ng/dL is an indication of in utero stimulation of the immune system and stimulation by the rubella virus, the cytomegalovirus, syphilis, or toxoplasmosis.

Decreases in:
- Agammaglobulinemia
- Lymphoproliferative disorders (certain cases)
- Lymphoid aplasia
- IgG and IgA myeloma
- Chronic lymphoblastic leukemia.

Immunoglobulin A

Increases in:
- Certain stages of collagen and other autoimmune disorders such as rheumatoid arthritis and lupus erythematosus
- Chronic infections not based on immunologic deficiencies
- IgA myeloma.

Decreases in:
- Immunologic deficiency states (e.g. dysgammaglobulinemia, congenital and acquired agammaglobulinemia, and hypogammaglobulinemia)
- Malabsorption syndromes
- Lymphoid aplasia
- IgG myeloma
- Acute lymphoblastic leukemia
- Chronic lymphoblastic leukemia

Immunoglobulin D

Increases in:
- Chronic infections
- IgD myelomas.

Immunoglobulin E

Increases in:
- Atopic skin diseases such as eczema
- Hay fever
- Asthma
- Anaphylactic shock
- IgE-myeloma.

Decreases in:
- Congenital agammaglobulinemia
- Hypogammaglobulinemia due to faulty metabolism or synthesis of immunoglobulins.

CHAPTER 40

ABO Blood Group System

Learning Objectives
- The ABO system is regarded as the most important blood-group system in transfusion medicine because, this is the only blood group system in which antibodies are consistently, predictably, and naturally present in the serum of people who lack the antigen.
- This chapter explains characteristics of ABO antigens and antibodies, inheritance of red cell antigens, production of A, B and H antigens and importance of blood grouping.
- ABO blood grouping system has 20 subgroups. This chapter has information on determination of subgroups and its importance.

Keywords
Landsteiner, ABO antigens and antibodies, Homozygous, Heterozygous, Dominant, Recessive, Transferases, Bombay Blood Group, Transfusion recipients, Transplant candidates and donor compatibility, Prenatal patients, Paternity testing, Subgroups A1 and A2, Determination and importance of subgroups

INTRODUCTION

A blood type (also called a blood group) is a classification of blood based on the presence or absence of inherited antigenic substances on the surface of red blood cells (RBCs). These antigens may be proteins, carbohydrates, glycoproteins or glycolipids, depending on the blood group system, and some of these antigens are also present on the surface of other types of cells of various tissues. Several of these red blood cell surface antigens that stem from one allele (or very closely linked genes), collectively form a blood group system.

There are nearly 300 blood group systems so far discovered. Of these ABO and Rh are major, universally adapted and medically important of all the blood groups.

ABO Blood Group

The ABO blood group was discovered in 1900 at the University of Vienna by Karl Landsteiner. All humans and many other primates can be typed for the ABO blood group. There are four principal types: A, B, AB, and O. There are two antigens and two antibodies that are mostly responsible for the ABO types. The specific combination of these four components determines an individual's type in most cases. The presence of antibiotics in plasma follows the Landsteiner's law which states that "the corresponding antibody is never present in serum of an individual when the antigen is present on his red cells."

Table 40.1 shows the possible permutations of antigens and antibodies with the corresponding ABO type.
- *A blood group*: People with blood group A blood will have the A antigen on the surface of their red cells. As a result, anti-A

TABLE 40.1: Presence/absence of antigens and antibody in ABO blood group.

ABO blood type	Antigen A	Antigen B	Antibody Anti-A	Antibody Anti-B
A	✓	×	×	✓
B	×	✓	✓	×
O	×	×	✓	✓
AB	✓	✓	×	×

antibodies will not be produced by them because they would cause the destruction of their own blood. Instead anti-B antibody will present in their plasma.
- *B blood group*: People with blood group B blood will have the B antigen on the surface of their red cells and anti-A antibody in their plasma.
- *O blood group*: People with blood group O blood will not have any of the antigen (A and B) on the surface of their red cells. The plasma of these people will have both the antibodies (anti-A and anti-B antibodies).
- *AB blood group*: People with blood group AB blood will have both the antigens (A and B) on the surface of their red cells. The plasma of these people will not have any of the antibodies (neither anti-A nor anti-B antibodies).

Characteristics of ABO Antigens

ABO antigens are glycolipid in nature, meaning they are oligosaccharides attached directly to lipids on red cell membrane. These antigens stick out from red cell membrane and there are many antigen sites per red blood cell (approximately 800,000).

Besides their presence on red blood cells, soluble antigens can be present in plasma, saliva, and other secretions. These antigens are also expressed on tissues other than red cells. This fact is important to consider in organ transplantation.

ABO antigens are only moderately well developed at birth. Therefore, ABO-HDN is not as severe as other kinds of hemolytic disease of the newborn.

Characteristics of ABO Antibodies

- These are expected naturally occurring antibodies that occur without exposure to red cells containing the antigen.
- These are immunoglobulin M antibodies, predominantly.
- They react in saline and readily agglutinate.
- Their optimum temperature is less than 30°C, but reactions do take place at body temperature.
- Not only are these antibodies expected and naturally occurring, they are also commonly present in high titer, 1/128 or 1/256.
- They are absent at birth and start to appear around 3–6 months as result of stimulus by bacterial polysaccharides.
- Besides humans, ABO antibodies are found in many animal species like sheep, goat, buffalo, pig, snails, chicken and also in the plant seeds (lectins).

Inheritance of Red Cell Antigens

To understand the inheritance of red cell antigens, it is important to know the terminology of inheritance:

Gene: It determines specific inherited trait (e.g. blood type).

Chromosome: It is a unit of inheritance. It carries genes. There are 23 pairs of chromosomes per person, carrying many genes. One chromosome inherited from mother, one from father.

Locus: It is site on chromosome where specific gene is located.

Allele: It is alternate choice of genes at a locus (e.g. A or B; C or c, Lewis a or Lewis b).

Homozygous: The alleles are same for any given trait on both chromosomes (e.g. A/A).

Heterozygous: The alleles for a given trait are different on each chromosome (e.g. A/B or A/O).

Phenotype: It is observed inherited trait (e.g. group A or Rh positive).

Genotype: It is actual genetic information for a trait carried on each chromosome (e.g. O/O or A/O).

Dominant: The expressed characteristic on one chromosome takes precedence over the characteristic determined on the other chromosome (e.g. A/O types as A).

Codominant: The characteristics determined by the genes on both chromosomes are both expressed—neither is dominant over the other (e.g. A/B types as AB).

Recessive: The characteristic determined by the allele will only be expressed if the same allele is on the other chromosome also (e.g. can type as O only when genotype is O/O).

The antigenic characters of red cells are inherited. The Mendelian laws of inheritance are applicable in the transfer of the antigen from the parent to offspring.

■ BIOCHEMISTRY OF THE ABO SYSTEM

The ABO antigens are terminal sugars (glycoproteins) found at the end of long sugar chains (oligosaccharides) that are attached to lipids on the red cell membrane. The A and B antigens are the last sugar added to the chain. The "O" antigen is the lack of A or B antigens, but it does have the most amount of next to last terminal sugar that is called the H antigen.

■ PRODUCTION OF A, B, AND H ANTIGENS

The production of A, B and H antigens are controlled by the action of transferases. The H, A, or B genes each produce a different transferase, which adds a different specific sugar to the oligosaccharide chain.

The procedure of formation of A, B and H antigens follows sequence of events:

1. Precursor chain of sugars is formed most frequently as either Type 1 or Type 2 depending on the linkage site between the N-acetylglucosamine (G1cNAc) and Galactose (Gal).

Type 1
Gal — G1cNAc $\beta1\to3$ Gal
$\beta1\to3$ linkage

Type 2
Gal — G1cNAc $\beta1\to3$ Gal
$\beta1\to4$ linkage

2. H gene causes L-fucose to be added to the terminal sugar of precursor chain, producing H antigen/substance (shown in below diagram of a Type 2 H antigen saccharide chain).

H antigen
Gal $\beta1\to4$ GlcNAc $\beta1\to3$ Gal
$\alpha1\to2$
Fuc

3. A gene causes N-acetyl-galactosamine to be added to H substance, producing A antigen (shown in below diagram).

A antigen
G1cNAc $\alpha1\to3$ Gal $\beta1\to4$ G1cNAc $\beta1\to3$ Gal
$\alpha1\to2$
Fuc

4. B gene causes D-galactose to be added to H substance, producing B antigen.

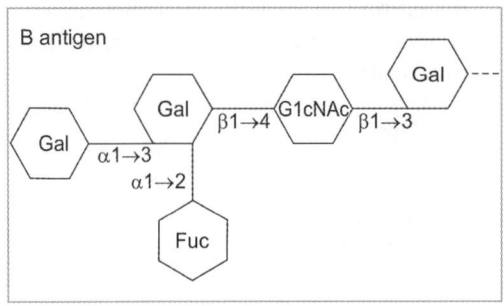

5. If both A and B genes present, some H-chains converted to A antigen, some converted to B antigen.
6. In absence of A/B gene, H antigen is not converted to A/B antigen. This results into O blood groups with H antigen.
7. If H gene is absent (extremely rare); no H substance can be formed. Therefore, A or B antigens are also not produced. Anti-H antibodies are present in serum. Result is Bombay blood group.

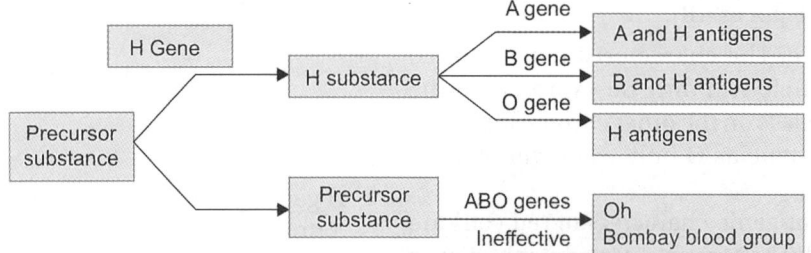

Importance of Blood Grouping

ABO grouping is required for all of the following individuals:
- *Blood donors*: Since we need to know the donor blood is ABO compatible with patient.
- *Transfusion recipients*: Since it can be life-threatening to give the wrong ABO group to the patient.
- *Transplant candidates and donors*: ABO antigens are found in other tissues as well. Therefore, the transplant candidates and donors must be compatible.
- *Prenatal patients*: To determine whether the mothers may have babies who are suffering from ABO-HDN. It is also beneficial to know the ABO group to prevent hemolysis.
- *Newborns (sometimes)*: If the baby is demonstrating symptoms of hemolytic disease of the newborn, the ABO group needs to be determined along with Rh and others.
- *Paternity testing*: Since the inheritance of the ABO blood group system is very specific, this serves as one of the first methods to determine the likelihood that the accused father is the biological father or not.

SUBGROUPS

The ABO blood grouping system has about 20 different known subgroups. The majority subgroups are of blood type 'A'. Among these, medically important are A1 and A2.

In 1911, Hirszfeld showed that there are two types of A antigen. The anti-A contains anti-A and anti-A1 *Dolichos biflorus*. The cells which are agglutinated by anti-A, but not by anti-A1 are A2 antigen cells and those agglutinated by both are A1 antigen cells. A2 cells can totally absorb anti-A from group B serum.

Thus, considering subgroups of A, there will be total six blood groups of ABO system: A1, A2, A1B, A2B, B and O.

TABLE 40.2: Difference between A1 and A2 subgroups.	
A1	A2
A1 makes about 80% of A blood type population	A2 makes about 20% of A blood type population
A1 red cells have about one million A antigens per cell	A2 red cells have only 2,50,000 A antigens per cell
A1 antigen have Type 2A, Type 3A and Type 4A antigens	A2 antigen has Type 2A antigens only
A1 red cells have less H antigens	A2 red cells have much more H antigens
Optimum pH for A1 transferases is 6	Optimum pH for A1 transferases is 7

A1 and A2 are qualitatively as well as quantitatively different **(Table 40.2)**.

Determination of Subgroups

This is most simply done by using the anti-A lectin, *Dolichos biflorus*. In the undiluted state, the lectin extract of *Dolichos biflorus* reacts as anti-A, since it agglutinates both A1 and A2 cells. When prepared at an appropriate dilution, however, the lectin reacts directly with A1 and A1B but not A2 or A2B red cells. If the red cells agglutinate, the person is subgroup A1. If no agglutination takes place, the blood is not A1, and most probably is group A2.

Other A Subgroups

A3 is a fairly rare subgroup (1/1000). The main distinguishing feature of A3 red cells is MFA (mixed field agglutination) with anti-A and anti-A, B.

AO(Ax): This is a rare subgroup (1/40,000). The main distinguishing features of AO cells are: the A antigen is so weak it may only be detectable by using anti-A,B; and anti-A1 is usually present in the serum. If anti-A,B is not used, AO cells may be mistyped as group O.

Am is a very rare subgroup. The main distinguishing features of Am cells are: no reaction with anti-A or anti-A, B in routine testing, and anti-A1 is not present in the serum.

Some of the other A subgroups are named A4, Abantu, Afinn, Aint (A1–A2 intermediate), Ael, Acl (various genotypes—AO1, AO1var, AO2), Aend, Ay, and Aweak.

Importance of Subgroups

The subgroups are important in blood transfusion. Anti-A1 may be present in A2 persons and also, weaker subgroups can be mistyped as O (relatively rare). If this mistyped group O blood is transfused to group O recipients whose serum contains anti-A, a transfusion reaction may occur.

Occurrence of A2 blood group is rare. The A2 antigen may give only a weak reaction with the usual anti-A serum. A special agglutinin obtained from seeds (lectin) with the specificity of anti-A1 will agglutinate all A1 cells but not A2 cells. Thus in a reverse grouping if the serum of an A blood group individual shows the presence of anti-A, agglutinating A cells the presence of anti-A1 may be suspected.

The group B also has similar weaker variants which are much less common. These are: B2, B int, B3, B x, B m.

CHAPTER 41

Rhesus Blood Group System

Learning Objectives
- The Rhesus system is regarded as the second most important blood-group system in transfusion medicine as it is an inherited protein responsible for hemolytic disease of newborn (HDN).
- This chapter describes Rhesus factor, characteristics of Rh antigens and antibodies, concept of universal donor and acceptor, CDE nomenclature and Wiener nomenclature.
- Information on Rhesus system inheritance and Rh variant is also included in this chapter.

Keywords
Rhesus factor, Alleles, Universal donor, Universal acceptor, HDN, Fisher-Race (CDE) nomenclature, Wiener nomenclature, Rh type mother-fetus incompatibility, Rh variant D^u

■ INTRODUCTION

The Rh (Rhesus) blood group system is clinically the second most important blood group system in the humans (after ABO).

The Rh system was named after Rhesus monkey (Rhesus macaque), since they were initially used in research to make antiserum for typing blood samples. In 1937 (published in 1940), Karl Landsteiner and Alexander S Wiener transfused the red cells of Rhesus monkey into the rabbit. The rabbit produced antibodies (anti-Rh) that were capable of agglutinating the red cells from Rhesus monkeys and also from many humans.

The term Rhesus blood group system refers to the five main Rhesus *antigens* (C, c, D, E and e) as well as the many other less frequent Rhesus antigens. The terms Rhesus factor and Rh factor are equivalent and refer to the Rh D antigen only.

■ RHESUS FACTOR

Individuals either have, or do not have, the Rhesus factor (or Rh D antigen) on the surface of their red blood cells. This is usually indicated by 'RhD positive' (does have the RhD antigen) or 'RhD negative' (does not have the antigen). This is often combined with ABO type and written as suffix to the ABO blood group. This suffix is often shortened to 'D pos'/'D neg', 'RhD pos'/'RhD neg', or +/−. The later is generally not preferred in research or medical situations, because it can be altered or obscured accidentally. The group O positive are most common in India.

Rh Antigens

There are five principal antigens that may be found in most individuals. They are:
1. D found in 85% of the population
2. C found in 70% of the population
3. E found in 30% of the population
4. c found in 80% of the population
5. e found in 98% of the population

(d) which has never been identified individually but refers to the 15% of the population who has no D antigen.

There are over 50 Rh antigens that have been identified including those that are either combinations of these antigens or weak expressions of the above antigens, but most Rh problems are due to D, C, E, c or e.

Alleles

The common alleles are:
- C and c are alleles with C^w occasionally seen as a weaker expression of C.
- E and e are alleles although E is seen only a third as often as e. The e antigen is referred to as a high incidence antigen since it is found in 98% of the population.
- D and the lack of D (or d) are alleles.

Characteristics of Rh Antigens

The Rh antigens are proteolipids and lack carbohydrates. These are made up of proteins of 417 amino acids. These proteins cross the red cell membrane 12 times. There are only small loops of the protein on the exterior of the cell membrane.

Therefore, the Rh antigens are not as available as to react with their specific antibodies and there are fewer antigen sites than ABO. Unlike the ABO system the Rh antigens are not soluble and are not expressed on the tissues. They are well developed at birth and, therefore, can easily cause hemolytic disease of the newborn, if the baby has an Rh antigen that the mother lacks. These are very good immunogens. This is especially true to D, which is the most immunogenic after A and B antigens. The Rh antigens are inherited.

Rh Antibodies

Characteristics

Anti-Rh is an IgG immunoglobulin of lower molecular weight. They are not naturally occurring and, therefore, are formed by immune stimulus due to transfusions. These are capable of crossing placenta and can cause hemolytic disease of newborn in an Rh-negative mother, bearing an Rh-positive fetus. Optimum visible immunologic reaction of these antibodies with the corresponding antigen takes place at 37°C in the presence of protein.

Although all Rh-negative individuals would be capable of producing anti-Rh, about 50–75% of the individuals will form anti-Rh when immunized with Rh-positive cells. These individuals are known as responders. The presence of anti-D in Rh-negative individuals creates problems during blood transfusion. For these persons, transfusion of Rh-negative blood is essential.

Importance of Rh Blood Group

The Rh blood group system is clinically very important because of two main reasons:
1. An Rh-negative individual if transfused with Rh-positive blood will form Rh antibodies in the majority (50–75%) of instances, which could lead to subsequent hemolysis.
2. Hemolytic diseases of newborn occur as a result of Rh incompatibility of the mother (Rh-negative) and the fetus (Rh-positive).

UNIVERSAL DONOR AND UNIVERSAL ACCEPTOR

Individuals with type O blood have red blood cells with neither antigen, but produce antibodies against both types of antigens. Therefore, a person with type O-negative (absence of Rh D) blood can safely donate to a person with any ABO blood type and is called a "universal donor". However, an O-negative person can only receive blood from another O-negative person.

Individuals with type AB blood have red blood cells with both antigens A and B, and do not produce antibodies against either antigen in their serum. Therefore, a person with type AB-positive (presence of Rh D) blood can safely receive any ABO type blood and is called a "universal recipient". However, an AB-positive person cannot donate blood except to another AB-positive person.

However in practice, transfusion with same blood group is indicated. Only in emergencies, one may practice this concept.

Rh Nomenclature

The Rhesus system has two sets of nomenclatures, one developed by Doctors Fisher and Race and one by Dr Wiener.

1. *The Fisher–Race (CDE) nomenclature*: This is more commonly in use today. It utilizes the CDE nomenclature. This system originally postulated that there are three closely linked genes on each chromosome. The genes were designated as D and its hypothetical allele d; C and its allele c, E and its allele e. Each gene was supposed to control the product of the corresponding antigen (i.e., D gene produces D antigen, etc.) However, the d gene was hypothetical, not actual.

   In this type of nomenclature, one gene codes for the protein carrying D expression; the other codes for the proteins carrying C or c and E or e expression. Rh-positive individuals have both a D and a CE gene while Rh-negative individuals have only a CE gene. Depending on which genes are present on a chromosome, eight common antigen combinations or haplotypes are possible: Dce, DCe, DcE, DCE, dce, dCe, dcE, dCE. Since every human being will contain any two of these eight genes, 36 possible genotypes combination could occur. D antigen is the most important Rh antigen. Presence of a single D antigen confers upon an individual the designation Rh-positive; its absence means that the person is Rh-negative. The letter d is commonly used to indicate the lack of D in Rh-negative individuals, but neither d antigen nor anti-d has been detected.

2. *The Wiener nomenclature*: The Wiener system used the Rh-Hr nomenclature. This system theorised that there was one gene at a single locus on each chromosome of the pair which controls production of multiple antigens. Wiener is convenient because it uses a single letter, R or r, with superscripts to name a 3 locus haplotype. It is possible to translate from one nomenclature to the other by remembering a few rules:

   In the Wiener system, D is indicated by an uppercase R and the absence of D is indicated by lower case r. The superscripts or numbers are used to indicate which Cc or Ee genes are present. Numbers are used with R and primes are used with r. The Dd position is numbered 0, Cc position is 1 and Ee position is 2.

   In the Fisher–Race system, loci are lined up in the order Dd, Cc, Ee (e.g., DCE).

   The Wiener superscript of 0, 1, and 2 indicates which of the Fisher Race loci is in its uppercase form (D, C, or E). For example, 1 or prime indicates that C is capitalized, while a 2 or double prime indicates that E is capitalized **(Table 41.1)**.

   DNA testing has shown that both theories are partially correct. There are in fact two linked genes, on chromosome 1, one with multiple specificities and one with a single specificity. Thus, Wiener's postulate that a gene could have multiple specificities (something many did not give credence to originally) has been proven correct. On the other hand, Wiener's theory that there is one

TABLE 41.1: Rh nomenclature and Rh D status.

Fisher race	Wiener	Rh D status
Dce	R^0	Positive
DCe	R^1	Positive
DcE	R^2	Positive
DCE	R^z	Positive
dce	r	Negative
dCe	r'	Negative
dcE	r''	Negative
dCE	r^y	Negative

	Father	
	D	D
Mother d	Dd	Dd
d	Dd	Dd

	Father	
	D	d
Mother d	Dd	dd
d	Dd	dd

Figs. 41.1A and B: (A) 100% RH⁺ children; (B) 50% RH⁺ children.

gene has proven incorrect, as has the Fischer-Race theory that there are three genes.

Notations of the two theories are used interchangeably in blood banking [e.g., Rho(D)]. Wiener's notation is more complex and cumbersome for routine use. Because it is simpler to explain, the Fisher–Race theory is more widely used. However, an abbreviated version of the Wiener system is useful to describe Rh genotypes.

■ RHESUS SYSTEM INHERITANCE

The Mendelian law of inheritance is applicable in the transfer of Rh antigen from parent to offspring. Inheritance of Rh group is independent of ABO group. Approximately 95% of the Indian populations are Rh-positive and 5% are Rh-negative. Among the Rh-negative, the frequency of cde is higher, while the other types are rare.

The Rh(D) antigen is inherited on one locus (on the short arm of the first chromosome, 1p36.13-p34.3) with two alleles, of which RH⁺ is dominant and Rh⁻ recessive. The gene codes for a polypeptide on the red cell membrane. Rh⁻ individuals (dd genotype) do not produce this antigen, and may be sensitized to RH⁺ blood, e.g., Rh negative mother and Rh positive father.

In the United States, 1 out of 1000 babies is born with this condition.

Rh type mother-fetus incompatibility occurs only when an RH⁺ man fathers a child with an Rh⁻ mother. Since an RH⁺ father can have either a DD or Dd genotype, there are two mating combinations possible as shown in **Figures 41.1A and B**.

Only the RH⁺ children (Dd) are likely to have medical complications. When both the mother and her fetus are Rh⁻ (dd), the birth will be normal.

The first time an Rh⁻ woman becomes pregnant; there usually are not incompatibility difficulties for her Rh⁺ fetus. This is because normally, anti-Rh⁺ antibodies do not exist in the first-time mother unless she has previously come in contact with RH⁺ blood. Therefore, her antibodies are not likely to agglutinate the red blood cells of her RH⁺ fetus. However, the second and subsequent births are likely to have life-threatening problems. The risk increases with each birth.

Placental blood vessels rupture normally at birth so that some fetal blood gets into the mother's system, stimulating the development of antibodies to RH⁺ blood antigens. As little as one drop of fetal blood stimulates the production of large amounts of antibodies. When the next pregnancy occurs, a transfer of antibodies from the mother's system once again takes place across the placental boundary into the fetus. The anti-RH⁺ antibodies that she now produces react with the fetal blood, causing many of its red cells to burst or agglutinate.

Rh Variant D^u

D^u is the weak expression of D antigen. The cells which are not immediately agglutinated by anti-D sera cannot be easily classified as D negative, because some of these agglutinate after addition of antiglobulin sera (Coombs' sera). This weak reactivity is termed as D^u. The genetically transmissible D^u is transmitted in Mendelian dominant pattern of inheritance. The gene in this case appears to be Ro (cDe) and this is referred as low grade D^u. The more commonly occurring D^u represents CDe gene which is referred as high-grade Du.

The D^u positive cells are likely to elicit an immune response in D negative individuals and the Du cells could be destroyed if the recipient is already immunized. Therefore, D^u positive donor is treated as D positive, and a recipient is treated as D negative. Hemolytic disease of the newborn has also been reported in the D negative mother with D antibodies due to earlier D^u positive baby.

CHAPTER 42

Other Blood Group System

Learning Objectives
- Besides ABO and Rh, eight other blood group systems are considered to be clinically significant as these are known to cause hemolytic transfusion reactions (HTR) and hemolytic disease of fetus and newborn (HDFN).
- Discoverer, location, alleles and characteristics of these eight antigens are interpreted in this chapter.
- This chapter also includes information on Bombay blood group.

Keywords
Lewis system, P system, MNS system, Kell system, Duffy system, Kidd system, Lutheran (Lu), Ii system, Public and private antigens, Bombay blood group

■ INTRODUCTION

The ABO and Rh dominate the human blood group systems, with A, B and D antigens. There are however more than 17 blood group systems and 400 red cell antigens recognized. Each blood group system consists of various antigens, and the majority of blood group systems inherit independently of other blood group systems.

■ OTHER TYPES OF BLOOD GROUPING

The more commonly encountered blood group systems include—Lewis (Le), P, MNSs, Kell (K), Duffy (Fy), Kidd (JK), Luthern (Lu), and Ii. These blood groups are not routinely determined in the blood bank except in the investigation of difficult cross matches and transfusion reactions. They are also clinically significant because the antibodies to some of these groups can be naturally present (e.g. anti-P) while others will develop following incompatible transfusion (e.g. anti-K). Some of them are also implicated in hemolytic disease of the newborn (HDN).

1. *The Lewis system*: The Le gene is present on chromosome no. 19. This system was focused on a single locus with two antigens, Le a and Le b. These antigens do not form an integral part of the red cell membrane, but are soluble antigens which may be present in body fluids and secretions. They are adsorbed on to the surface of red cells if they are present in the plasma in sufficient amounts. There are only three phenotypes: Le (a-b-); Le (a+b-); and Le (a-b+). Lewis phenotypes may change during pregnancy. Examples of Le (a+b+) are only transient. Lewis antibodies are only found in Le (a-b-) individuals, and are almost entirely naturally acquired IgM. They are the only blood group antibodies which have never been implicated in HDN.

2. *The P system*: This system was discovered by injecting animals with human red cells. P1 is the most common antigen which has

variable strength of expression. Anti-P1 may be naturally occurring. It is most often an IgM antibody. Individuals lacking P1 antigen but show to possess P antigen are called as P2 (P+P1-). All individuals are either P1 or P2 and complexities of P group are explained on similar basis are subgroups of A into A1 and A2. Anti-P1 is found in normal individuals with P2 phenotype and is active at 37°C. It does not cause clinically significant hemolytic reaction. Anti-P is the major antibody in P1k and P2k phenotypes and can cause hemolytic transfusion reactions (HTR).

Anti-PP1Pk (anti-Tja) is found in individuals with p phenotype and is usually (IgM types). This may cause HTR and its presence increases the risk of abortion in pregnant mothers.

Auto anti-P is found in the serum of the patients of paroxysmal cold hemoglobinuria.

3. *The MNSs system*: This system was discovered by Landsteiner and Levine (in 1927) by injecting animals with human cells. There are two loci—M/N and S/s. The antigens are M, N, S and s. The MN antigens are situated on glycophorin A and Ss antigens are situated on glycophorin B, respectively.

The antigens M and N are codominant alleles that are closely linked to the S and s antigens, which are also codominant. The homozygous individuals (MM/NN) show stronger agglutination than heterozygotes (MN) thus showing a dosage effect. Chromosome 4 contains these linked genes. These antigens are inherited by a complex pattern similar to the Rh system. The Ms and Ns linkage is more common than the MS and NS linkage. The U antigen is also related to Ss antigen as U negative individuals are also Ss negative.

Anti-M is naturally occurring antibody and is found more commonly than anti-N. Anti-M is predominantly IgM and Anti-N is IgG. Anti-M and anti-N are not usually clinically significant but HDN and HTR are known to occur. Anti-N has been traced in dialysis patients. The Ss antibodies may be either IgM or IgG type antibodies. These are clinically significant antibodies, formed in response to prior blood transfusion. These can cause HDN as well as HTR. The U antibody is known to cause HDN and rarely autoimmune hemolytic anemia in Ss negative U positive individuals.

4. *Kell system*: This system is named after the family of antibody producer Mrs. Kellacher. There are three pairs of alleles within the Kell system. Each pair has a high frequency and low frequency gene that are co-dominate if present. The three pairs are as follows:
   i. K (Kell), or K1, and k (Cellano), K2
   ii. Kp^a (K3) and Kp^b (K4)(Penney)
   iii. Js^a (K6) and Js^b (K7)(Sutter)

K, Kp^a and Js^a are low frequency antigens and k, Kp^b and Js^b are high frequency antigens. There is a Kell phenotype, K null (K_o or K5), is very rare and K, k, Kp^a, Kp^b, Js^a, Js^b antigens are not expressed.

The Kell systems antigens are found in only small amounts on the red cell carried on a single protein. K has approximately 3500 sites and k has between 2000 and 5000. The function of this protein is unknown.

Anti-Kell is the most clinically significant antibody within this system. The Kell antigen is considered the next most antigenic after the D antigen of the Rh system. Individuals lacking the K antigen can make anti-Kell after only two exposures to Kell-positive blood. These antibodies are IgG, can cause HDN and HTR (delayed) and does not show dosage (homozygous KK and heterozygous Kk cells react with the same strength).

5. *Duffy (Fy)*: This system is named after the family of antibody producer, Duffy. The Duffy antigens Fy^a and Fy^b are a pair of

codominant alleles found on chromosome 1. Biochemically the Duffy antigens are glycoproteins that have an external loop. This external loop can be destroyed by enzymes such as ficin, papain, and trypsin. The Fy^a and Fy^b antigens are receptors for the malarial parasite, *Plasmodium vivax*. Therefore individuals that are phenotypically Fy(a–b–) have a resistance to malaria. This particular phenotype is found up to 100% of western Africa. Four different types of phenotype are defined Fy(a+b+), Fy(a+b–), Fy(a–b+) and Fy(a–b–) in decreasing order of frequency. Duffy antigens are thermolabile and are inactivated by heating at 56°C for 10 minutes. Enzymes markedly reduce the activity of Fya and Fyb. Duffy antibodies are usually of IgG type and bind with complement to produce transfusion reactions. Anti-Fy2 is the most frequent antibody induced by red cell exposure which may cause delayed hemolytic transfusion reactions. Fyb antigen is a weak antigen and anti-Fyb is a rare antibody.

The Duffy antibodies are detectable only by indirect antiglobulin test and antibody reacts more strongly with homozygous cells as compared to heterozygous cells. The activity is enhanced by LISS and reduced pH of the suspending media. Both anti-Fya and anti-Fyb are known to cause HTR and HDN.

6. *Kidd (JK)*: Two antigens Jk^a and Jk^b are inherited on chromosome 18 where urea transport mechanisms are located. Three common phenotypes are Jk(a+b–), Jk(a+b+) and Jk(a–b+). Cells that are Jk(a–b–) (very rare) are less likely to lyse in the presence of high concentration of urea. These antigens are inherited by the codominant alleles Jk^a and Jk^b that are high frequency antigens. The kidd antigens are thought to be grouped very close together in clusters on the red cell membrane. Due to the close proximity of the antigens when the antibodies are attached complement can be activated. The activation of complement can cause intravascular transfusion reactions. Both anti-JK^a and anti-Jk^b are hard to detect and identify since they are very weak and are detected primarily at the antiglobulin phase of testing. These antibodies are usually low titer as well as being weak reactions. The antibodies disappear rapidly from circulation and also in stored serum since their recognition is enhanced if complement is present. These antibodies will often show dosage. Enzyme can enhance the reaction as well as PEG enhancement solution. These antigens are immunologically weak but are significant in clinical practice. JUdd antibodies are immune in nature and found in low titer for short duration after antigen stimulation. These antibodies may be either IgG or IgM which can bind complement and are detected by the antiglobulin test using polyspecific anti-human globulin. These may lead to delayed HTR and can cause HDN.

7. *Lutheran (Lu)*: Two common antigens Lua (Lul) and Lub (Lu2) are controlled by Lutheran gene located on chromosome 19 which is linked to secretor gene. Lu antigens are present at birth. Most common phenotypes are Lu (a–b+), Lu (a+b+) and Lu (a+b–). Lu (a–b–) phenotype is rarely encountered. The incidence for Lua antigen in India is 1: 200 and Luh is a high frequency antigen. Lutheran antibodies are uncommon and occur in low titre.

Anti-Lua may be IgG or IgM type which cannot cause significant HTR. It could be naturally occurring or produced by immunization. Anti-Lub is a rare antibody which reduced the survival of transfused red cells is reported to IgA in nature and may cause delayed transfusion reactions. These are found in Lu (a–b–) individuals following blood transfusion or pregnancy.

8. *Ii*: I antigen is present on the red cells in adults in varying strength and is expressed weakly on cord blood cells. The i antigen is

expressed strongly on cord blood cells and in neonatal red cells. The expression of i antigen decreases with age as the I antigen increases during first 18 months of age. Anti-I antibodies are IgM type and present in low titers in all individuals. The naturally occurring antibody is active at cold temperature and is not clinically significant. Anti-i may be found in patients suffering from lymphoma or infectious mononucleosis.

Many other blood group systems have been described, such as Xg, Ina, Bg, Diego (Di), cartwright (Yt), chido (Ch) and Roger (Rg), etc.

High Frequency Antigens (Public Antigens)

Antigens with a frequency of >99% on human red cells, e.g. Kph, Jsh, Lub, k, vel, Ge, etc.

Low Frequency Antigens (Private Antigens)

Antigens with a frequency of <1% of human red cells, e.g. SW9, Js9, Kpa, etc.

■ BOMBAY BLOOD GROUP

This is an extremely rare ABO group. It was first reported among some people in Bombay (now Mumbai) after which, it is called Oh or Bombay blood group. It is discovered in the year 1952 by Dr Bhende, Dr Bhatia and Dr Deshpande. It is also found in East Indians, Caucasians and Japanese, etc.

The red cells of the Bombay blood group peoples lack ABH antigens and their sera contain anti-A, anti-B, and anti-H antibodies.

The H antigen is a precursor to the A and B antigens. This is biochemically produced by the binding of fucose to the surface of glycoproteins, the process being catalysed by fucosyl transferase. The absence of the H antigen in the Bombay blood group attributed to the deficiency of the enzyme fucosyl transferase. As the H antigen is a precursor to the A and B antigens, there absence of A and B antigens.

Patients who test as type O may have the Bombay phenotype if they have inherited two recessive alleles of the H gene. Their blood group is Oh and their genotype is "hh" (homozygous for the silent h allele of the H substance) and so do not produce "H". Thus, both parents that carry this recessive allele are required to transmit this blood type to their children.

If proper blood grouping or testing practices is not followed, it can lead to people with Bombay blood group not being detected. During cell grouping or routine grouping, Bombay Blood Group would be categorized as O group because they would not show any reaction to anti-A and anti-B antibodies just like a normal O group. When a cross matching with different blood bags of O group is done, then it would show cross-reactivity or incompatibility. Therefore, reverse grouping or serum grouping has to be performed to detect the Bombay blood group.

Individuals with Bombay phenotype blood group can only be transfused with blood from other Bombay phenotype individuals. The incompatible blood transfusion can lead to a hemolytic transfusion reaction, which can be fatal and lead to death.

Around 179 persons in India with a frequency of 1 in 10,000 have "Bombay blood group" and registered at Institute of Immunohematology (IIH) for the further studies as well as for the information regarding donors of this group.

CHAPTER 43

Preparation and Preservation of Antisera

Learning Objectives
- Antiserum is a serum that contains immunoglobulin from blood of human or animals inoculated with an antigenic material or from those that recovered from a disease when they naturally developed certain antibodies against particular antigens.
- Antisera are used to determine which antigens are on the red cells. Antiserum is also used as an antitoxin or antivenom to treat envenomation in individuals bitten by a venomous snake.
- This chapter describes step wise preparation of antisera. It also has information on monoclonal and polyclonal antibody, and hybridomas.

Keywords
Antisera from lectin, Monoclonal and polyclonal antibody, Hybridomas

■ ANTISERA

A complete antisera is the serum of an animal, immunized by injection of serum from other animal.

Antisera in use are available commercially but can be prepared easily in laboratory from collected blood of immunized donors.

When collecting blood for antisera, collect blood in a sterile container without anticoagulant. Incubate at 37°C for 1 hour. to get good clot retraction. Leave the clotted blood at 4°C overnight to allow absorption of cold agglutinins on the red cells. Centrifuge the container and separate the serum in a second sterile container. If plasma pheresis is carried out, add one mL of 1 M $CaCl_2.6H_2O$ for every 100 mL of plasma to be defibrinated. Incubate at 37°C for 15-30 min allowing clot to form and retract. Separate the clear serum. To prevent bacterial contamination, use sterile procedures, add bacteriostatic sodium azide to achieve final concentration of 0.1% (0.5 mL of 20% sodium azide for every 100 mL of plasma) and store at 4°C.

This human serum is used to immunize animals to prepare antisera. For this, rabbit, goat, sheep, horse, donkey and chicken are in use. Rabbits being small and easy to handle are preferred, though goat gives 10 times more antiserum.

The inoculated animals produce antisera against human's serum. These antisera require standardising procedures, such as absorption to remove unwanted antibodies and dilution to adjust prozone.

Some of the antisera can also be prepared from the plants. Lectins are the saline extracts made from seeds that have ability to agglutinate the red cells. They are highly specific for known red cell antigens and hence are useful as grouping reagents.

The various lectins available with their specific activity are as follows:

Dolichos biflorus—agglutinates A_1 cell, *Ulex europaeus* is anti-H, *Vicia graminea* and *Bauhinia purpurea*—anti-N, *Iberis amara*—

anti-M, *Arachis hypogea*—anti-T and *Salvia sclarea*—anti-T. The extracts are easy to make, but the seeds may be difficult to obtain.
1. Grind seeds until course
2. Add 3–4 times their volume of saline
3. Incubate at room temperature for 4–12 hours stirring occasionally
4. Centrifuge supernatant for 1 minute and filter
5. Determine the activity

Dolichos extracts agglutinates A_1 and A_1B cells but not the A_2B or B cells. If all cells agglutinate add enough saline to dilute so that specific agglutination is achieved. The strength of agglutination of seeds extract is in following order: A_2, B, A_1, A_1B.

Store the extracts at 4°C. The shelf life is 1 year at least.

Monoclonal and Polyclonal Antibody

The antibody produced has a single specificity is called monoclonal antibody. The antibodies pooled from several immunized individuals having heterogeneous character are called as polyclonal antibody.

The monoclonal reagents are commonly in use for ABO, Rho (D) and antihuman globulin tests.

■ HYBRIDOMAS

The monoclonal antibody technique devised by Kohler and Milstein has proved useful in producing high-titer and specific antibodies. Laboratory animals, usually mice are immunized for the production of monoclonal antibody. After suitable immune response, mouse spleen cells containing antibody-secreting lymphocytes are fused to neoplastic plasma cells of infinite reproductive capacity from a mouse (i.e., myeloma cells). The resulting hybridomas are screened for antibody with the required specificity and affinity. The antibody-secreting clones may then be propagated in tissue culture or by inoculation into mice, in which case the antibody molecules produced by a clone of hybridoma cells are identical in terms of antibody structure and antigen specificity. Once one antibody-secreting clone of cells has been established, antibody with same specificity and reaction characteristics will be available for sure. These will be available indefinitely.

Selection of Antisera

There is broad variety of antisera available in market. Following points should be considered while selecting antisera for laboratory use:
- Antisera must be of high quality with a shelf life of at least one year of use and should be received in cold chain
- Should contain a preservative to minimize contamination
- Should be stored in the refrigerator at 2–8°C
- Should be used according to manufacturer's instructions
- Should be clearly labeled with batch number, expiry date, and storage temperature
- Appearance reagent must be clear. No turbidity, precipitate, particles on visual inspection
- Must comply with the standards laid down for potency (titer and avidity) and specificity
- Specificity is clear-cut reaction with RBC bearing the corresponding antigen(s)
- Titer is the highest dilution of the antisera at which the macroscopic agglutination is seen at strength of 1+
- Avidity means the overall strength of reaction between antigen and antibody. It is measured by the time duration in seconds for the appearance of macroscopic agglutination.

New reagents should not be introduced into routine work until internal QC testing have confirmed that they are satisfactory.

CHAPTER 44

Technique of Blood Grouping and Crossmatching

Learning Objectives
- A blood grouping is a classification of blood, based on the presence and absence of antibodies. Crossmatching is a test done to check if donor's blood is compatible to recipient or not.
- In this chapter, principle and procedure of both methods—tube method and slide method of blood grouping are explained.
- Interpretation of procedure of crossmatching, its importance and limitations are discussed here.

Keywords
Anti sera-A, Anti sera-B, Agglutination, Forward and reverse grouping, Rh blood typing, Anti sera-D, Major crossmatch, Minor crossmatch, Reasons for blood typing and crossmatching, Limitations of crossmatching, Coomb's crossmatch

ABO BLOOD GROUPING

Introduction

A person's ABO blood group—A, B, AB, or O is based on the presence or absence of the A and B antigens on his red blood cells. The A blood type has only the A antigen and the B blood type has only the B antigen. The AB blood type has both A and B antigens, and the O blood type has neither A nor B antigen.

By the time a person is six months old, he naturally will have developed antibodies against the antigens his red blood cells lack. That is, a person with A blood type will have anti-B antibodies, and a person with B blood type will have anti-A antibodies. A person with AB blood type will have neither antibody, but a person with O blood type will have both anti-A and anti-B antibodies. Although the distribution of each of the four ABO blood types varies between racial groups, O is the most common and AB is the least common.

The ABO grouping is the first test done on blood when it is tested for transfusion.

Principle

This ABO grouping test is based on the principle of hemagglutination reaction. Hemagglutination of red cells occur when the red cell antigens (agglutinogens) react with corresponding antibody—(a) positive agglutination is observed by the clumping of red cells as seen on slide or by button formation in the test tube, (b) negative reaction is observed by uniform distribution of red cells on slide and lack of button formation in test tube.

Procedure

There are two basic methods to observe the hemagglutination reactions in ABO blood grouping—(i) slide method and (ii) test tube method. Former is easier to perform and the latter is more sensitive. Many laboratories of developing countries perform the tube test only in case the result of the slide test is doubtful. However, tube method is recommended for reliable results as per FDA approved guidelines.

Slide Method

Requirement

Glass slides, pastuer pipettes, applicator sticks and centrifuge.

Reagents

- **Anti-A sera (blue color):** Human polyclonal or murine monoclonal.
- **Anti-B sera (yellow color):** Human polyclonal or murine monoclonal.
- **Normal saline:** 0.9 g/dL sodium chloride in distilled water.

Specimen

Clotted blood is generally used. Centrifuge the clotted blood at 1500 rpm for few minutes to separate serum. With the help of Pastuer pipette, separate the red cells from the clot and suspend them in saline. Anticoagulated blood with proper anticoagulant like EDTA can be used. Store the specimen at 2–8°C if there is any delay in examination.

Blood obtained by finger puncture may be tested directly by the slide method. To avoid clotting of the collected blood (on the slide), it should be mixed quickly with antisera.

Procedure

1. Prepare a 10% suspension of red blood cells in normal saline as follows: (i) Mix 0.05 mL (5 drops) of sedimented red cells with 2 mL of normal saline, (ii) Centrifuge at 1,500 rpm for 1 to 2 minutes. Discard supernatant, (iii) Add 2 mL of normal saline to the sedimented red cells. Mix well. This gives a 10% suspension of red cells.
2. On one-half of a glass slide, place 1 drop of anti-A sera.
3. On the other half slide, place 1 drop of anti-B sera.
4. Using Pastuer pipette add one drop of the red cell suspension to each half of the slide.

TABLE 44.1: Reaction of antisera with respective blood group.

Reaction: Anti-A	Reaction: Anti-B	Blood group	Agglutination pattern
+	–	A	
–	+	B	
+	+	AB	
–	–	O	

+, Agglutination present; –, No agglutination
(For color version See Color Plate 8)

5. With separate applicator sticks, mix each cell serum mixture well.
6. Tilt the slide back and forth and observe for agglutination.

Interpretation

- Tests that show no agglutination within two minutes are considered negative **(Table 44.1)**
- Do not interpret peripheral drying or fibrin stands as agglutination.

Tube Method

Requirements

- Test tubes (10 × 75 mm or 12 × 75 mm)
- Microscope

Procedure

1. Prepare a 5% suspension of red blood cells in normal saline as follows: (i) Mix 0.05 mL (5 drops) of sedimented red cells with 2 mL of normal saline, (ii) Centrifuge at 1,500 rpm for 1 to 2 minutes. Discard supernatant, (iii) Add 4 mL of normal saline to the sedimented red cells. Mix well. This gives a 5% suspension of red cells.
2. To a small test tube, add one drop of anti-A sera.

TABLE 44.2: Agglutination reaction in cell and serum grouping.

Cell grouping			Serum grouping			Interpretation
Anti-A	Anti-B	Anti-AB	A cells	B cells	O cells	
+	–	+	–	+	–	A
–	+	+	+	–	–	B
+	+	+	–	–	–	AB
–	–	–	+	+	–	O
–	–	–	+	+	+	Bombay blood group

+, Agglutination present; –, No agglutination

3. To a second test tube, add one drop of anti-B sera.
4. Using a Pasteur pipette, add one drop of 5% red cell suspension to each of the two test tubes.
5. Mix well and centrifuge both the tubes at 1,500 rpm for one min or incubate at room temperature for one min.
6. Examine for agglutination: If the tube is centrifuged red cell sediment will be seen at the bottom of the tube, which is called a button. Gently tap the button from the tube by a spring action of right index finger and dislodge the cell button.
   If, red cells form one or more clumps wih clear supernatant fluid, the agglutination is present.
   If, red cells re-suspend easily, without any visible clumping, agglutination is absent.
7. In case of any doubt, take a drop of the suspension on a slide and observe under the 10× objective for agglutination.

Forward and Reverse Grouping

To determine ABO blood group, there are two ways:
1. When the individuals red cells are tested with a known anti-A and anti-B sera, this procedure (as described above) is called forward grouping or front typing or cell typing.
2. When the individuals serum is tested with known group A cells and group B cells, the procedure is called reverse grouping or back typing or serum typing **(Table 44.2)**.

RH BLOOD TYPING

Rh typing (also called as Rh blood grouping) is next important to ABO blood grouping. It detects only the presence of Rh antigen (or D antigen) out of all Rh factors on the red cells.

Principle

It is based on the principle of hemagglutination that the red cells with Rh antigen (D antigen) will clump with anti-D antiserum at room temperature in presence of protein. The technique is similar to ABO blood grouping and hence, Rh typing is done along with ABO blood grouping.

Procedure

The Rh typing can also be done by two methods: (i) Slide method and (ii) Tube method.

Slide Method

Requirements

Same as that of ABO slide method.

Reagents

- Anti-D sera (human polyclonal or human monoclonal).
- Normal saline

Specimen

Same as that of ABO method.

Procedure

1. On a pre-warmed glass slide, place one drop of anti-D serum.

2. By using a Pastuer pipette add one drop of 10% suspension of red blood cells (in case of anemic patients, use one drop of sedimented red cells).
3. With an applicator stick, mix cell–serum mixture well.
4. Tilt the slide back and forth and observe for agglutination.
5. Tests that show no agglutination within two minutes are considered negative.

Tube Method

Requirements

Same as that of ABO tube method.

Reagents

- Anti-D sera (human polyclonal or human monoclonal).
- Normal saline.

Specimen

Same as that of ABO method.

Procedure

1. Prepare a 5% suspension of red blood cells in normal saline.
2. To a test tube add one drop of anti-D serum.
3. Add one drop of cell suspension with the help of Pastuer pipette.
4. Mix well and centrifuge both the tubes at 1,500 rpm for one min. or incubate at room temperature for one min.
5. Examine the agglutination reaction in each tube by dislodging the button gently. If necessary, use a magnifying hand lens.
6. Interpretation: Agglutination will be recognised by the formation of small clumps in a clear liquid. As the bottom of the test tube is tapped, the clumps whirl up and then settle down. This will be marked as positive reaction and the cells are identified as Rh-positive. If the red cells resuspend homogeneously with no visible clumps, it should be marked as negative reaction and the cells are identified as Rh-negative.
7. All the Rh negative cells must be tested for D^u.

■ CROSSMATCHING

Crossmatching is the final step in the pretransfusion testing. It is commonly referred to as compatibility testing.

For the safe transfusion, blood group of donor and recipient must be same and match according to the antigen and antibody in blood (*in vivo*). If the blood groups are matched (*in vitro*), there are 99% chances of their compatibility. However, there are some occasions, in which though, blood groups are matched, but crossmatching is incompatible. These are—(a) The donor may have unexpected antibodies in his serum or (b) The patient may have unexpected antibodies in his serum or (c) There may have been a mistake in performing, reading or recording of the blood grouping and Rh typing results.

Considering all these possibilities, a compatibility test is essential before all transfusions.

This procedure is performed in two parts:
1. *Major crossmatch*: The donors cells are mixed with the patient's serum. This brings reaction of donors red cells with patients serum or plasma to detect antibodies that could destroy donors red cells **(Fig. 44.1A)**.
2. *Minor crossmatch*: The patient's cells are mixed with the donor's serum/plasma. This brings reaction of patients' red cells with donor serum or plasma to detect antibodies that would destroy patients' red cells **(Fig. 44.1B)**.

Requirements

- Small test tubes (10 × 75 mm)
- Pasteur pipettes
- Normal saline
- Centrifuge.

Specimen

- Patient's blood and serum
- Donor's blood and serum/plasma.

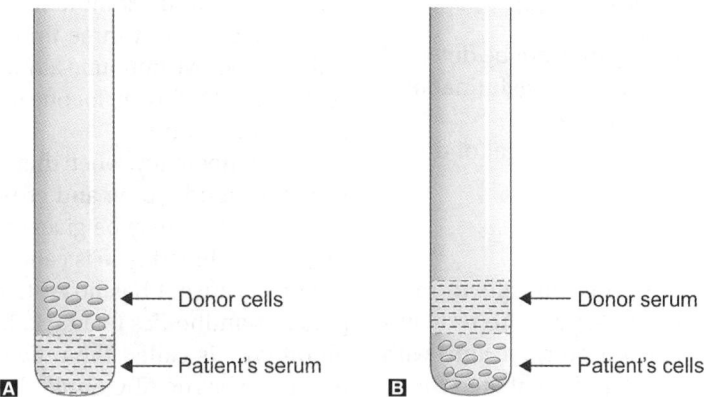

Figs. 44.1A and B: (A) Major crossmatch; (B) Minor crossmatch.

Procedure

1. Prepare 5% cell suspensions of patient's blood (P) and donor's blood (D) in two separate tubes.
2. To the patient's tube (P), add two drop of patient's serum and one drop of donor cell suspension (major crossmatch).
3. To the donor's tube (D), add two drops of donor's serum and one drop of patient's cell suspension (minor crossmatch).
4. Mix the contents of the tubes gently and keep the tubes at room temperature for 30 minutes. Centrifuge at 1500 rpm for one minute.
5. Examine for the agglutinations both macroscopically and also microscopically.

Interpretation

1. Blood which shows a major incompatibility should never be transfused.
2. The minor crossmatch results are also important. But in an emergency it is possible to use blood which is minor incompatible, (but not major incompatible) without leading to a transfusion reaction. This is because of the fact that, in patient's body the 'minor side" would be the donor plasma (about 200–300 mL). This may contain the antibodies. But these antibodies will get mixed and diluted with about 2500 mL of patient's serum so that there will not be a major reaction. Only following two conditions may show significant incompatibility:
   i. High titer of donor antibodies and
   ii. Multiple transfusions of minor incompatible blood.

The saline tube method requires longer incubation but weak reactions are detected better by this method.

Reasons for Blood Typing and Crossmatching

- Avoid a transfusion reaction in a previously sensitized patient.
- Prevent formation of isoantibodies which may cause a delayed transfusion reaction and subsequent haemolytic anemia.
- Provide maximum survival of transfused cells.
- Prevent sensitization of recipient to future incompatible transfusions.
- Avoid sensitization of future breeding stock and subsequent hemolytic disease of newborns through receiving colostral antibodies.

Limitations of Crossmatching

- Hemolyzing antibody may not be detected in a crossmatch looking for agglutination.
- Will not detect clinical errors.
- Does not guarantee the survival of donor cells.

Coombs' Crossmatch

For faster results, use the red cells in thermophase with protein. Where the red cells are suspended in the antibody (serum) with 22% albumin (protein) and incubated for 30 minutes at 37°C. Now centrifuge at 1500 rpm for one min and examine for agglutination. If negative, wash it three times with normal saline to remove unbound albumin. Add AHG, centrifuge at 1500 rpm for one minute and look for agglutination.

In an emergency, when there is not enough time for blood typing and crossmatching, O red blood cells may be given, preferably Rh-negative. O blood type is called the universal donor because it has no ABO antigens for a patient's antibodies to attack. In contrast, AB blood type is called the universal recipient because it has no ABO antibodies to attack the antigens on transfused red blood cells.

CHAPTER 45

Coombs' Test

Learning Objectives
- Coombs tests are done to find certain antibodies that attack red blood cells. This is very helpful to diagnose hemolytic anemia.
- This chapter has explanation of principle and stepwise description of procedure of direct and indirect Coomb's test.
- Determination of D^u and principle and procedure of antibody titration is also explained in this chapter.

Keywords
Direct Coomb's test (DCT) Antihuman globulin (AHG), Hemagglutination, Autoimmune hemolytic anemia, Erythroblastosis fetalis, Hemolytic disease, D^u factor, Antibody titration, Avidity

▌ INTRODUCTION

The Coombs' test was first described in 1945 by Cambridge immunologists Robin Coombs (after whom it is named), Arthur Mourant and Rob Race. Historically, it was done in test tubes. Today, it is commonly done using microarray and gel technology.

The two Coombs tests are:
1. Direct Coombs test (also known as direct antiglobulin test or DAT).
2. Indirect Coombs test (also known as indirect antiglobulin test or IAT).

▌ DIRECT COOMBS' TEST

The direct Coombs' test is (DCT) used to detect autoantibodies on the surface of red blood cells. Many diseases and drugs (quinidine, methyldopa, and procainamide) can lead to production of these antibodies. These antibodies sometimes destroy red blood cells and cause anemia. This test is sometimes performed to diagnose the cause of anemia or jaundice.

Principle

The direct Coombs' test is a test of whether IgG antibodies are already attached directly to the patients red cells. The test is based on the fact that, serum containing anti-human IgG, is added to patients red cell. The anti-human antibodies are produced by immunizing laboratory animals (e.g., rabbit, sheep, goat, horse, donkey and chicken) with human serum. The mixture is observed for agglutination. If human IgG antibody has already attached to the patient's red cells in vivo (in the bloodstream), then the addition of anti-human IgG will cause the cells to agglutinate.

This is a positive direct antihuman globulin test (DAT) or a positive direct Coombs test.

Requirements

Test tubes, centrifuge

Reagents

- Antihuman globulin (AHG) reagent
- Presensitized red cells (Coombs' control cells)
- Saline

Procedure

1. Wash the red cells suspected of being sensitized, 3 to 4 times in large volume of saline. Complete removal of free globulin is important.
2. Add two drops of antihuman globulin serum to the sedimented cells.
3. Mix well and centrifuge at 1500 rpm for 1 minute.
4. Examine agglutination by holding against a lighted background and tapping the bottom of the tube.
5. If the agglutination is not seen, leave the tube at room temperature for 10 minutes then re-centrifuge and read. A weaker reacting antibody will show delayed reaction. Consider this as positive **(Fig. 45.1)**.
6. If hemagglutination is not seen in step 5, add one drop of presensitized red blood cells (5% suspension is saline). This should result in hemagglutination of presensitized cells indicating that the AHG is reactive and the result is valid.

Interpretation

Hemagglutination of red cells with the addition of AHG (positive) indicates that the cells are sensitized inside the body.

Positive Coombs' test means patient have antibody that acts against his own RBC. This may be due to:

- Autoimmune hemolytic anemia without another underlying cause.
- Drug-induced hemolytic anemia (many drugs have been associated with this complication).
- Erythroblastosis fetalis (hemolytic disease of the newborn)
- Infectious mononucleosis
- Mycoplasmal infection
- Syphilis

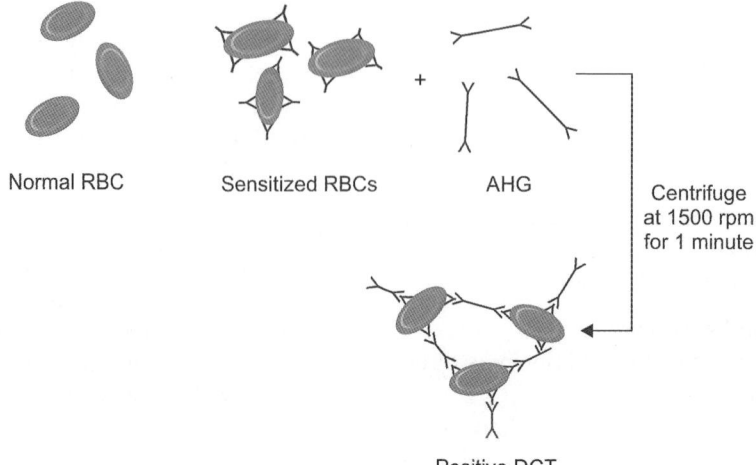

Fig. 45.1: Positive direct Coombs' test.

- Chronic lymphocytic leukemia or other lymphoproliferative disorder.
- Systemic lupus erythematosus or another rheumatologic condition.
- Transfusion reaction, such as one due to improperly matched units of blood.

■ INDIRECT COOMBS' TEST

The indirect Coombs' test (ICT) looks for anti-RBC antibodies that flow freely in blood serum. The indirect Coombs' test is only rarely used to diagnose a medical condition. More frequently, it is used to determine a reaction.

Principle

The indirect Coombs' test determines whether there are free IgG antibodies in the patient's serum, as opposed to being on the red cells. The test is called indirect because, in this test the red cells are first sensitized in laboratory and then detected by direct Coombs' test.

When a person's serum is suspected to be having some 'incomplete antibodies', such serum is mixed with cell-suspension of cells known to have antigen corresponding to the suspected antibody. After incubation at a temperature appropriate for the suspected antibody for an appropriate time the cells are washed and direct Coombs' test is performed.

Requirements and Reagents

Same as that of direct Coombs' test.

Procedure

1. Prepare a 4% saline suspension of the test cells.
2. Add two drops of cell suspension to a small test tube.
3. Add two drops of antiserum to the cell suspension.
4. Incubate in a water bath at 37°C for 30 minutes.
5. Remove the tube from the water bath and wash 3–4 times with large volume of saline. Decant completely after last washing.
6. Add immediately two drops of antihuman globulin (AHG) and mix well.
7. Centrifuge at 1500 rpm for 1 minutes.
8. Examine for hemagglutination **(Fig. 45.2)**.
9. In case of negative hemagglutination, add presensitized reagent cells or Coombs'

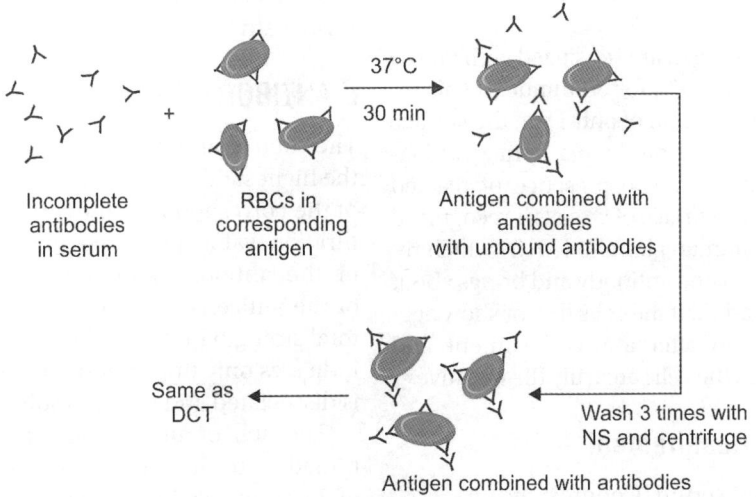

Fig. 45.2: Positive indirect Coombs' test.

control cells to test the reactivity of AHG. Agglutination must be seen with the addition of Coombs' control cells.

Positive indirect Coombs' test means patient have antibodies that the body views as foreign. This may be due to:
- Erythroblastosis fetalis hemolytic disease.
- Incompatible blood match (when used in blood banks).
- Autoimmune or drug-induced hemolytic anemia.

Precautions while performing the test:
- *Proportion of serum to cells*: 1 drop of 2.5% cells + 2 drops of serum.
- *Incubation temperature*: Optimum reacting temperature for antibody is 37°C.
- *Incubation time*: 30–40 minutes for 1 drop of 5% cells with two drops of serum.
- *Cell wash*: It is must to prevent neutralization of AHG by free antibody in serum.

■ DETERMINATION OF D^u

Indirect Coombs' test is applied in D^u testing. D^u factor is variant of D antigen present on the red cells of individuals of D^u blood type.

Principle

Cells with D^u antigen are sensitized with anti-D by incubating at 37°C for 30 minutes. This results in the adsorption of anti-D on the surface of the cell without producing hemagglutination (sensitization). The presence of reacted antibody on the surface of D^u cells is recognized by using antihuman globulin (AHG) which reacts with the coated antibody and brings about hemagglutination. If the cells do not show agglutination, even after anti-D treatment and AHG reaction, the cells are truly Rh-negative.

Additional Requirement

- Antihuman serum (Coombs' serum)
- Bovine albumin, 22% (control)
- Incubator or water bath (37°C)

Procedure

1. Prepare 5% suspension of red blood cells in isotonic saline.
2. Label one tube as 'T' and add in it one drop of anti-D serum (test).
3. Label second tube as 'C' and add in it one drop of 22% bovine albumin reagent (control).
4. By using a Pasteur pipette, add one drop of the cell suspension to each of the test tubes, mix well.
5. Incubate the test and the control for at least 15 minutes at 37°C.
6. After incubation, wash the cells in each tube three times with fresh normal saline (for each washing add test tube full of normal saline).
7. Decant the tubes completely after the last washing.
8. To each tube, add two drops of antihuman serum (containing anti-IgG).
9. Mix the contents of the tube gently and centrifuge at 1,500 rpm for 1 minute.
10. Resuspend the cells by gentle agitation and examine macroscopically and confirm the results microscopically.

Interpretation: Agglutination indicates Rh-positive cells and absence of agglutination is Rh-negative cells.

■ ANTIBODY TITRATION

The titer of an antibody is the reciprocal of the highest dilution that causes agglutination of the corresponding antigen cells. Thus, the titration value gives the quantitative value of the antibody and the relative strength of the antigens in the cells. But it is not the total strength of the antibody in the serum. It indicates only the amount of antibody which is dissociated and is free in solution.

The titer of an antibody is usually determined by testing the serial two-fold dilution of the serum against appropriate red cells.

To obtain exact titration results, maintain meticulous pipetting, optimum incubation time and temperature. Use freshly drawn and prepared red cell suspension and evaluate entire series of the tubes.

Specimen

Serum (antibody) to be titered.

Reagents

- Red blood cells that express the antigen(s) corresponding to the antibody specificity (ies) in a 5% saline suspension. Uniformity of cell suspension is very important to ensure compatibility results.
- Normal saline (dilutions may be made with 6% albumin if desired).

Procedure (Double Dilution)

- Label a row of test tubes, according to the serum dilution, usually 1:1 through 1:512.
- Add 0.1 mL of saline to all tubes except the first tube.
- Add 0.1 mL of serum to tubes 1 and 2 (dilution 1:1 and 1:2).
- Mix the contents of the tube 2 with a clean pipette and then transfer 0.1 mL of the mixture to tube 3 (1:4 dilution).
- Continue the same technique, through all dilutions and remove 0.1 mL from dilution tube with dilution of 1:512 and discard or save for further dilution if required.
- Add 0.1 mL of 5% saline suspension of appropriate red cells to each tube.
- Incubate at the appropriate temperature according to the antibody being tested. In case of anti-A and anti-B, incubate at room temperature for 30–45 minutes.
- Gently dislodge the red cells and observe macroscopically for agglutination. The agglutination titer is recorded. Results are expressed as the reciprocal of the highest serum dilution that causes macroscopic agglutination. Thus, a serum which gives visible agglutination at 1:256 is said to have titer of 256. In describing the titer of the serum, it is usual to ignore the diluting effect of the cell suspension.

Note

- For IgG antibody titer add 0.1 mL of bovine albumin 22% or papain cysteine after step 5.
- Incubate at 37°C for 30–40 minutes.
- Observe for the agglutination.
- IgG antibody titer can also be done by IAT.

Avidity

Speed and strength of agglutination is termed as avidity. The test is done by mixing two drop of anti-serum with one drop of 40–50% cell suspension on a slide and rocking gently at room temperature. The time for clearly visible reaction (+1) and then for strong reaction (+4) reaction to occur are recorded with the help of stop watch.

Grading of Agglutination Reaction

- +4 single clump of agglutination with no free cells
- +3 three or four individual clumps with few free cells
- +2 many fairly large clumps with many free cells
- +1 fine granular appearance visually, but definite small clumps (10–15 cells) per low power field
- +W 2 to 3 cells sticking together per low power field, uneven distribution. Visually no agglutination
- – All cells are free
- Hemolysis (partial or total) must be interpreted as positive.

CHAPTER 46

Blood Transfusion Technique

Learning Objectives
- A blood transfusion is a life-saving procedure to replace blood that is lost due to injury, infection or surgery. This chapter has detailed explanation of transfusion techniques.
- Preparation and properties of anticoagulant, different criteria for donor selection, equipments and chemicals needed in donor room, procedure of phlebotomy are described in this chapter.
- This chapter also has information on care of collected blood unit, care of donor, storage of blood and changes in blood after storage.

Keywords
Citrate, Oxalate, EDTA, Heparin, SAGM (Saline adenine glucose mannitol), Donor selection, Autologus blood transfusion (ABT), Apheresis, Label on blood bag, Venepuncture, Care of collected blood unit, Care of donor, Storage of blood, Changes in blood after storage

INTRODUCTION

Approximately, 8% of the body weight is blood. Thus, a person weighing 50 kg would have about 4,000 mL blood. The average adult has about 5,000 mL of blood.

Blood transfusion is the process of transferring blood or a blood component from one person, the donor, to another person, the recipient. Blood transfusions are given to increase the blood's ability to carry oxygen, to restore the body's blood volume when there has been a great blood loss, to improve the blood's clotting ability, and to improve a recipient's immunity to infection. Depending upon the recipient's needs, a doctor may order a whole blood transfusion, or a blood component. Blood components include red blood cells, white blood cells, platelets, immunoglobulins, or fresh frozen plasma.

Loss of blood	Replacement fluid needed
< 20% of blood volume	None
20–30% of blood volume	Crystalloids/colloids
30–40% of blood volume	RBCs and crystalloids
> 40% of blood volume	Whole blood/RBCs and crystalloids

PREPARATION AND PROPERTIES OF ANTICOAGULANT

An anticoagulant is a substance that prevents coagulation of blood.

Collection of blood for transfusion purpose requires anticoagulants to keep the blood in a liquid state. Anticoagulants used for laboratory service commonly are:
1. Citrate
2. Oxalate
3. EDTA
4. Heparin.

The criteria for selection of anticoagulant in blood bank are:
- It should efficiently prevent clotting of blood with minimum quantity.
- It should not be toxic and produce any deleterious effects on the recipient.
- It should not alter any of the functions of the components of the collected blood.
- It should help to increase the stability of the collected blood when stored in the refrigerator.

The ratio of blood and anticoagulant should be maintained.

The common anticoagulants which suits the above criteria are: Citrate or heparin. Therefore, these are commonly used in blood bank.

- *Citrate*: Citrate prevents coagulation by removing ionized calcium. The citrate can be used in two forms:
  a. *Acid citrate dextrose (ACD)*: The composition of ACD is as follows:
     - Glucose: 24.50 g
     - Trisodium citrate: 22.0 g
     - Citric acid: 8.9 g
     - Distill water: 1000 mL
     - pH: 5.0–5.5

     Addition of glucose to anticoagulant provides nutrition to red cells and helps longer storage. ACD solution can be stored for 21 days at 4°C (± 2°C).
     For every 100 mL of blood, 15 mL of ACD is used.
  b. *Citrate phosphate dextrose (CPD)*: The composition of CPD is as follows:
     - Dextrose: 25.50 g
     - Trisodium citrate: 26.30 g
     - Citric acid: 3.27 g
     - Sodium phosphate: 2.22 g
     - Distill water: 1000 mL
     - pH: 5.6–5.8

     In this anticoagulant solution, the citrate is dissolved in phosphate buffer which maintains the blood pH much more accurately than ACD solution. The dextrose present in this provides nutrition to the red cells. The storage period with this anticoagulant is 28 days. For every 100 mL of blood, 14 mL of CPD is used.

     The disadvantage is that, this is costly, and it is difficult to prepare and adjust the pH.
  c. *Citrate phosphate dextrose adenine (CPDA)*

     The constituents of CPDA solution are exactly same as for CPD solution except, for the addition of 27.5 mg of adenine per liter of the solution. Adenine provides ATP molecules for the maintenance of red blood cells. This prolongs the lifespan of red cells and blood can be stored upto five weeks (35 days) in this anticoagulant. For every 100 mL of blood, 14 mL of CPDA is used.

     A simple solution of 3% trisodium citrate as an anticoagulant is very useful if a fresh blood transfusion is contemplated, which does not permit any storage. This anticoagulant is more economical than other citrate solution.

- *Heparin*: Heparin is a biological substance, usually made from pig intestines. It works by activating antithrombin III, which blocks thrombin from clotting of blood.

  Heparin as an anticoagulant for blood collection is very useful when fresh blood transfusion is contemplated to a patient of bleeding disorders and cardiovascular operations.

  The blood collected in heparin can be used only within two days of collection when stored at 4°C (± 2°C).

Other anticoagulants less frequently used in blood bank are oxalate and EDTA:
  a. *Oxalate*: The composition of oxalate is,
     - Ammonium oxalate: 12 g
     - Potassium oxalate: 8 mL
     - Distill water: 1000 mL

     A 10 mL of anticoagulant is required for 100 mL of blood. The blood collected in oxalate can be used for 14 days of

collection when stored at 4°C (± 2°C). It prevents coagulation by precipitating calcium.

b. Ethylenediaminetetraacetic acid (EDTA): The composition is:
   - EDTA: 10 g
   - Distill water: 1000 mL

The storage period of EDTA is two days. It prevents coagulation by binding or chelating calcium in the form of potassium or sodium salt.

The whole blood without anticoagulant, i.e., clotted blood can be stored for 14 days at 4°C (± 2°C).

Anticoagulant with additives: SAGM/ADSOL
The latest and widely used anticoagulant with maximum benefits is—**SAGM (Saline Adenine Glucose Mannitol)**.

Composition

- *Sodium chloride*: Provides isotonicity
- *Adenine*: Maintains ATP for red cell viability
- *Glucose*: Supports red cell metabolism
- *Mannitol*: Helps reduce red cell lysis.
  - Dextrose (monohydrate): 9.00 g
  - Sodium chloride: 8.77 g
  - Adenine: 0.169 g
  - D-Mannitol: 5.25 g
  - Distill water: 1000 mL

A combination of constituents in SAGM additive solution provides optimum red cell viability. SAGM additive solution benefits blood banks, transfusion services and patients in several ways:

- Allows preparation of RBC units with a final hematocrit of about 60%
- Increase plasma yield for optimum production of platelets, plasma and cryoprecipitate, reduces metabolic burden to patients because of reduced glucose load
- Extends red cell dating for utilization in predeposit autologous blood program
- Improves inventory management with 42-day red cell storage
- Increase flow rates for easier transfusion and eliminates predilution of red cells
- 3–5 days platelet storage.

■ DONOR SELECTION

To collect blood for storage and use in blood bank is an important function of transfusion service.

The person from whom blood is collected for transfusion is called as 'donor' and the patient who is going to receive this blood is called as 'recipient'. Any adult male and female can donate the blood. Men once in three months and women every four months can donate the blood. Good health of donor fully ensured. This is important for donor as well as recipients health.

The universally accepted criteria for donor selection are:

- Age between 18 and 60 years
- Hemoglobin: Not less than 12.5 g/dL
- Pulse: Between 80 and 100/minute with no irregularities
- Blood pressure: Systolic 100–180 mm Hg and diastolic 50–100 mm Hg
- Temperature: Normal (oral temperature not exceeding 37.5°C)
- Body weight: Not less than 45 kg (if 350 mL of blood is to be drawn) and not less than 50 kg (if 450 mL of blood is to be drawn).

General Condition

The donor should appear healthy. He/she should not be on empty stomach. Do not donate blood within 1 hour after the last meal (30 minutes in case of light snacks). The donor should have had proper rest during the past 24 hours before blood donation.

Health Conditions

- Past one year not been treated for rabies, had jaundice, tested positive for hepatitis B virus or received hepatitis B immune globulin.

- Past six months—a tattoo, ear or skin piercing or acupuncture, received blood or blood products, serious illness or major surgery, contact with a person with hepatitis or yellow jaundice.
- Past three months—donated blood or been treated for malaria.
- Past one month—had any immunizations.
- Past 48 hours—taken any antibiotics or any other medications (Allopathic or Ayurveda or Sidha or Homeopathic).
- Past 24 hours—taken alcoholic beverages.
- Past 7 hours—had dental work or taken Aspirin.
- Present—suffering from cough, flue or sore throat, cold, pregnancy or breastfeeding.
- Free from diabetes, not suffering from chest pain, heart disease or high BP, cancer, blood clotting problem or blood disease, unexplained fever, weight loss, fatigue, night sweats, enlarged lymph nodes in armpits, neck or groin, white patches in the mouth, etc.
- Ever had TB, bronchial asthma or allergic disorder, liver disease, kidney disease, fits or fainting, blue or purple spots on the skin or mucous membranes, received human pituitary-growth hormones, etc.

Only after satisfactorily fulfilling the laid down basic criteria, the blood donors will be selected.

The following categories of people should avoid giving blood:
- Pregnant or lactating women or those who have recently had an abortion.
- Persons who are on steroids, hormonal supplements or certain specified medication.
- Persons with multiple sexual partners or those who are addicted to drugs.
- Persons who have had an attack of infection like jaundice, rubella, typhoid or malaria.
- Persons who have undergone surgery in the previous six months.
- Persons who have consumed alcohol in the 24 hours prior to donation.

- Women should avoid donation during their menstruating period.
- Those who have undergone various vaccinations should avoid donation for the corresponding period specified below:

Type of vaccine	The period in which donation should be avoided
Hepatitis B	6 months
Live vaccines	2 weeks
Killed vaccines	48 hours
Rabies	1 year

Donors for Babies

A small percentage of adults may donate blood to small children in emergency rooms, newborn babies, and fetuses. To ensure the safety of blood transfusion to pediatric patients, including those in whom the immune systems are not fully developed, hospitals are taking every precaution to avoid infection and prefer to use specially tested pediatric blood units that are guaranteed negative for cytomegalovirus (CMV), because the consequences of CMV infection for newborns or low weight infants may be severe or even fatal. Additionally, for pediatric patients with certain disorders or in emergency, when there is no time to perform crossmatching, only O/Rh negative blood can be used for neonatal transfusion. Potential baby donors are less than 1 in 200.

Screening test for donor: When donor comes to blood banks, he is questioned by a medical officer regarding his medical history and lifestyle. Further, the screening tests performed to select donor are:
- Hemoglobin
- Body weight
- Blood pressure
- Blood group
- Test for transfusion transmitted diseases. These include:
  - Viral diseases: HIV I and II, HbsAg, and HCV by ELISA

- Bacterial infection: VDRL—for *Treponema pallidum*
- Protozoa infection: MP—for *Plasmodium* species.

In India, a person can donate blood only when he/she clear all the above tests. The list of screening tests of donor varies country wise.

Autologous Blood Transfusion

Autologous blood transfusion (ABT) is a unique approach of providing the patient with his own blood. In other words, autologous blood transfusion refers to the procedure of transfusing blood or blood components that have been donated by the intended recipient. ABT in all its forms has now gained a prominent role in transfusion medicine and modern medical practice. Besides ensuring the availability of compatible blood (especially important for patients with rare blood types), this procedure also eliminates the risk of disease transmission from infected donors. Autologous donation is sometimes done by the hospital instead of a community blood bank. Eligibility requirements are relaxed for autologous donors, as the blood is not used for anyone else. Generally, any patient who is eligible for elective surgery is eligible for autologous donations, though there are some exceptions, particularly history of heart disease.

Apheresis

Rather than donating whole blood, a donor sometimes has the option to donate only some blood components while retaining others. This process is known as apheresis, and is time consuming, and requires more specialized equipment. The benefit is that more of the desired components can be concentrated and removed, and the donor is usually able to donate significantly more frequently than if whole blood had been removed. In some cases, the usefulness of the removed components is not as sensitive to blood type considerations.

The typical method of apheresis is to draw whole blood from the donor, then centrifuge the blood to separate its components. The desired components (e.g. platelets, plasma) are removed and then the remaining components are returned to the donor.

■ BLOOD COLLECTION (PHLEBOTOMY)

Phlebotomy is a practice of drawing blood. The word phlebotomy is derived from Greek phlebo means vein and tomy means to make incision. Phlebotomy is one of the important functions of the blood bank.

Personnel involved in donor blood collection should be polite, courteous and friendly, as well as efficient and professional. Blood collection is done in closed plastic collection bag system which is now commercially available. The glass bottles are totally replaced by blood bags for the blood collection due to the risk of breakage and infection.

The labels on every bag containing blood and/or component shall contain the following particulars:
- Donors name, age, date of birth and sex
- The proper name of the blood product in a prominent place and in bold letters on the bag
- Name and address of the blood bank
- License number
- Serial number
- The date on which the blood is drawn and the date of expiry
- A colored label shall be put on every bag containing blood. The following color scheme for the said label is universally accepted for different groups of blood **(Table 46.1)**
- The Rh group
- Any other antigen or antibody if present
- The results of the tests for hepatitis B surface antigen, and hepatitis C virus antibody,

TABLE 46.1: Colors of labels according to blood groups.

Blood group	Color of the label
O	Blue
A	Yellow
B	Pink
AB	White

syphilis, freedom from HIV I and HIV II antibodies and malarial parasite
- Total volume of blood, the preparation of blood, nature and percentage of anticoagulant.

Donor Room

The phlebotomy room should be separate, clean, well-aerated and air-conditioned. The height of the donor beds should be 3 feet.

Equipment and Chemicals Needed in Donor Room

- Blood collection bags with anticoagulant (the bags should be designed to prevent contamination. Plastic bags with CPD/CPDA-1 are most commonly used. The bags are with needle and a collection tube).
- Weighing scale to weigh the blood bag during collection.
- Sphygmomanometer.
- Weighing machine, thermometer, artery forceps.
- Sterile cotton swabs, Savlon, iodine and methylated spirit (each of these must be placed in clean labeled containers).
- Tube sealer with clips.
- Medicated dressing (band-aid).
- Emergency kit, intravenous fluids, ampoules of adrenaline, dexamethasone, calcium gluconate, mephentamine, oxygen. cylinder with regulator and mask.
- Test tubes stand by bedside to hold tubes.
- Blood bag shaker is required when components like platelets to be manufactured from whole blood unit.

Identification of Donor

Before starting the phlebotomy, identify the donor by donor name and number. Attach the donor number to the blood bag and pilot tubes. The date of collection and expiry; and the blood group of donor if tested, should be written on the blood bag label.

Inspection of the Bag

All blood bags must be inspected before starting the blood collection procedure. The anticoagulant must be clear. Look for any leaks, breaks, turbidity or any change in color of the anticoagulant, fungal growth over the bag, or under the label or an abnormally large air bubble. Check the intact ports and a sealed needle.

Volume of Blood

The volume of blood collected is proportionate to the anticoagulant (49 mL of CPDA-1 for 350 mL blood and 63 mL CPDA-1 for 450 mL blood).

Procedure of Venepuncture

- Make the donor lie down comfortably.
- Selecting the vein
  - Inspect both arms in the antecubital fossa (first left and then right) to select a suitable vein. The selected vein should be large and firm, but not very superficial, slippery or mobile.
  - Apply a sphygmomanometer cuff and inflate to 80–100 mm Hg to select a vein. Ask the donor to make a fist which will help in selecting the vein. Release the cuff pressure and ask the donor to loosen the tight fist, after selecting the vein.
- Clean about 4–5 cm of area around the selected vein in a concentric centrifugal (spiral) pattern starting from the venepuncture site as the center.
  - Apply 15% chlorhexidine (Savlon) as the antiseptic and detergent solution to remove the dirt from the donor arm.

- Remove the foam with a dry, sterile swab and apply tincture iodine. Allow the solution to dry.
- Remove the iodine with methylated spirit.
- Do not touch the cleaned area after preparation.
- Apply local anesthetic agent (2% lignocaine). This is optional depending upon the donor acceptability to the venepuncture.
- Put a loose knot just near the needle end of the tubing, which enables the needle to be easily disconnected from the tubing after blood collection.
- Raise the cuff pressure to 60 mm Hg, break the seal and insert the needle held at an angle of 45° with bevel upwards into the vein. Push a little way into the vessel lumen to avoid displacement. Anchor the needle hub with a plaster on the donor arm.
- Never leave the donor unattended during the process of blood collection.
- Ask the donor to open and close the fist to increase the blood flow during collection of blood.
- Mix the blood and anticoagulant gently and periodically during collection of blood either manually or using automated mixing equipment.
- Monitor the volume of blood being drawn using a balance (1 mL blood = 1.05 g, 350 mL blood = 367 g and 450 mL = 472 g + weight of empty bag). Monitoring of volume alone with mixing of anticoagulant with the blood may also be done by automated blood mixer.

When the appropriate amount has been collected, clamp the tubing with artery forceps and deflate the cuff. Place a sterile swab at puncture site and withdraw the needle.

CARE OF COLLECTED BLOOD UNIT

- Take the bag and pilot tubes to another table.
- Release the artery forcep and allow blood from the tubing to drain into one of the numbered pilot tubes.
- Clamp the tubing after it has emptied, mix the blood and anticoagulant by gently agitating the bag for 15–20 seconds.
- Open the clamp again and allow anti-coagulated blood to run into the second numbered pilot tube.
- Seal the tubing at minimum four places by using the tube-sealing machine. Ensure that the tubing contains blood in these sealed parts. Also ensure the each sealed part of the tubing has the serial number printed by the manufacturers. This blood in a tube is used for crossmatching.
- Refrigerate the bag between 4°C and 6°C immediately. Do not refrigerate if platelet concentrate is to be prepared from this unit, but keep at temperature between 22°C and 24°C (in the 'platelet incubator').
- Enter the time of completion of blood collection in the space provided on the donor form.

Care of the Donor

The resting period of 15–20 minutes after blood collection is actually the time to observe the donor for any donor reaction. When the oozing stops, apply a medicated dressing such as band-aid.

Ask the donor to sit up on the donor bed and if he does not feel giddy in sitting position lead him to the recovery bed, make him sit there and have the refreshments, like tea or coffee with biscuits.

Check the phlebotomy site to ensure that there is no bleeding from the vein puncture site. Put a medicated adhesive tape (previously cut to about 1 square centimeter).

Thank the donor for his donation and encourage him to donate again.

Instructions to the Blood Donors

(After leaving the blood donor room)
- Do not smoke for 30 minutes
- Do not drive a vehicle for 2 hours

- Drink more fluids than usual for the next 4 hours
- Avoid strenuous exercise for next 24 hours
- If there is bleeding from phlebotomy site raise the arm above your head and apply pressure on the site till bleeding stops (usually 2 to 3 minutes)
- Do not remain hungry
- If feeling faint or dizzy either lie down or sit with head between your knees. If symptoms persist ask for help, or consult a doctor.

Storage of Blood

Blood is collected into a plastic bag for blood collection and storage which contains anticoagulant/buffers, etc., which allow storage of blood. These include citrate-phosphate dextrose (CPD), acid-citrate dextrose (ACD), ACD or CPD with adenine to prolong red cell storage, and other preservative solutions like SAGM, etc. If red cells are preserved in SAGM solution then their life goes upto 42 days. The CPD solution preserves whole blood for 21 days whereas CPDA solution preserves blood for 35 days. The material of the bag is biocompatible with blood cells and allows diffusion of gases permitting optimal cell preservation. The blood is stored in refrigerators at 4–6°C.

Each unit of whole blood normally is separated into several components. Red blood cells may be stored under refrigeration for a maximum of 42 days, or they may be frozen for up to 10 years. Cryopreservation of red blood cells is done to store special, rare red blood cells for up to 10 years. The cells are first incubated in a 40% glycerol solution which acts as a cryoprotectant ('antifreeze') within the cells. The units are then placed in special sterile containers in a deep freezer at less than –60°C.

Platelets are stored at 22–24°C and may be kept for a maximum of five days. Fresh frozen plasma, used to control bleeding due to low levels of some clotting factors, is usually kept in the frozen state (–30°C or lower) for up to one year. Cryoprecipitated AHF, which contains only a few specific clotting factors, is made from fresh frozen plasma and may be stored frozen for up to one year. Granulocytes are sometimes used to fight infections, although their efficacy is not wellestablished. They must be transfused within 24 hours of donation.

Changes in Blood after Storage

- Stored RBCs develop complex and multiple membrane changes leading to increased osmotic fragility (due to shape change), decrease in the level of 2,3-DPG (increasing the oxygen affinity of hemoglobin), reduced ATP levels, loss of potassium ions with seeping in of sodium ions, loss of deformability of RBCs and reduced lifespan
- Loss of about 25% viability
- Loss of platelet functions in 24 hours
- Disappearance of 30% of coagulation factor VIII
- Increase in plasma potassium
- Increase in plasma hemoglobin
- Increase in blood ammonia
- Increase in lactic acid.

47 CHAPTER

Transfusion Reactions

Learning Objectives
- Transfusion reactions are the adverse events associated with the transfusion of whole blood or one of its components.
- This chapter reveals information on immediate and delayed transfusion reactions. Cause, symptom, immediate management, and preventions are discussed for various transfusion reactions.
- This chapter also throws light on post-transfusion purpura and transfusion transmitted diseases.

Keywords
Febrile nonhemolytic transfusion reaction, Allergic transfusion reactions, Anaphylactic reactions, Hemolytic transfusion reactions, Bacterial contamination, Circulatory overload (hypervolemia), Microembolization, Delayed hemolytic reaction, RBC alloimmunization, Platelets alloimmunization, Graft vs Host reaction, Post-transfusion purpura, Transfusion transmitted diseases

INTRODUCTION

Blood transfusions, when used with caution, and clear indication are useful and life saving. In spite of precautions and preventive measures, in some cases certain unfavorable reactions happen to the recipient. A transfusion reaction is any adverse event which occurs because of blood transfusion. These can vary from allergic reaction, transfusion related infections or may be some times to fatal complications. The risk of a transfusion reaction must always be balanced against the anticipated benefit of a blood transfusion.

TYPES OF TRANSFUSION REACTIONS

Transfusion reactions are divided into two categories:
a. Those which result immediately
b. Delayed transfusion reactions.

Those which Result Immediately

These reactions occur during transfusion or immediately after transfusion. For any such reactions, immediately stop the transfusion and send the sample for investigation.

Febrile Nonhemolytic Transfusion Reaction

Cause

Usually due to pyrogen, may be due to leukocyte or platelet antibody. More recently, these reactions have been postulated to stem from the formation of cytokines during the storage of the blood.

Symptoms

They occur between 1 and 6 hours of transfusions and are associated with the nonspecific symptoms of fever (increased >1°C), chills, and malaise. Some patients may complain of dyspnea. This is usually mild in nature and subsides within few hours. The frequency is one per two million unit transferred.

Immediate management
Provide warmth (use blankets) and aspirin.

Prevention
Use proper anticoagulant, ACD solution and transfusion sets/blood collecting bags must be checked for pyrogen. Avoid repeated blood transfusion.

Allergic Transfusion Reactions
Cause
These types of reactions are thought to be due to allergy to some ingredients in donor plasma to which recipient is sensitized. The specific allergen is not identified.

Symptoms
These are characterized by local erythema, urticaria and itching.

Immediate management
Transfusion can be stopped and 25–50 mg of antihistaminic can be given orally or parenteraly. After relief of symptoms, the transfusion is continued slowly.

Prevention
Ask for history of allergic reaction to patient, so that patient can be pre-medicated with antihistamine. Use of washed or preglycerolized frozen cells may be helpful in preventing these reactions.

Anaphylactic Reactions
Cause
Anaphylactic reactions most often are observed in those patients with a hereditary immunoglobulin A (IgA) deficiency. Some of these patients have developed complement-binding anti-IgA antibodies that cause anaphylaxis when exposed to donor IgA.

Symptoms
The symptoms usually start with transfusion. These include—chills, vomiting, dyspnea, diarrhea, flushing of skin and hypotension.

Immediate management
Transfusion should be stopped—0.4 mL of epinephrine 1:1000 should be given subcutaneously, and 100 mg of hydrocortisone may also help.

Prevention
Use of IgA deficient blood or washed cells is indicated.

Hemolytic Transfusion Reactions
Cause
The basic cause of hemolytic transfusion reaction is, destruction of transfused red cells due to incompatible transfusion or transfusion of blood hemolyzed in vitro. The incompatibility may be due to—clerical error (e.g. mislabeled samples, misidentified patient), technical error (e.g. weak reactions, incomplete cross-matching), some drugs, etc. Blood may be hemolyzed in vitro due to—exposure to 5% dextrose, contamination, overheating, freezing or mishandling.

Symptoms
The symptoms are fever and chills, sometimes with back pain and pink or red urine (hemoglobinuria). The major complication is that hemoglobin released by the destruction of red blood cells can cause acute renal failure and disseminated intravascular coagulation (DIC). In unconscious or obtunded patients, the diagnosis of hemolysis is suggested by development of—hypotension, dark urine, oozing from an IV or other puncture sites.

Immediate management
The treatment should aim to prevent shock and increase renal blood flow, thereby avoiding renal failure. Intravenous fluids should be started. Osmotic diurectic agent (like mannitol) which increase blood volume,

and intravenous furosemide which improve renal blood flow will be helpful. If DIC sets in, patients need heparinization. Use of vasopressor agents may also help.

Prevention

Ensure prevention of human errors. Employ sensitive techniques for crossmatching, prefer autologous transfusion.

Bacterial Contamination

Cause

Bacteria may enter the blood product container if it is opened at any time from collection from the donor until transfusion to the recipient. Bacteria on the donor's skin may enter the container if the needle entry site on the donor's skin is sterilized incompletely. Some donors implicated in septic reactions have low concentrations of bacteria (e.g. *Yersinia enterocolitica*) in their blood (i.e. bacteremia) that are not associated with a fever or other signs at the time of collection. If such contaminated blood is stored for a few days at room temperature (e.g. platelets) or for a few weeks at refrigerated temperature (e.g. red cells), bacteria may grow and elaborate endotoxin, which is a major adverse factor in such reactions. Blood may contaminate during storage due to small cracks or pinholes in bags.

Symptoms

This reaction is characterized by high fever with chills, vomiting, diarrhea, marked hypotension and shock.

Immediate management

Intravenous administration of antibiotics and steroids may help to combat septicemia and vasopressor agents may control shock.

Prevention

The phlebotomy and blood storage should follow a proper aseptic procedure. Proper sealing of plastic bags and pilot tubes is also important. For separation of components, proper aseptic precautions must be taken. Use blood within the expiry limits. Put regular blood cultures for quality control of stored blood bags.

Circulatory Overload

Causes

Increase in fluid volume in susceptible patients including those with cardiovascular compromise, elderly patients, and small children result in circulatory overload. This may be due to high rate of transfusion. This is also called as transfusion associated circulatory overload (TACO) or hypervolemia.

Symptoms

In this, the volume becomes too great for heart to pump. It leads to edema, dyspnea (shortness of breath), coughing, cyanosis and raised systemic blood pressure.

Immediate management

Stop transfusion. Prop up the patient in sitting proportion, keep the patient warm, administrate oxygen and diuretics or use exchange transfusion.

Prevention

A usual rate of transfusion is 2–2.5 mL/kg per hour in at risk patients, the rate can be slower. Overloading may be avoided by use of packed cells and transfusion of small aliquots at a time.

Microembolization

Cause

This is due to aggregates of leukocytes, platelets, fibrin and other particulate matter such as pieces of rubber bungs or skin fragments are likely and more common in stored blood.

Symptoms

The small particle can block pulmonary capillaries and cause respiratory failure—shock lung syndrome.

Immediate management

Stop the transfusion; give patient intravenous saline to dilute the blood.

Prevention

A filter must be incorporated in the administration set. A standard filter has pore size 170 µ. When there are chances of microembolization, like in case of massive transfusion, patients with pulmonary disorder or when large quantity of stored blood is needed, use filter with smaller pore size, i.e. 40 µ.

Delayed Transfusion Reactions

These reactions occur after about 48 hours of transfusion. It include:

Delayed Hemolytic Reaction

Cause

This could be due to alloimmunization, i.e. formation of antibody against antigen of transfused cells.

Symptoms

Symptoms starts after 3–7 days after transfusion. It shows fever, jaundice, lower than expected hemoglobin after transfusion (in case of RBC alloimmunization) and lower than expected platelet count after transfusion (in case of platelet alloimmunization).

RBC Alloimmunization

Patients experiencing alloantibody formation are asymptomatic. The alloantibody is discovered at the time of pretransfusion testing. Appropriate antigen negative blood will be supplied.

Prevention

Alloimmunization to the D and K (Kell) antigens is prevented by the provision of Rh(D) negative and Kell negative blood for Rh(D) negative, Kell negative patients. This is important for females with child-bearing potential as these antibodies can cause severe hemolytic disease of the newborn during pregnancy.

At risk groups

Patients with sickle cell disease or major hemoglobinopathy syndromes who are chronically transfused are at greatest risk of alloantibody formation.

Platelets Alloimmunization

Cause

Immunological causes include the development of antibodies to human leukocyte antigens (HLA) or human platelet antigens (HPA).

Management

Immunological refractoriness can be managed by the provision of HLA or HPA matched platelets.

Prevention

Leukocyte reduction of blood products to levels less than 106/unit reduces the likelihood of alloimmunization. This can be achieved through the use of prestorage or bedside leukocyte reduced blood products.

Grafts vs Host Reaction

Cause

It is rare complication. The mitotically active lymphocytes survive in stored blood for 17–20 days. This blood when transfused to immunosuppressed patient, leads to temporary engraftment of bone marrow by immunocompetent lymphocytes. This develops a graft vs host reaction.

Symptoms

These donor lymphocytes proliferate and damage target organs especially bone marrow, skin, liver and gastrointestinal tract. The clinical syndrome comprises fever, skin rash, pancytopenia, abnormal liver function and diarrhea and is fatal in over 80% of cases. The usual onset is 8–10 days post-transfusion, with a longer interval between transfusion and onset of symptoms in infants.

Prevention

Gamma irradiation of cellular blood products (whole blood, red blood cells, platelets, granulocytes) for at risk patients.

Post-transfusion Purpura

It occurs in some patients who develop an anti-platelet antibody usually Platelet Allomunization (PLAI) which destroys the platelets in circulation leading to thrombocytopenia and resulting in purpura.

TRANSFUSION TRANSMITTED DISEASES

A variety of infectious agents may be transmitted by transfusion **(Table 47.1)**. Definitive evidence of transmission by transfusion requires demonstration of seroconversion or new infection in the recipient and isolation of an agent with genomic identity from both the recipient and the implicated donor.

TABLE 47.1: List of transfusion transmitted diseases.

Viral	Bacterial	Parasitic
Cytomegalovirus	Syphilis	Babesiosis
Hepatitis		Chagas disease
HTLV I and II (human T lymphotropic virus)		Malaria
West Nile virus		Toxoplasmosis
Epstein-Barr virus		Leishmaniasis
Human herpesvirus 6		
TT virus		
SEN virus		

Although, the list of transfusion transmitted diseases (TTD) is long, the frequency is lowered because of donor selection and antibody screening tests.

CHAPTER 48

Hemolytic Disease of Newborn

Learning Objectives
- Hemolytic disease of the newborn is also called erythroblastosis fetalis. This condition occurs when there is an incompatibility between the blood types of the mother and baby.
- This chapter unfolds causes, clinical features, symptoms, diagnosis, treatment and preventive measures of the disease.
- This chapter also has information on ABO incompatibility of HDN.

Keywords
Erythroblastosis fetalis, DD and Dd genotype, Bilirubin, Kernicterus, Hydrops fetalis, Amniocentesis, RhoGAM

■ INTRODUCTION

Hemolytic disease of the newborn (HDN) is a syndrome resulting from hemolytic destruction of circulating fetal red cells in uterus, and after delivery. Hemolytic disease of the Newborn is also called erythroblastosis fetalis ("hemolytic" means breaking down of red blood cells, "erythroblastosis" refers to making of immature red blood cells, "fetalis" refers to fetus). This condition occurs when there is an incompatibility between the blood types of the mother and baby.

■ CAUSES

HDN most frequently occurs when an Rh-negative mother has a baby with an Rh-positive father. When the baby's Rh factor is positive, such as the father's, problems can develop if the baby's red blood cells cross to the Rh-negative mother. This usually happens at delivery when the placenta detaches. However, it may also happen anytime blood cells of the two circulations mix, such as during a miscarriage or abortion, with a fall, or during an invasive prenatal testing procedure (i.e., an amniocentesis or chorionic villus sampling).

The mother's immune system sees the baby's Rh-positive red blood cells as "foreign." The immune system responds by developing antibodies to fight and destroy these foreign cells. The mother's immune system then keeps the antibodies in case the foreign cells appear again, even in a future pregnancy. The mother is now "Rh sensitized;" for example, Rh-negative mother and Rh-positive father.

Rh type mother-fetus incompatibility occurs only when an Rh^+ man fathers a child with an Rh^- mother. Since, an Rh^+ father can have either a DD or Dd genotype, there are two mating combinations possible as shown in **Figures 48.1A and B**.

Only the RH^+ children (Dd) are likely to have medical complications. When both the mother and her fetus are Rh^- (dd), the birth will be normal.

In a first pregnancy, Rh sensitization is not likely. Normally, anti-RH^+ antibodies do not exist in the first-time mother unless she has previously come in contact with RH^+ blood.

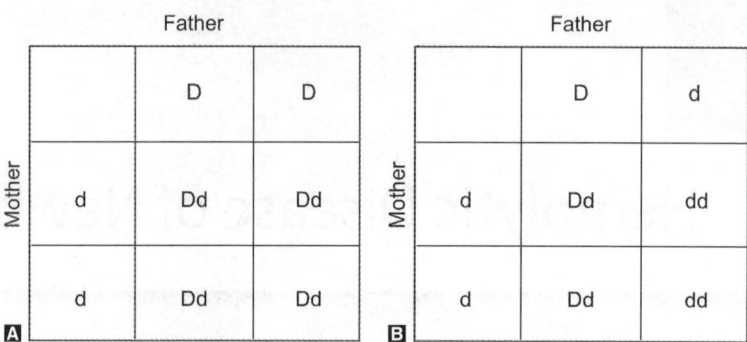

Figs. 48.1A and B: 100% RH⁺ children; (B) 50% RH⁺ children.

Therefore, her antibodies are not likely to agglutinate the red blood cells of her RH⁺ fetus.

Placental ruptures do occur normally at birth so that some fetal blood gets into the mother's system, stimulating the development of antibodies to RH⁺ blood antigens. As little as one drop of fetal blood stimulates the production of large amounts of antibodies. When the next pregnancy occurs, a transfer of antibodies from the mother's system once again takes place across the placental boundary into the fetus. The anti-RH⁺ antibodies that she now produces react with the fetal blood, causing many of its red cells to burst or agglutinate. This is called erythroblastosis fetalis during pregnancy. In the newborn, the condition is called hemolytic disease of the newborn. Therefore, the second and subsequent births are likely to have life-threatening problems. The risk increases with each birth.

■ CLINICAL FEATURES

When the mother's antibodies attack the red blood cells, they are broken down and destroyed (hemolysis). This makes the baby anemic. Anemia is dangerous because it limits the ability of the blood to carry oxygen to the baby's organs and tissues. As a result:
- The baby's body responds to the hemolysis by trying to make more red blood cells very quickly in the bone marrow and the liver and spleen. This causes these organs to get bigger. The new red blood cells, called erythroblasts, are often immature and are not able to do the work of mature red blood cells.
- As the red blood cells break down, a substance called bilirubin is formed. Babies are not easily able to get rid of the bilirubin, and it can build up in the blood and other tissues and fluids of the baby's body. This is called hyperbilirubinemia. Because bilirubin has a pigment or coloring, it causes a yellowing of the baby's skin and tissues. This is called jaundice.

Complications of hemolytic disease of the newborn can range from mild to severe. The following are some of the problems that can result:

During Pregnancy

- *Mild anemia, hyperbilirubinemia, and jaundice*: The placenta helps rid some of the bilirubin, but not all.
- *Severe anemia with enlargement of the liver and spleen*: When these organs and the bone marrow cannot compensate for the fast destruction of red blood cells, severe anemia results and other organs are affected.
- *Hydrops fetalis*: This occurs as the baby's organs are unable to handle the anemia. The heart begins to fail and large amounts of fluid buildup in the baby's tissues and organs. A fetus with hydrops is at great risk of being stillborn.

After Birth

- *Severe hyperbilirubinemia and jaundice*: The baby's liver is unable to handle the large amount of bilirubin that results from red blood cell breakdown. The baby's liver is enlarged and anemia continues.
- *Kernicterus*: Kernicterus is the most severe form of hyperbilirubinemia and results from the buildup of bilirubin in the brain. This can cause seizures, brain damage, deafness, and death.

Symptoms

The following are the most common symptoms of HDN. However, each baby may experience symptoms differently. During pregnancy symptoms may include:
- With amniocentesis, the amniotic fluid may have a yellow coloring and contain bilirubin.
- Ultrasound of the fetus shows enlarged liver, spleen, or heart and fluid build-up in the fetus' abdomen.

After birth, symptoms may include:
- A pale coloring may be evident, due to anemia.
- Jaundice or yellow coloring of amniotic fluid, umbilical cord, skin, and eyes may be present. The baby may not look yellow immediately after birth, but jaundice can develop quickly, usually within 24–36 hours.
- The newborn may have an enlarged liver and spleen.
- Babies with hydrops fetalis have severe edema (swelling) of the entire body and are extremely pale. They often have difficulty in breathing.

▌DIAGNOSIS

Because anemia, hyperbilirubinemia, and hydrops fetalis can occur with other diseases and conditions, the accurate diagnosis of HDN depends on determining if there is a blood group or blood type incompatibility.

Sometimes, the diagnosis can be made during pregnancy based on information from the following tests:
- Testing the presence of Rh-positive antibodies in the mother's blood (positive indirect Coombs' test).
- *Ultrasound:* To detect organ enlargement or fluid buildup in the fetus. Ultrasound is a diagnostic imaging technique which uses high-frequency sound waves and a computer to create images of blood vessels, tissues, and organs. Ultrasound is used to view internal organs as they function, and to assess blood flow through various vessels.
- *Amniocentesis:* To measure the amount of bilirubin in the amniotic fluid. Amniocentesis is a test performed to determine chromosomal and genetic disorders and certain birth defects. The test involves inserting a needle through the abdominal and uterine wall into the amniotic sac to retrieve a sample of amniotic fluid.
- Sampling of some of the blood from the fetal umbilical cord during pregnancy to check for antibodies, bilirubin, and anemia in the fetus.

Once a baby is born, diagnostic tests for HDN may include the following:
- Testing of the baby's umbilical cord blood for blood group, Rh factor, red blood cell count, and antibodies
- Testing of the baby's blood for bilirubin levels.

Treatment

During pregnancy, treatment for HDN may include:
- Intrauterine blood transfusion of red blood cells into the baby's circulation. This is done by placing a needle through the mother's uterus and into the abdominal cavity of the fetus or directly into the vein in the umbilical cord. It may be necessary to give a sedative medication to keep the baby from

moving. Intrauterine transfusions may need to be repeated.
- Early delivery if the fetus develops complications. If the fetus has mature lungs, labor and delivery may be induced to prevent worsening of HDN.

After birth, treatment may include:
- Blood transfusions (for severe anemia)
- Intravenous fluids (for low blood pressure)
- Help for respiratory distress using oxygen or a mechanical breathing machine (ventilator).

Exchange transfusion to replace the baby's damaged blood with fresh blood. The exchange transfusion helps increase the red blood cell count and lower the levels of bilirubin. An exchange transfusion is done by alternating giving and withdrawing blood in small amounts through a vein or artery. Exchange transfusions may need to be repeated if the bilirubin levels remain high.

Prevention

Fortunately, HDN is a very preventable disease. Because of the advances in prenatal care, nearly all women with Rh-negative blood are identified in early pregnancy by blood testing. If a mother is Rh-negative and has not been sensitized, she is usually given a drug called Rh immunoglobulin (RhIg), also known as RhoGAM. This is especially developed blood product that can prevent an Rh-negative mother's antibodies from being able to react to Rh-positive cells. Many women are given RhoGAM around the 28th week of pregnancy. After the baby is born, a woman should receive a second dose of the drug within 72 hours.

ABO incompatibility HDN

Mother-fetus incompatibility problems can result with the ABO system also. However, they are very rare—less than 0.1% of births are affected and usually the symptoms are not as severe. It most commonly occurs when the mother is type O and her fetus is A, B, or AB. The symptoms in newborn babies are usually jaundice, mild anemia, and elevated bilirubin levels. These problems in a baby are usually treated successfully without blood transfusions.

The ABO incompatibility of the mother and baby is observed in the following situations:

Mother's blood type	O	A	B
Baby's blood type	A or B	B	A

49 CHAPTER

Exchange Transfusion

Learning Objectives
- Exchange transfusion is the simultaneous removal of a patient's blood and replacement by donated blood. It is used in treating serious conditions such as hemolytic disease of the newborn.
- Selection of blood for exchange transfusion, types of exchange transfusion and exchange transfusion techniques are discussed in this chapter.
- This chapter also throws light on risks associated with exchange transfusion.

Keywords
Partial exchange transfusion, Single blood volume exchange, Double volume exchange, Isometric exchange, Push-Pull exchange, Infusion method

INTRODUCTION

Exchange transfusion is a potentially lifesaving procedure performed to counteract the effects of serious jaundice or changes in the blood form (for example, sickle cell anemia). The procedure involves the incremental removal of the patient's blood and replacement with fresh donor blood or plasma.

In infants, the conditions in which exchange transfusion may be needed include:
- Hemolytic disease of the newborn (Rh disease)
- Sickle cell crisis (severe)
- Severe disturbances in body chemistry
- Toxic effects of certain drugs
- Polycythemia
- Severe neonatal hyperbilirubinemia (jaundice) in a newborn baby, which does not respond to phototherapy (treatment with light).

SELECTION OF BLOOD FOR EXCHANGE TRANSFUSION

Blood should be as fresh as possible (48-hour-old) but should not be more than five days old. The Rh factor negative is preferred. **Table 49.1** shows selection of blood group for exchange transfusion.

In order to perform an exchange transfusion, it is essential to have the ability to both remove and replace blood. In most cases, this involves the insertion of more than one intravenous (or arterial) catheter. The exchange transfusion proceeds in cycles, each generally of a few minutes duration.

The patient's blood is slowly withdrawn (usually in increments of 5–20 mL depending on the patient's size and the severity of illness), and an equal amount of fresh, pre-warmed blood or plasma is transfused. This cycle is repeated until a predetermined volume of blood has been replaced.

The exchange transfusion should be done under a radiant warmer using sterile

TABLE 49.1: Selection of ABO group blood for exchange transfusion in Rh–HDN.

Baby's blood group	Mother's blood group	Blood selected for exchange transfusion
A	A	A or O
	B	O
	AB	A or O
	O	O
B	A	O
	B	B or O
	AB	B or O
	O	O
O	O	O
AB	A	A or O
	B	B or O
	AB	AB, A, B, O
	O	O
O	A	O
	B	O
	AB	O
	O	O

technique. The donor blood should be warmed using the blood warmer to a temperature not exceeding 37°C. The infant's blood pressure, respiratory rate, heart rate and general condition should be monitored during the exchange transfusion according to standard nursing protocol.

TYPES OF EXCHANGE TRANSFUSION

- *Partial exchange transfusion*: It consists of removing whole blood and replacing it with albumin, plasma or saline. The partial exchange transfusion is often done for polycythemia (Hct >65%) to lower, Hct approximately 55%.

  For example: If the serum bilirubin concentration is at a dangerous level and the blood for exchange transfusion is not yet ready, consider priming the infant with 1 g/kg (4 mL/kg) of a 25% solution of salt-poor albumin to bind additional bilirubin and keep it in the circulation until the exchange can be accomplished.

- *Single blood volume exchange*: In this type of exchange, 80–100 mL/kg of blood is exchanged. It is usually performed for anemia with heart failure.
- *Double volume exchange*: In this type of exchange, 160–200 mL/kg of blood is exchanged. It is usually done through umbilical venous catheter taking 5–10 mL/kg of blood out at a time and replacing it by fresh blood.

EXCHANGE TRANSFUSION TECHNIQUES

There are a variety of techniques for exchange transfusion. That chosen will depend on the vascular access available and the choice of the specialist supervising the exchange.

- *Isovolumetric exchange*: In this type, blood is removed from an artery while infusing through a vein at the same rate.

	In	Out
	Umbilical vein	Peripheral artery
or	Umbilical vein	Umbilical artery
or	Peripheral vein	Peripheral artery
or	Peripheral vein	Umbilical artery

- *Push-pull*: This can be done through an umbilical venous catheter. Exceptionally, an umbilical artery catheter can be used. Withdraw blood over 2 minutes, infuse slightly faster. Aim to exchange 180 mL/kg over 1½–2 hours. If using a 2-catheter push-pull method, withdraw the blood at the same time that blood is given.
- *Infusion method*: In this type, blood is removed by syringe or infusion pump.

  Ideally, blood (or colloid in the event of a partial volume exchange) should be infused through a peripheral vein at a rate equal to blood withdrawal from the UVC. If the "push-pull" (single catheter) technique is utilized, no more than 5 mL/kg body weight should be withdrawn at any one time. The exchange volume is generally twice the infant's blood volume (generally estimated to be 80 mL/kg). The total volume exchange should not exceed one adult unit of blood (450–500 mL). A standard two-volume exchange will remove approximately 85% of the red cells in circulation before the exchange and reduce the serum indirect bilirubin level by one-half. The exchange of blood should require a minimum of 45 minutes. At the end of an exchange transfusion blood should be sent for sodium, glucose, calcium, total and direct bilirubin, hemoglobin and hematocrit. Feedings may be attempted two to four hours after the exchange transfusion.

The need for exchange transfusion has been reduced due to improved bilirubin surveillance, phototherapy, immunoprophylaxis with anti-RhIG, and intrauterine transfusion of non-maternal RBCs. Exchange transfusion is done when other methods to reduce bilirubin have failed, and rate of rising in bilirubin is approaching dangerous levels (risk of kernicterus).

RISKS ASSOCIATED WITH EXCHANGE TRANSFUSION

General risks are the same as with any transfusion. Other possible complications include:
- Heart and respiratory problems
- Shock due to inadequate replacement of blood
- Infection (greatly decreased risk due to careful screening of blood)
- Clot formation
- Alterations in blood chemistry (high or low potassium, low calcium, low glucose, change in pH).

Convalescence

The infant may need to be monitored for several days in the hospital after the transfusion, but the length of stay generally depends on the condition for which the exchange transfusion was performed.

CHAPTER 50

Transfusion-Transmitted Diseases

Learning Objectives
- This chapter discusses the various diseases transmitted by blood transfusion. These may cause prolonged illness or death.
- Transfusion transmitted diseases (TTD) can be caused by viruses, bacteria or parasites.
- Causative agents of these diseases and possible mode of infections are discussed in this chapter.

Keywords
Hepatitis A virus (HAV), Hepatitis B virus (HBV), Hepatitis C virus (HCV), Hepatitis E virus (HEV), Hepatitis G virus, Human T lymphotropic virus I, II, West Nile Virus, Epstein–Barr virus, Human herpes virus 6, TT virus, SEN virus, Bacteremia, Leukodepleted, Syphilis, Babesiosis, Chagas disease, Malaria, Toxoplasmosis, Leishmaniasis

INTRODUCTION

Transfusion of blood is not without risks. The most important hazard of blood transfusion is the risk of transmission of blood-borne diseases. It is the worst fact that in an attempt to save life, blood and blood products having transmissible infections are transfused. Many of these infectious agents may cause death or prolonged illness. The blood-borne infection has following characteristics:
- Long incubation period
- Carrier or latent state in donor
- Ability to cause asymptomatic/subclinical infection
- Viability and stability in stored blood or plasma.

Knowledge of the infectious agents, with special emphasis on the diseases endemic in a particular region, is essential in understanding the strategies to prevent the transmission of these infections.

Provision of safe blood is of paramount importance and its responsibility lies solely with the blood transfusion service.

The three groups of microorganisms, viruses, bacteria and protozoa, have been reported to transmit by blood transfusion.

The infections transmitted through blood can be divided into:
- Exogenous
- Endogenous

Exogenous infections are those which are introduced into a blood unit from an external source. This is generally as a result of bacterial contamination at various stages of blood collection and transfusion.

Endogenous infections are those transmitted from the donor's blood to the recipient.

The infectious agents known to be transmitted through blood can be:
- *Viruses*: Cell-associated and plasma-associated.
- Bacteria.
- Protozoa.

Endogenous microbiological agents transmitted by blood transfusion have certain characteristics which makes it likely to be transmitted by transfusion.

VIRUSES

Viruses are most commonly transmitted by transfusion, majorly because they have property of latency. Following is the list of important viruses that can be transmitted by blood transfusion.

- *Human immunodeficiency virus (HIV)*: HIV infection together with acquired immunodeficiency syndrome (AIDS) caused by HIV are important public health problems. HIV is a RNA virus with a special enzyme called reverse transcriptase having ability to convert RNA to DNA so that viruses can replicate or integrate itself in the cells DNA. HIV is transmitted through sexual contact, sharing of HIV contaminated needles and/or syringes, transfusion of blood components, and nosocomial exposure to HIV contaminated blood or bodily fluids, and can be passed vertically from a mother to her infant. HIV I and II antibodies are detected by ELISA. Confirmatory test is Western blot. An HIV antibody test for serologic screening of blood donors was implemented in 1985. Since then, the risk of transmission of HIV through blood transfusion has been reduced substantially. Transfusion medicine specialists are continually researching new technologies to further reduce the transmission of HIV. Examples of technologies on the horizon include methods to kill viruses in donated blood (called viral inactivation) and blood component substitutes.
- *Cytomegalovirus (CMV)*: Cytomegalovirus is a virus belonging to the herpes group that is rarely transmitted by blood transfusion. It is known to be carried in WBC; therefore, blood components containing WBC are most likely to transmit CMV infections. CMV infection is usually mild, but it may be serious or fatal in those who are immunocompromised. Particularly at risk are low-birth weight infants and bone marrow and organ transplant patients.
- *Hepatitis*: Hepatitis was the first documented transfusion-transmitted disease.

    Hepatitis viruses, which infect the liver, fall primarily into two groups: viruses with a chronic course that can readily be transmitted by blood transfusion (hepatitis B and C) and viruses that cause only acute disease and are rarely transmitted by transfusion (hepatitis A and E).
    - *Hepatitis A virus (HAV)*: Hepatitis A infection is rarely transmitted through blood transfusion; it is usually spread by contaminated food and water, i.e., fecal–oral mode of transmission.
    - *Hepatitis B virus (HBV)*: Transmission of hepatitis B virus is rare because of routine testing of blood for the HBsAg and hepatitis B core antibody, donor screening and deferral for risk of HBV infection, and the use of only altruistic volunteer blood donors. HBV is a major cause of acute and chronic hepatitis.
    - *Hepatitis C virus (HCV)*: Hepatitis C, formerly known as non-A, non-B hepatitis, was discovered in the late 1980s, and all blood donations have been screened for it since 1990. Acute hepatitis C virus (HCV) is a relatively mild infection, and most people are unaware they have become infected; however, HCV becomes chronic in 80% of those infected of which, 10–20% may progresses to cirrhosis and liver cancer.
    - *Hepatitis E*: Hepatitis E is an acute infection caused by hepatitis E virus (HEV) and is endemic in parts of Asia and Africa. The clinical presentation of hepatitis E is similar to that of hepatitis A. It is possible that the virus has been transmitted through blood transfusion

in hepatitis E endemic areas. The solvent-detergent method and heat method for viral inactivation are used to reduce the amount of HEV in pooled plasma.
- *Hepatitis G virus/GB virus C*: The acute infection of hepatitis G (HGV) or GB virus C (GBV-C) is mostly asymptomatic. This virus also causes chronic infection and viremia. HGV/GBV-C is primarily transmitted through blood transfusion, but it can also be spread by organ transplantation, hemodialysis, homosexual and bisexual activities, and injection drug use, and can also be transmitted vertically from mother to fetus. Currently, no screening assays have been approved to test blood donors for serologic markers of HGV/GBV-C infection.
- Human T lymphotropic virus I, II (HTLV-I, II): HTLV-I and II are viruses that are not related to HIV. HTLV-I is found mainly in Southwestern Japan and Caribbean islands. The viruses can cause blood or nervous system diseases in a small number of infected people (<5% lifetime risk). HTLV-II is endemic in the Americas and also may infrequently cause slightly increased susceptibility to infections. Tests specifically designed to detect both viruses are now available and are used by blood centers to screen every donation.
- *West Nile virus (WNV)*: West Nile virus is spread by the bite of an infected mosquito. WNV was first detected in the United States in 1999 and has since been detected in many parts of the US. The first documented cases of WNV transmission through organ transplantation and transfusion were noted in 2002. The most common symptoms of transfusion-transmitted cases of WNV were fever and headache.
- *Epstein-Barr virus (EBV)*: Epstein-Barr virus infection is common in the general population. It is usually asymptomatic in children, although in adults the infection often results in clinical symptoms such as fever and sore throat.

Transmitted primarily through person-to-person contact via saliva, EBV can also be spread through blood transfusion. The prevalence of antibodies to EBV among blood donors is as high as 90%, therefore, it is not practical to screen and eliminate all seropositive blood units through donor serologic screening tests. On the other hand, leukodepletion may be an effective way to reduce EBV transmission through blood transfusion.
- *Human herpes virus 6 (HHV-6)*: Human herpes virus 6 has been described as the causative agent of the sixth disease. This disease features high and persistent fever and affects primarily children between 3 months and 3 years of age. HHV-6 has been described as a potential threat to transfusion safety because of its persistent infection and the high prevalence of antibodies to HHV-6 among blood donors.
- *TT virus (TTV)*: TT virus is also a newly identified virus. Infection with TTV is common throughout the general population, particularly in recipients who have received multiple transfusions and in injection drug users. Blood units are not routinely screened for serologic markers of TTV infection.
- *SEN virus (SEN-V)*: SEN virus was discovered in 1999. The prevalence of antibodies to SEN-V is higher among individuals infected with HIV, HBV or HCV than in the general population. SEN-V is transmitted through blood transfusion and injection drug use. Currently, there are no specific measures to prevent SEN-V transmission through blood transfusion.

BACTERIAL CONTAMINATION

Transfusion-transmitted bacterial reaction has been identified as the most common and severe infectious complication associated with transfusion. Approximately 57% of all transfusion-transmitted infections and 16% of transfusion-related deaths have been associated with bacterial contamination. Blood components may be contaminated with bacteria throughout many stages of preparation, including blood collection, processing, pooling, and transfusion. Bacteria may enter into blood components through several sources: donors' bacteremia, exposure to donor skin bacteria by venepuncture, and contaminated bags and environment in blood banks or hospitals.

The load of bacteria is determined by the storage time. Platelet units that are stored over 5 days and red cell units that are stored over 42 days are strongly associated with an increased risk of bacterial reactions.

In addition, age and underlying diseases in recipients may also play an important role in determining the severity of a bacterial reaction.

Measures have been implemented to prevent and reduce bacterial contamination and its associated transfusion reactions. Phlebotomy sites on donors' skin are carefully prepared using an improved skin disinfected method. All red blood cell units and platelet units are leukodepleted to further remove bacteria from blood components.

Syphilis

The causative agent of syphilis is *Treponema pallidum*. Syphilis is transmitted primarily through sexual contact with an infected individual. Transmission of syphilis by blood transfusion has become extremely rare after implementation of the serologic test for antibodies to *T. pallidum*—the first infectious disease marker tested in blood donors. A positive VDRL test in donor reflects increased risk for other STD in donor.

PARASITIC INFECTION

Babesiosis

Babesiosis is a parasitic infection carried by the white-footed mouse and transmitted by tick bites. About 30 transfusion-associated cases have been reported in the US. While babesiosis is often quite mild, some patients, including those without a spleen, the elderly, or the immunocompromised, may be at risk of serious illness. There are no useful tests available for screening blood donors. All donors must be asked if they have a history of babesiosis. Those individuals with a history of the disease are permanently deferred from donating blood.

Chagas' Disease

A Brazilian doctor, Carlos Chagas, discovered Chagas' disease almost 100 years ago. This disease is caused by a parasite that infects as many as 18 million people worldwide. Permanently prohibit blood donation from anyone who has had Chagas' disease, and tests are being developed and screening strategies discussed.

Malaria

It is caused by the bite of female anopheles mosquito and the causative parasite is *Plasmodium* species. These cases were most likely caused by donations from people who felt well and were not aware that they were carrying malaria. Temporarily defer blood donations for three months from malarial patients.

Toxoplasmosis

Toxoplasmosis is a zoonosis caused by *Toxoplasma gondii*, a parasite that is hosted in cats and dogs. *T. gondii* is transmitted through several routes: ingestion of *T. gondii* oocysts, eating undercooked contaminated pork or beef, direct contamination of open wounds, and vertical transmission from mother to infant. In addition, the agent has been reported to be transmitted through blood transfusion and organ transplantation. Nevertheless, the risk of *T. gondii* transmission through blood transfusion is extremely low, and serologic testing of antibodies to *T. gondii* in blood donors appears to be unnecessary.

Leishmaniasis

Caused by *Leishmania donovani*, leishmaniasis affects approximately 12 million people in tropical and subtropical areas. Transmitted primarily by the bite of an infected vector: the sand fly, *L. donovani* can also be transmitted through blood transfusion and cause clinical disease in newborns or immunosuppressed recipients.

CHAPTER 51

Blood Component Transfusion

Learning Objectives
- The whole blood which is a mixture of cells, colloids and crystalloids can be separated into different blood. Each blood component is used for a different indication; thus the component separation has maximized the utility of one whole blood unit.
- Separation procedure of different Blood components by centrifugation and sedimentation technique is explained in detail.
- This chapter also has information about conditions in which different blood components are used for transfusion, required volume of the component, its storage and shelf life.

Keywords
Relative centrifugal force (RCF), Packed red blood cells, Saline washed red cells, Leukocyte poor cells, Frozen cells, Neocytes, Platelet pheresis, Fresh frozen plasma, Cryoprecipitate, Granulocyte, Leukopheresis

INTRODUCTION

This is an era of blood component transfusion. Transfusion of whole blood is very rare today. The blood components are transfused separately or in combinations, depend upon the need of patients.

Transfusion of blood components should be preferred over the transfusion of whole blood. This is due to following reasons:

- Separation of blood into components allows optimal survival of each constituent.
- It is possible to transfuse blood component as per the need of patient. This avoids the use of other unnecessary component, which could harm the patient.
- By using blood components, several patients can be treated with the blood from one donor, giving optimal use of every unit of donated blood.

Thus, blood component transfusion achieves a most effective way of optimum, safe and economical use of blood. The various blood components that can be separated and transfused are shown in **Table 51.1**.

TABLE 51.1: Various blood components that can be separated and transfused.

Cellular components	Plasma components	Plasma derivatives
Red cell concentrate	Fresh frozen plasma	Albumin 5% and 25%
Leukocytes-reduced RBC	Single donor plasma	Plasma protein fractions
Platelet concentrate (PC)	Cryoprecipitate	Factor VIII concentrate
Leukocytes-reduced PC	Cryopoor plasma	Immunoglobulins
Platelet apheresis		Fibrinogen
Granulocytes apheresis		Other coagulation factors

These components have highly specific and regulated preparation and storage requirements. Blood group compatibility between the components and patients is considered during transfusion. Each component carries the same risk of transfusion transmitted diseases as that of the whole blood. In contrast, plasma derivatives (fractions) such as albumin, immune serum globulins, and concentrated coagulation factors, etc. have more flexible storage requirements and are given without regard to ABO compatibility. These fractions also carry a decreased risk of transfusion transmitted diseases. Plasma derivatives are prepared by biochemical or other manufacturing conditions in well-equipped plasma fractionation laboratory.

Preparation of Blood Components

- Multiple plastic packs system
- Refrigerated centrifuge
- Different specific gravity of cellular components
  - Red cells specific gravity: 1.08–1.09
  - Platelet specific gravity: 1.03–1.04
  - Plasma specific gravity: 1.02–1.03

Due to different specific gravity of cellular components, they can be separated by centrifuging at different centrifugal force in gravity (g) for different time.

Centrifugation for Blood Component Preparation

Refrigerated centrifuge, rotor speed and duration of spin are critical in preparing components by centrifugation. Each centrifuge should be calibrated for optimum speeds and times of spin for the preparation of each component. Times given here include only the time of acceleration and its speed, not the deceleration time.

The blood components are prepared by centrifuging at different relative centrifugal force in g at different time. Conversion of relative centrifugal force (RCF) to rpm depends upon the radius of centrifuge rotor. It can be calculated by:
1. Nomogram for computing relative centrifugal force and speed.
2. By any one of the formulae:
   (i) Relative centrifugal force in g = 28.38 R (rpm/1000)^2
   R = radius of centrifuge rotor in inches
   (ii) Relative centrifugal force in g = 118 × 10^{-7} × r × N^2
   R = radius of centrifuge rotor in cm
   N = speed of rotation (rpm)

Relative Centrifugal Force in g (RCF × g) for Preparing Components

Components	Spin RCF and Time
Red cells	
Plasma heavy spin	
Platelet concentrate	5000 × g for 5 minutes
Cryoprecipitate	
Platelet-rich plasma	Light spin 2000 × g for 3 minutes

Calculations:
RCF = 28.38 × R × (RPM/1000)^2
Or
RPM = $\sqrt{[RCF/(28.38 \times R)]}$ × 1000
RCF = Relative centrifugal force (X g)
R = Radius in inches
RPM = Revolutions per minute

Precautions to be observed in preparing components:
In blood collection:
- Proper donor selection and vein puncture to minimize bacterial contamination and tissue trauma.
- Correct amount of blood in proper anticoagulant and mixed properly.
- The blood should be collected in primary bag that has satellite bags attached with integral tubings.
- Triple packs system with two attached bags makes it possible to make red cells, platelet concentrate and fresh frozen plasma. While

quad packs system with three attached bags are used for preparing red cells, platelet concentrate, cryoprecipitate (factor VIII) and cryopoor plasma. Double bags are used for making red cells and plasma only.

In centrifugation:
- Opposing cups with blood bag and satellite bags must be equal in weight to avoid irregular wear and tear and eventual breakage. If any abnormal vibration is observed till required speed is attained, stop the centrifuge and check the weight of the opposite cups with bags. Rubber disks should be used for balancing.
- The bags should be so placed that its broad side faces the outside wall of the cup.
- Correct speed of centrifugation and time must be maintained.

Centrifuges used for separation are calibrated to produce highest product yield in the shortest time at the lowest possible spin so as to cause the least trauma to each product and at the same time maintaining optimal temperature for component viability. In a unit of blood, the centrifuged products settle in layers, starting from bottom—red blood cells, white blood cells, and platelet rich plasma.

■ WHOLE BLOOD

Whole blood contains 450 + 45 ml or 350 + 35 ml of donor blood plus anticoagulant solution. The name of the anticoagulant is used with the name of the product, e.g. citrate-phosphate-dextrose solution with adenine (CPDA).

Whole blood has a hematocrit of 30-40%. Minimum 70% of transfused red cells should survive in the recipient's circulation 24 hours after transfusion. Stored blood has no functional platelets and no labile coagulation factors V and VIII.

■ RED CELL

The red blood cells can be transfused in following different forms described here.

Packed red blood cells: When red cells are separated from the plasma and used for transfusion, they are called packed red cells.

There is a need to transfuse packed red blood cells in case of—(i) Decreased bone marrow production like aplastic anemia and leukemia. (ii) Decreased red cell survival—such as hemolytic anemia and thalassemia. (iii) In bleeding patients—surgical or traumatic bleeding. The packed red cell transfusion is specially used in cases with congested cardiac failure to reduce the load on the heart by reducing the volume.

Also the packed red cell transfusion lessens severity and incidence of allergic reactions. It is proved that, packed cells are equally effective as whole blood when used for transfusion in elective surgery, saving the plasma for fractionation. In case of emergency, or group specific shortage, when O blood group is used, it is advantageous to use packed cells, as the plasma with antibody is removed, minimizing the risk of hemolytic reactions due to anti-A and anti-B.

The packed red cells are obtained from whole blood either by centrifugation or by gravitational sedimentation, where it is allowed to sediment during storage.

Sedimentation

The blood after collection is kept upright in refrigerator at 2-6°C, the red cells settle down and the clear supernatant plasma is transferred into a satellite bag. The sedimented RBCs have 30% plasma and all original leukocytes and platelets.

Centrifugation

- Collect appropriate volume of donor blood in CPDA double or triple bag.
- Store at 2-6°C till processed.
- Place bags in the buckets of refrigerated centrifuge and balance the opposite bags accurately.
- Centrifuge at heavy spin (5000 × g) for 5 minutes at 2-6°C.

- Express approximately three-fourth of the plasma into the satellite bag.
- Double seal the tube between primary and satellite bags with plasma. Separate the satellite bag with plasma and keep at –30ºC or below.
- Keep the red cells at 2–6ºC.
- This sedimented RBCs have 15% plasma and all original leukocytes and platelets.

The increased viscosity of packed red cells may result in significantly reduced infusion rate and a poor cell survival in storage. To reduce the viscosity and also prolong the red cell shelf life, circle packs with additive systems (SAGM, ADSOL, etc.) or addition of 50–100 ml normal saline just prior to the transfusion may be helpful.

From a single unit of packed cells, the hemoglobin is raised by about 1.0 g/dL and Hct by about 3% of total pretransfusion Hct value. Provided patient is not bleeding from any site.

Saline washed red cells: The saline washed RBCs are free of almost all traces of plasma, most WBCs and platelets. They are generally given to the patients who have severe reactions to plasma like severe allergies, paroxysmal nocturnal hemoglobinuria or IgA immunization. To prepare this, red cells are first separated without the buffy coat and then washed with saline in order to remove most of the remaining white cells. Washing of the cells can be done manually or with the use of machines (hemonetic cell washing machine). The packed red cell should be diluted and mixed with saline, centrifuged and the saline supernatant is removed. The procedure is repeated for three times. This procedure removes 70–95% of leukocytes and effectively removes plasma proteins and microaggregates. The washed red cells have to be used within 24 hours. The process is done with aseptic precautions under laminar flow.

Leukocyte poor red cells (WBC depleted RBCs): The leukocyte poor red cell transfusion is needed in case of multitransfused and multiparous patients like thalassemia, leukemia, aplastic anemia, and immunosuppressed or immunodeficient patients. These patients get a febrile reaction with any transfusion of packed cells and hence require a leukocyte poor red cell preparation. This implies that nearly 70% of leukocytes are removed and over 70% of red cells are retained. This can be prepared by inverted centrifugation, washing or freezing cells and by use of leukocyte filters (of pore size 20–40 micron). These filters can remove approximately 99.99% of WBCs with little loss of RBC. They are indicated for patients who have experienced nonhemolytic febrile transfusion reactions, or for exchange transfusion. The inverted centrifugation is also simple and helps to reduce the number of leukocytes by avoiding the buffy coat from the packed cell preparation. In this method, the red cells are centrifuged in an inverted position, so that the red cells can be transferred into a satellite bag, leaving buffy coat, some red cells and plasma in primary bag. This method reduces leukocytes by 70–80% and sacrifices 20% RBCs. It is also laborious method; therefore, it is mostly replaced by filters.

The leukoreduction can be done at three different points:
1. Prestorage leukoreduction.
2. After storage leukoreduction in blood bank, before issue.
3. Bed side filteration.

Frozen cells: Frozen cells improve cell survival and increase shelf life to 5 years and above. They are useful in storage of rare blood group cells and blood for autologous transfusion. Frozen cells prevent alloimmunization.

The disadvantage is its enormous cost, and the time and labor involved. For freezing, red cells are used within 6 days of collection. The widely used high glycerol technique employs a final glycerol concentration of 40% w/v. To a standard unit of packed cells—100 ml glycerol is added at room temperature with constant mixing. After 5 minutes equilibration another 200 ml glycerol is added. The unit is kept in metal or cardboard canister and stored at

−65°C or lower. The storage period for routine use is limited to 3 years. For use, the unit is thawed at 37°C in a waterbath with agitation. About 12% NaCl solution is added and mixed for 5 minutes, and then NaCl in the descending grades is used for washing cells. The final cell concentrate is suspended in 0.9% NaCl with 0.2% dextrose. This deglycerolized unit has a shelf life of only 24 hours.

Neocytes: Neocytes are the young red cells. The transfusion of these is desirable in young patients with severe chronic anemia (e.g. thalassemia patients) who require repeated transfusion. Each ml of RBC contains about 1 mg of iron, which theoretically can be deposited in tissues and cause hemosiderosis. If neocytes, with an average 90-day lifespan, are transfused instead of conventional RBC, with an average 60-day lifespan, RBC transfusion requirements and the chance of inducing hemosiderosis may be reduced. The younger cells are larger and less dense and hence the collection of the upper half of the unit may contain more of younger cells. This can be procured more effectively with the use of a cell separator machine. Because of the high cost of neocyte preparation and the time consuming laborious procedure the initial enthusiasm is now dwindling.

PLATELET TRANSFUSION

Platelets are primarily important to maintain normal hemostasis. The need of platelet transfusion is:

Indications for Platelet Transfusion

- Platelet count is <5000/µl regardless of clinical condition.
- Platelet count is 5000–10,000/µl, if there is increased risk of bleeding due to hematological malignancies, sepsis, severe aplastic anemia or patient undergoing bone marrow transplant.
- Platelet count is 10,000–20,000/µl, if thrombocytopenic bleeding is present.

Thrombocytopenic bleeding (microvascular bleeding) is:
- Bleeding from the mucous membrane
- Oozing from the surgical incision
- Bleeding from the venepuncture site
- Scattered petechiae
- Ecchymoses.

- Chemotherapy for malignancy (decreased production), if platelet count <20,000/µl.
- DIC (increased destruction), if platelet count < 50,000/µl.
- Massive transfusion (platelet dilution), if platelet count <50,000/µl.
- In major surgery if the platelet count is <70–80,000/µl.
- In addition, platelets are indicated prophylactically for patients who have platelet count <20,000 µl to prevent bleeding.

Two platelet products are available for transfusion: Platelets obtained from whole blood, known as platelets or random donor platelets, and platelets obtained by apheresis, known as platelets, pheresis or single-donor platelets. Random donor platelets are whole-blood-derived platelets obtained by centrifugation of whole blood within 6–8 hours after collection. The blood is subjected to a low centrifugal force (light spin – 2000 × g for 3 minutes) at room temperature (20–22°C) to obtain platelet-rich plasma. This plasma is then separated from the red blood cells in a satellite bag and the unit is recentrifuged at a high centrifugal rate (heavy spin – 5000 × g for 5 minutes) to concentrate the platelets. The majority of the plasma is expressed into a separate bag (platelet poor plasma), leaving a residual volume of approximately 50 ml plasma in which to resuspend the concentrated platelets (platelet rich plasma). Platelets may also be prepared after centrifugation to create a buffy coat containing the platelets, leukocytes, and some red blood cells, a method used mainly in Europe. The buffy coat is then centrifuged at a low centrifugal force to concentrate the platelets. Store platelets at 20–22°C under constant agitation, in platelet incubator with agitator, till used. A random donor platelet preparation should contain at least 5.5×10^{10} platelets per 50 ml unit and have a pH of 6.0 or higher. The shelf life of this product is currently 5 days.

One unit of platelet concentrate should elevate the platelet count by approximately 5000 to 10,000/(mu) L in a recipient weighing 70 kg.

Platelet Pheresis

The advent of apheresis instruments has facilitated the collection of a product from a single donor. Platelets pheresis yields a product equivalent to 10 random units. Platelets collected by pheresis should contain at least 3.0×10^{11} platelets suspended in approximately 300 ml plasma and are stored in the same manner and have the same shelf life as random donor platelets, provided the integrity of the system has not been compromised.

Calculation of Platelet Yield

Number of platelet in whole blood = Platelet per $mm^3 \times 1000 \times$ volume of whole blood (ml)

Number of platelet in PRP = Platelet per $mm^3 \times 1000 \times$ volume of PRP (ml)

Number of platelet in PC = Platelet per $mm^3 \times 1000 \times$ volume of PC (ml)

Calculation

% of platelets yield in PRP =

$$\frac{\text{Number of platelet in PRP} \times 100}{\text{Number of platelet in whole blood}}$$

% of platelets yield in PC =

$$\frac{\text{Number of platelet in PC} \times 100}{\text{Number of platelet in PRP}}$$

Fresh Frozen Plasma (FFP)

Fresh frozen plasma is an unconcentrated source of all clotting factors except platelets. It is prepared from whole blood and is frozen within 6–8 hours of collection.

Indications

- Correction of bleeding secondary to factor deficiencies for which specific factor replacements are unavailable,
- Multifactor deficiency states [e.g. massive transfusion, disseminated intravascular coagulation (DIC), liver failure] and
- Urgent warfarin reversal.

FFP can supplement RBCs when whole blood is unavailable for exchange transfusion. FFP should not be used simply for volume expansion.

Procedure

To prepare fresh frozen plasma, centrifuge the whole blood collected with anticoagulant at heavy spin (5000 × g for 5 minutes) at 4ºC. Remove about two-third volume of plasma into the satellite bag. Seal the tube and separate the bag. The bag should be rapidly frozen (within 1 hour). It can be achieved by spreading the plasma in a thin layer (bags laid flat not vertical) in freezer at –70ºC or placing the bags protected by plastic over wrap at –70ºC in ethanol dry ice bath. Once frozen, it can be stored at or below –30ºC and can be used up to one year.

The formation of cryoprecipitate (containing factor VII 1c, fibrinogen and fibronectin) should be avoided during thawing as it would reduce the expected clotting properties. Thaw it in a plasma defroster (microwave) or place the bag in a plastic over wrap and put in a 37°C circulating water bath (the entry ports of the bag should remain above the water).

The FFP should be administered as soon as possible after thawing, and in any event within 12 hours if kept at 2–6ºC. The most common dosage of FFP is 10 ml/kg of body weight.

Cryoprecipitate

Cryoprecipitate are precipitated proteins of plasma, rich in factor VIII and fibrinogen, obtained from a single unit of fresh plasma (approximately 200 ml) by rapid freezing within 6 hours of collection. It is rich in factor

VIII, von Willebrand factor, fibrinogen (factor XIII) and fibronectin.

Indications

- For hemophilia and von Willebrand's disease.
- Cryoprecipitate is currently used as a source of fibrinogen in acute DIC with bleeding.
- Treatment of uremic bleeding.
- Cardiothoracic surgery (fibrin glue).
- Obstetric emergencies such as abruptio placentae and HELLP (hemolysis, elevated liver enzymes, and low platelet count) syndrome.
- Rare factor XIII deficiency.

Several factors which improve the yield of factors VIII in cryoprecipitate are:
1. Clean, single vein puncture at the first attempt.
2. Rapid flow of blood, donation of blood (450 ml) obtained in less than 8–10 minutes should be used.
3. Adequate mixing of blood and anticoagulant.
4. Rapid freezing of plasma as soon as possible after collection in any case within 6–8 hours after collection as done for preparing FFP.
5. Rapid thaw at 4°C in circulating water bath.
6. Use of siphon technique which prevents thawed plasma remaining in contact with the cryoprecipitate.

Procedure

1. Prepare fresh frozen plasma (FFP), as described under FFP, for processing into cryoprecipitate.
2. Freeze the plasma at –70°C in freezer or in ethanol dry bath.
3. Thaw frozen plasma either at 4°C in a cold room (air thaw) or at 4°C in circulating water bath.
   - If FFP is thawed in cold room, hang the bag in an inverted position with ports lower most and place the second satellite bag on a lower shelf. Observe the pack frequently to make sure the thawed plasma is flowing into the satellite bag and not accumulating in the primary bag. When 10–15 ml of plasma remain with cryoprecipitate seal the tubing and separate bags.
   - If FFP is thawed in 4°C water bath, centrifuge the bag when the plasma is slushy at 5000 × g for 5 minutes at 4°C. Then supernatant cryopoor plasma is siphoned out in the satellite bag, leaving 10–15 ml plasma with cryoprecipitate. Seal the tubing and separate the bags, label bags.
4. Store the bag with cryoprecipitate at 30°C or lower and bag with cryopoor plasma in the second satellite bag is stored at 20°C or below.

Storage and shelf life of cryoprecipitate: One year at –30°C or below.

Reconstituting Cryoprecipitate
(Thawing and issue of cryoprecipitate)

Reconstitute cryoprecipitate before issue by placing in an over wrap in a 30°C water bath until the cryoprecipitate has dissolved. Cryoprecipitate should be resuspended thoroughly by gentle kneading. After thawing pool the cryoprecipitate from all thawed bags into one bag under laminar flow by means of bag-to-bag connector. Wash the empty bags with 10 ml of normal saline to dissolve residual cryoprecipitate and add to pooled cryoprecipitate. Once thawed, cryoprecipitate should be kept at 2–6°C and administered within 4 hours. It should not be frozen.

One bag of cryoprecipitate contains on an average 80–120 units of factor VIII in 15–20 ml of plasma.

■ GRANULOCYTES

These may be transfused when sepsis occurs in a patient with profound persistent neutropenia

TABLE 51.2: Blood Components and their uses (Summary).

Components	Composition	Approx. volume	Indications	Shelf life
Whole blood	RBC (Hct 40%), WBC and some platelets, plasma deficient in factors V, VIII	500 mL	Increase red cells and plasma volume	35 days or 42 days with SAGM/ADSOL
Red blood cells	RBC (Hct 75%), WBC and some platelets, reduced plasma	250 mL	Increase red cells mass in symptomatic anemia	35 days or 42 days with SAGM/ADSOL
Washed RBCs	RBC (Hct 75%) WBC $<5 \times 10^8$ and no plasma	180 mL	Increase red cells mass, reduce risk of allergic reactions to plasma proteins	24 hours
Platelet concentrate	Platelets 5.5×10^{10}/unit, few RBCs, WBC, plasma	50 mL	Bleeding due to thrombocytopenia or thrombocytopathy	5 days
Platelet pheresis	Platelet $>3 \times 10^{11}$/unit, WBC $< 5.5 \times 10^6$, plasma and minimal RBCs	300 mL	Bleeding due to thrombocytopenia or thrombocytopathy. HLA matched	5 days
Fresh frozen plasma	Plasma having all coagulation factors	220 mL	Coagulation disorders if PT >18 sec., aPTT >60 seconds (>1.5–1.8 times of controls)	1 year
Cryoprecipitated AHF (factor VIII)	Factor VIII, von Willebrand's factor XIII, fibrinogen	15 mL	Hemophilia A, von Willebrand's disease, deficiency of fibrinogen and factor XIII	1 year

(WBCs <500 µl) who is unresponsive to antibiotics. These can be obtained by centrifugal leukopheresis and filtration leukopheresis.

These are stored at room temperature (22–24°C) and should be used within 24 hours of collection.

Different blood components and their uses are summarized in **Table 51.2**.

CHAPTER 52

Hemapheresis

Learning Objectives
- Hemapheresis refers to the selective removal of certain component(s) of the blood via machine, designed specifically for this purpose. The blood component may require removal due to a disease or excess
- This chapter has information on types of plasmapheresis, ways to separate plasma or the components of blood, and its clinical significance.

Keywords
Plasmapheresis, Cytapheresis, Erythropheresis, Leukapheresis, Plateletpheresis, Myasthenia Gravis, Autoimmune vasculitis, Centrifugal apheresis, Membrane filtration, Autologous plasmapheresis

Hemapheresis (heam-blood, apheresis- taking away) is the process of removal of normal or abnormal blood constituents such as plasma and various blood cells. By this technique, abnormal components from blood are separated and other components can be returned to patient. When it is applied for donation of normal, desired components, targeted components are separated and other components can be returned to donor. Hemapheresis can be divided into:
- *Plasmapheresis*: Removal of plasma from blood.
- *Cytapheresis*: Removal of cell components of blood.

Cytapheresis can be divided into three types:
1. *Erythropheresis*: Removal of red blood cells from blood.
2. *Leukapheresis*: Removal of white blood cells from blood.
3. *Plateletpheresis*: Removal of platelets from blood.

▌PLASMAPHERESIS

Three general types of plasmapheresis can be distinguished:
1. *Autologous*: It involves removing blood plasma, treating it in some way, and returning it to the same person, as a therapy.
2. *Exchange*: It involves removing blood plasma and exchanging it with blood products to be donated to the recipient. This type is called plasma exchange (PE, PLEX, or PEX) or plasma exchange therapy (PET). The removed plasma is discarded and the patient receives replacement with donor plasma, albumin, or a combination of albumin and saline (usually 70% albumin and 30% saline).
3. *Donation*: It involves removing blood plasma, separating its components, and returning some of them to the same person while holding out others to become blood products donated by the donor. In such a plasma donation procedure, blood is

removed from the body, blood cells and plasma are separated, and the blood cells are returned while the plasma is collected and frozen to preserve it for eventual use as fresh frozen plasma or as an ingredient in the manufacture of a variety of medications.

Plasma is removed from the apheresis patient/donor's blood by a special machine—a separator. The machine has an enclosed plastic system meant for one-time use, and it is hooked up to the donor using a needle. To keep the blood from clotting, an anticoagulant is added to the donor's blood. The plasma separated and collected in a sterile bag, and the remaining blood components are re-infused back into the patient/donor. The procedure will last for about 2 to 3 hours.

There are two ways to separate plasma or the components of blood:
1. *Centrifugation:* This process spins the blood, as a result, its components are separated according to their density. Centrifugal apheresis can be used to remove cellular components and is very efficient, achieving plasma extraction of nearly 80%. It requires lower blood flow rates and therefore can be performed using either peripheral or central venous access. Centrifugal apheresis usually uses citrate as an anticoagulant. Centrifugation can be intermittent or continuous.
   - *Intermittent flow centrifugation:* It involves the processing of small volumes of blood in cycles (a cycle consists of blood being drawn, processed, and re-infused). Typically, a 300 mL batch of blood is removed at a time and centrifuged to separate plasma from blood cells. The advantage of using an intermittent flow instrument includes use of single site venous access; however, the procedure time is longer and larger fluctuations in extracorporeal blood volume occur as compared with continuous flow centrifugation.
   - *Continuous flow centrifugation:* It involves the simultaneous removal, processing and re-infusion of blood components. Continuous flow instruments have the advantage of faster procedures, but require two sites of vascular access. This method is fast and requires slightly less blood volume out of the body at any one time.
2. *Membrane filtration:* Filtration involves passing the blood through a filter to separate plasma. These devices allow for the selective removal of high molecular weight proteins by altering pore sizes of membranes. Membrane filtration devices are not suitable for cytapheresis. These devices are less efficient as they have much lower plasma extraction (about 30%), use heparin as an anticoagulant and require much higher blood flow rates necessitating central vascular access.

Clinical Significance

Plasmapheresis is aimed to separate plasma from blood. This may be for donation purpose or for therapeutic purpose. For therapeutic purpose, unhealthy plasma is swapped for healthy plasma or a plasma substitute, before the blood is returned to the body.

The body has developed proteins called antibodies. These antibodies are in plasma. Normally, antibodies are programmed to identify cells and destroy them cells that may harm the body, such as a virus. In people with an autoimmune disease, however, antibodies will respond to cells inside the body that carry out important functions. For example, in multiple sclerosis, the body's antibodies and immune cells will attack the protective covering of nerves. That eventually leads to impaired function of muscles. Plasmapheresis can stop this process by removing the plasma that contains antibodies and replacing it with new plasma. Once the plasma has been removed, the remaining blood is returned to the patient along with plasma received from donor or plasma replacement, such as albumin or an albumin and saline mixture. Usually it is 70% albumin and 30% normal

saline. Other autoimmune diseases that can be treated with plasmapheresis are:
- Heparin induced thrombocytopenia- antibodies directed against platelets
- *Myasthenia gravis*: Antibodies bind to nerves and make them unable to stimulate muscles properly
- *Systemic lupus erythematosus*: Develop autoimmune antibodies that can attach to body tissues
- *Autoimmune vasculitis*: Happens when the immune system attacks blood vessels, and other conditions like Refsum's disease, Lambert-Eaton myasthenic syndrome, Guillian-Barre syndrome, etc.

It has also been used in case of organ transplant for recipient, to counter the effect of the body's natural rejection process. Plasmapheresis before transplant removes antibodies against the donor blood-type from the recipient, so it can't attack and damage the transplanted organ. This has solved an issue of compatibility to a great extent. It is also used to reduce cholesterol levels in patients with familial hypercholesterolemia.

CYTAPHERESIS

In cytapheresis, the cellular components of blood (e.g., RBCs, WBCs, platelets) are separated. This is often done on donated blood so that each component may be given to a different recipient. Cytapheresis also may be done therapeutically to remove excess or defective cellular components. Therapeutic cytapheresis removes cellular components from blood, returning plasma to patient's body.
- *Erythrocytapheresis*: It is the separation of erythrocytes from whole blood. It is most commonly accomplished using the method of centrifugal sedimentation. This process is used for red blood cell diseases such as sickle cell crises, other hemoglobin defects or severe malaria. The automated red blood cell collection procedure for donating erythrocytes is referred to as 'Double Reds' or 'Double Red Cell Apheresis.'

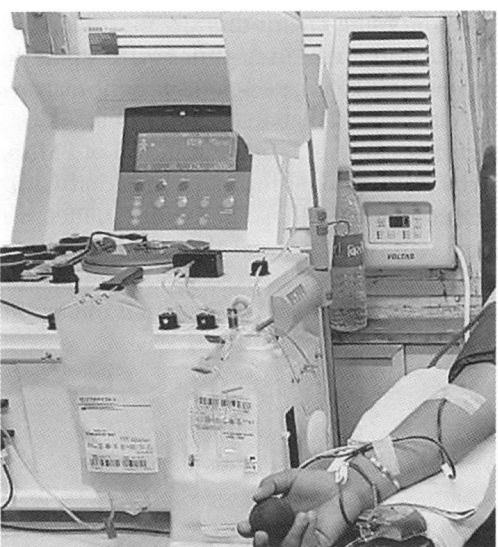

Fig. 52.1: Platelet apheresis.

- *Plateletpheresis (thrombapheresis, thrombocytapheresis)*: Plateletpheresis is a procedure of collecting platelets by apheresis. It involves directing the blood in the patient/donor's veins through tubing to a machine that separates the blood components. To remove platelets, a needle is placed in each arm. Blood flows through a needle into a machine that contains a sterile, disposable plastic kit specifically designed for this purpose. The platelets are isolated by means of centrifugation and channeled out into a collecting bag, while RBCs, WBCs and plasma components are reinfused back into the donor/patient through a needle in the opposite arm. There is also a platelet pheresis procedure that can be performed with a single needle **(Fig. 52.1)**. The entire procedure takes about 90 minutes. It is used for treating serious complications from bleeding and hemorrhage in patients who have disorders manifesting as thrombocytopenia (low platelet count) or platelet dysfunction. Or extraordinarily high platelet counts such as essential thrombocytosis. Platelet transfusions are traditionally given to those

undergoing chemotherapy for leukemia, multiple myeloma, those with aplastic anemia, AIDS, hypersplenism, bone marrow transplant, radiation treatment, etc.
- *Leukapheresis*: It is the removal of PMNs, basophils, eosinophils for transfusion into patients whose PMNs are ineffective or where traditional therapy has failed. Leukapheresis is used as treatment for leukostasis, where WBC count is increased up to 1 lac. This is very useful to treat various kinds of leukemia. The procedure is similar to plateletpheresis, it takes 3 to 4 hours to complete entire process.

Other uses of cytapheresis include collection of peripheral blood stem cells for autologous or allogeneic bone marrow reconstitution (an alternative to bone marrow transplantation).

CHAPTER 53

Recent Advances in Blood Banking

Learning Objectives
- With the advancement in technology, blood banking is becoming more and more life saving. This chapter aims to keep readers updated with latest technology and its benefits
- Stem cell transfusion is life saving, revolutionary discovery. This chapter has brief discussion different types of stem cell transplants, artificial blood, oxygen therapeutics, molecular typing, PCR (Polymerase chain reaction)
- Pathogen inactivation and some recent techniques of crossmatch are provided in this chapter.

Keywords
Stem cells, Umbilical cord, Stem cell transplant, Oxygen therapeutics, Perfluorocarbons (PFCs), Hemoglobin based products, Artificial blood, Volume expanders, Molecular typing, Polymerase chain reaction (PCR) and its application in transfusion medicine, Pathogen inactivation, Recent crossmatch techniques—Gel technique for crossmatch, Electronic crossmatch, Immediate spin crossmatch

■ STEM CELLS

Stem cells are primal cells found in all multicellular organisms. Stem cells have the remarkable potential to develop into many different cell types in the body. Serving as a sort of repair system for the body, they can theoretically divide without limit to replenish other cells as long as the person or animal is still alive. When a stem cell divides (mitotic cell division), each new cell has the potential to either remain a stem cell or become another type of cell with a more specialized function, such as a muscle cell, a red blood cell, or a brain cell.

Stem cells are one of the most fascinating areas of biology today. Research on stem cells is advancing knowledge about how an organism develops from a single cell and how healthy cells replace damaged cells in adult organisms. This promising area of science is also leading scientists to investigate the possibility of cell-based therapies to treat disease, which is often referred to as regenerative or reparative medicine.

The three broad categories of mammalian stem cells are: embryonic stem cells, derived from blastocysts, adult stem cells, which are found in adult tissues, and cord blood stem cells, which are found in the umbilical cord.

Embryonic Stem Cell

Embryonic stem cell lines are cultures of cells derived from the epiblast tissue of the inner cell mass (ICM) of a blastocyst or earlier morula stage embryos. A blastocyst is an early stage embryo—approximately 4-5 days old in humans and consisting of 50-150 cells. ES cells are pluripotent and give rise during development to all derivatives of the three primary germ layers: ectoderm, endoderm and mesoderm.

There exists a widespread controversy over stem cell research that emanates from the techniques used in the creation and usage of stem cells. Human embryonic stem cell research is particularly controversial because, with the present state of technology, starting a stem cell line requires the destruction of a human embryo and/or therapeutic cloning. However, recently, it has been shown in principle that embryonic stem cell lines can be generated using a single-cell biopsy similar to that used in preimplantation genetic diagnosis that may allow stem cell creation without embryonic destruction.

Opponents of the research argue that embryonic stem cell technologies are a slippery slope to reproductive cloning and can fundamentally devalue human life. Those in the pro-life movement argue that a human embryo is a human life and is therefore entitled to protection.

Contrarily, supporters of embryonic stem cell research argue that such research should be pursued because the resultant treatments could have significant medical potential. It is also noted that excess embryos created for in vitro fertilization could be donated with consent and used for the research.

After twenty years of research, there are no approved treatments or human trials using embryonic stem cells. Their tendency to produce tumors and malignant carcinomas, cause transplant rejection, and form the wrong kinds of cells are just a few of the hurdles that embryonic stem cell researchers still face.

Adult Stem Cells

The term adult stem cell refers to any cell which is found in a developed organism that has two properties: The ability to divide and create another cell like itself and also divide and create a cell more differentiated than itself. Also known as somatic (from Greek "of the body") stem cells, they can be found in children, as well as adults. Pluripotent adult stem cells are rare and generally small in number but can be found in a number of tissues including umbilical cord blood. Most adult stem cells are lineage-restricted (multipotent) and are generally referred to by their tissue origin (mesenchymal stem cell, adipose-derived stem cell, endothelial stem cell, etc.).

Adult stem cells have been identified in many organs and tissues. One important point to understand about adult stem cells is that there are a very small number of stem cells in each tissue. Stem cells are thought to reside in a specific area of each tissue where they may remain quiescent (non-dividing) for many years until they are activated by disease or tissue injury. The adult tissues reported to contain stem cells include brain, bone marrow, peripheral blood, blood vessels, skeletal muscle, skin and liver.

Scientists in many laboratories are trying to find ways to grow adult stem cells in cell culture and manipulate them to generate specific cell types so they can be used to treat injury or disease. Some examples of potential treatments include replacing the dopamine-producing cells in the brains of Parkinson's patients, developing insulin-producing cells for type I diabetes and repairing damaged heart muscle following a heart attack with cardiac muscle cells.

Adult Stem Cell Transplant: Bone Marrow Stem Cells

Perhaps the best-known stem cell therapy to date is the bone marrow transplant, which is used to treat leukemia and other types of cancer, as well as various blood disorders.

Successful treatment for leukemia depends on getting rid of all the abnormal leukocytes in the patient, allowing healthy ones to grow in their place. One way to do this is through chemotherapy, which uses potent drugs to target and kill the abnormal cells. When chemotherapy alone cannot eliminate them all, physicians sometimes turn to bone marrow transplants.

In a bone marrow transplant, the patient's bone marrow stem cells are replaced with those from a healthy matching donor. To do this, all of the patient's existing bone marrow and abnormal leukocytes are first killed using a combination of chemotherapy and radiation. Next, a sample of donor bone marrow containing healthy stem cells is introduced into the patient's bloodstream.

If the transplant is successful, the stem cells will migrate into the patient's bone marrow and begin producing new, healthy leukocytes to replace the abnormal cells.

Adult Stem Cell Transplant: Peripheral Blood Stem Cell Transplant

While most blood stem cells reside in the bone marrow, a small number are present in the bloodstream. These multipotent peripheral blood stem cells, or PBSCs, can be used just like bone marrow stem cells to treat leukemia, other cancers and various blood disorders. Since, they can be obtained from drawn blood, PBSCs are easier to collect than bone marrow stem cells, which must be extracted from within bones. This makes PBSCs a less invasive treatment option than bone marrow stem cells. PBSCs are sparse in the bloodstream; however, so collecting enough to perform a transplant can pose a challenge.

Umbilical Cord Blood Stem Cell Transplant

Newborn infants no longer need their umbilical cords, so they have traditionally been discarded as a by-product of the birth process. In recent years, however, the multipotent-stem-cell-rich blood found in the umbilical cord has proven useful in treating the same types of health problems as those treated using bone marrow stem cells and PBSCs.

Umbilical cord blood stem cell transplants are less prone to rejection than either bone marrow or peripheral blood stem cells. This is probably because the cells have not yet developed the features that can be recognized and attacked by the recipient's immune system. Also, because umbilical cord blood lacks well-developed immune cells, there is less chance that the transplanted cells will attack the recipient's body, a problem called graft versus host disease. Both the versatility and availability of umbilical cord blood stem cells makes them a potent resource for transplant therapies.

Cord blood can be collected during either vaginal delivery or cesarean section. Differing techniques include milking of blood from the clamped, cut umbilical cord and needle and syringe aspiration of the umbilical and placental veins. The anticoagulated specimens vary considerably in volume, and the greatest volume is associated with early cord clamping. Careful cleansing of the cord to avoid contamination by either bacteria or maternal blood is recommended. Maternal lymphocytes pose the theoretical risk of GVHD in the recipients, although the number of cells needed for this complication is uncertain. However, cord blood collected aseptically from the placenta after the birth of a healthy baby can be used safely as a blood substitute. It has a higher hemoglobin content and growth factors than normal blood from an adult, which has the potential to benefit patients in varying diseases.

■ ARTIFICIAL BLOOD

Blood substitutes, often called artificial blood, are used to fill fluid volume and/or carry oxygen and other blood gases in the cardiovascular system. Although commonly used, the term is not accurate since human blood performs many important functions. Red blood cells transport oxygen, white blood cells defend against disease, platelets promote clotting, and plasma proteins provide various functions. The preferred and more accurate terms are volume expanders for inert products, and oxygen therapeutics for oxygen-carrying products. Examples of these two "blood substitute" categories:

Volume expanders: Inert and merely increase blood volume. These may be crystalloid-based (Ringer's lactate), normal saline, dextrose 5% in water (D5W) or colloid-based (Haemaccel, Gelofusine).

Oxygen therapeutics: Mimic human blood's oxygen transport ability. Examples: Hemopure, oxygent, polyheme.

Artificial blood is also often used in movies.

Volume Expanders

When blood is lost, the greatest immediate need is to stop blood loss. The second greatest need is replacing the lost volume. This way remaining red blood cells can still oxygenate body tissue. Normal human blood has a significant excess oxygen transport capability, only used in cases of great physical exertion. Provided blood volume is maintained by volume expanders, a quiescent patient can safely tolerate very low hemoglobin levels, less than 1/3rd of a healthy person.

The body automatically detects the lower hemoglobin level and compensatory mechanisms start up. The heart pumps more blood with each beat. Since, the lost blood was replaced with a suitable fluid, the now diluted blood flows more easily, even in the small vessels. As a result of chemical changes, more oxygen is released to the tissues. These adaptations are so effective that if only half of the red cells remain, oxygen delivery may still be about 75% of normal. A patient at rest uses only 25% of the oxygen available in his blood. In extreme cases, patients have survived with a hemoglobin level of 2 g/dL, about 1/7th of normal, although these low levels are very dangerous.

With enough blood loss, ultimately red cell levels drop too low for adequate tissue oxygenation, even if volume expanders maintain circulatory volume. In these situations the only alternatives are blood transfusions, packed red cells, or oxygen therapeutics (if available). However, in some circumstances hyperbaric oxygen therapy can maintain adequate tissue oxygenation even if red cell levels are below normal life sustaining levels.

Volume expanders are widely available and are used in both hospitals and first response situations by paramedics and emergency medical technicians.

Oxygen Therapeutics

Unfortunately, oxygen transport (the function that distinguishes real blood from other volume expanders) has been very difficult to reproduce. There are two basic approaches to constructing oxygen therapeutic:

1. Perfluorocarbons (PFCs), a chemical compound which can carry and release oxygen. The specific PFC usually used is perfluorocarbon.
2. Hemoglobin derived from humans, animals, or artificially via recombinant technology.
   - *Perfluorocarbons:* Perfluorocarbons (PFC) are relatively large organic molecules that are chemically inert, nonimmunogenic, and not metabolized. They can dissolve 40–70% oxygen per unit volume, which is more than blood can. The amount of oxygen in PFC depends on the external environments oxygen concentration. Addition of surfactant, such as egg white lecithin or the synthetic polymer Pluronic F-68 causes the PFC to emulsify and thereby become miscible with blood. Because they do not carry carbon monoxide, PFC may be useful in carrying oxygen to the tissues during cases of carbon monoxide poisoning.

Because of their small size 1/70 that of an RBC, PFC can be used to deliver oxygen distal to partial vascular occlusion such as in an acute myocardial infarct, a stroke, or sickel cell crisis, PFC are also used to deliver oxygen to the interior of tumor to enhance subsequent treatment with ionizing irradiation. The FDA has approved the use of PFC for percutaneous transluminal coronary angioplasty.

The disadvantages of PFC are:
- The lack of affinity for oxygen.
- The necessity for the patient therefore to be in a high oxygen environment with the possible development of oxygen toxicity to the lungs.
- The potential for blockade of the reticuloendothelial system (RES) (clearing mechanism for PFC) and subsequent reduced clearing of pathogens.

For example: Oxygent is a solution used as an intravascular oxygen carrier to temporarily augment oxygen delivery to tissues and is currently being developed by Alliance Pharmaceutical Corp. Right now, the goal of the development of oxygent is simply to reduce the need for donor blood during surgery, but this product clearly has the potential for additional future uses. Perfluorocarbons surrounded by a surfactant called lecithin and suspended in a water based solution give oxygent its oxygen carrying capacity. The oxygent particles are removed from the bloodstream within 48 hours by the body's normal clearance procedure for particles in the blood. Namely, the lecithin is digested intracellularly and the PFC's are exhaled through the lungs. The fact that this blood substitute is completely man-made gives it certain distinct advantages over blood substitutes that rely on modified hemoglobin, such as unlimited manufacturing capabilities, ability to be heat-sterilized, and the PFCs' efficient oxygen delivery. Oxygent has done well in most clinical trials, but recently ran into some trouble, with participants in a cardiac surgery study slightly more likely to suffer a stroke if treated with oxygent rather than the standard care.

- *Hemoglobin based products:* These are either hemoglobin solutions or encapsulated hemoglobin.

Hemoglobin solutions: When a crude extract of hemoglobin is transfused, the red cell stroma infused acts as an antigen that can combine with the recipients antibodies and cause DIC with kidney failure. When the red cell stroma is removed, the hemoglobin solution becomes relatively non-toxic product.

The half-life of stroma free hemoglobin is short free hemoglobin remains in the circulation only two to four hours. Outside the RBC, the hemoglobin tetramer readily dissociates to dimers and monomers that are rapidly cleared by kidney. Hemoglobin is also bound by plasma proteins such as haptoglobin and cleared by RES.

Two methods are used to stabilize the hemoglobin molecule in solution. One is to use intramolecular crosslinks, which stabilize the tetramer, and the other is to employ intermolecular crosslinks which produce a high molecular weight polymer of hemoglobin. These processes can increase the intravascular half-life of hemoglobin to 15 to 30 hours. But the oxygen affinity remains high so that the oxygen is poorly released to the tissues.

Pyridoxylated hemoglobin is treated with pyridoxal-5-phosphate, an analogue of 2,3-DPG, to reduce the oxygen affinity for the hemoglobin, so that it more closely approximates that seen in RBC. Therefore, this product can better release oxygen to the tissues.

Because of the relatively short time free hemoglobin remains in the circulation, its usefulness may be limited only to emergency situations.

Encapsulated hemoglobin: Encapsulated hemoglobin can be made by surrounding hemoglobin molecules with liposomes comprising either non-immunogenic phospholipids or phospholipids and neutral fats. These liposomes are closed, spherical vesicles with an internal aqueous environment and a cell membrane—like outer layer consisting of lipids. When 2, 3-DPG is included in the internal compartment with the hemoglobin, the oxygen affinity is decreased to those levels seen with hemoglobin in the RBC.

Within a few HRS of intravenous administration, 50% of the liposomes are cleared from the circulation, primarily by the RES of the liver and some by RES of the spleen. Additional clearing mechanisms include irreversible binding to tissues and lysis by plasma lipoproteins. There is concern about this rapid V encapsulated hemoglobin clearance by the RES and its blockade by the liposomes, which might result in decreased immunity to pathogens.

Liposome technology has also been used to produce artificial platelets that can bind fibrinogen and agglutinate along with activated platelets.

The disadvantages of hemoglobin based products are: nausea, vomiting, fever, generalized discomfort, vasoconstriction, increased vascular pressure, and increased blood pressure. The vasoconstriction is due to free hemoglobin irreversibly binding endothelial nitrous oxide when hemoglobin leaks out from the vascular spaces.

For example: Hemopure is made by biopure, one of the leading companies in the development and manufacture of oxygen carrying solutions. It is biopure's first-in-class product for human use, and is a hemoglobin based oxygen carrying solution (HBOC). It is made of chemically stabilized, cross-linked bovine (cow) hemoglobin situated in a salt solution, and many safety measures are taken to ensure that the product is safe and free of pathogens, including herd control and monitoring. Hemopure molecules can be up to 1,000 times smaller than RBC's facilitating oxygen transport and off-loading to the tissues. Hemopure is currently in phase III clinical trials in the US, and is approved for use in South Africa for the use of surgical patients who are anemic, thereby reducing or eliminating the need for blood transfusions for these patients.

Need for Molecular Typing

- We routinely match RBCs for ABO and Rh with the intended patient by current serology procedures. There are more than 300 RBC antigens discovered so far. However, this means that minor RBC antigens are often incompatible, which can put the patient at risk for alloimmunization.
- Some clinically significant alloantibodies (Jka) will become senescent and less detectable with time, and can cause hemolytic events following even crossmatch compatible transfusions.
- Alloimmunization rates are highly variable depending on the patient population (range 1% to about 60%) Overall, the risk of delayed hemolytic transfusion reaction is estimated to be 1 in 2000 patients transfused, and the risk of a delayed serologic transfusion reaction 1 in.
- 2500 patients transfused (5), indicating that alloimmunization remains a fairly common occurrence.
    - Patients at high-risk of alloimmunization
    - Multiple transfused
    - Autoimmune hemolytic anemia
    - Multiparous females (female with many kids)
    - Transplant patients.

Disadvantages of Serology

- Typing sera not available for all RBC antigens
- Result interpretation can be subjective
- Patients with +DAT: No direct agglutinating sera available
- Antibody source variation: Poly vs monoclonal, human vs other may affect performance

- Transfused patients: Problematic!
- Advanced serological techniques not always available.

MOLECULAR TYPING

Antigens determined by multiple alleles are defined by DNA sequence variations. This allows prediction of the antigen phenotype.

A 38 RBC antigens and phenotypic variants can be detected through 24 DNA sequence variations.

Blood group	RBC antigens
Rh	C (RH2), c (RH4), E (RH3), e (RH5), V (RH10), VS (RH 20)
Kell	K (Kel 1), K (KEL 2), Kpa (KEL3), Kpb (KEL 4), Jsa (KEL 6), Jsb (KEL 7)
Duffy	Fya (FY1), Fyb (FY2), GATA (FY-2), Fyx (FY2W)
Kidd	Jka (JK1), Jkb (JK2)
MNS	M (MNS1), N (MNS2), S (NS3), S (MNS4), Uvar (MNS-3,5W), Uneg (MNS-3,-4,-5)
Lutheran	Lua (LU1), Lub (LU2)
Dombrock	Doa (DO1), Dob (DO2), Hy (DO4), Joa (DO5)
Landsteiner-Wiener	LWa (LW5), LWb (LW7)
Diego	Dia (DI1), Dib (DI2)
Colton	Coa (CO1), Cob (CO_2)
Scianna	Sc1 (SC1), Sc2 (SC2)

Knowledge of the molecular bases to blood group provides a means to predict blood group phenotype with a high degree of accuracy.

Common Terms used in Molecular Biology

- *Gene:* Sequence of nucleotides in the DNA that provides the coded instructions for.
- RNA synthesis, which translated into protein, leads to expression of a blood group.
- *Locus:* The place a gene occupies on a chromosome
- *Allele:* Mutually exclusive forms of the same gene, usually arising through mutation, that are responsible for variation in the blood group.
- *Exon:* The region of a gene that contains the code for producing protein. Each exon codes for a specific portion of the complete protein. Exons are separated by introns, regions of DNA that have no function.
- *Polymorphism:* The presence of two or more distinct phenotypes in a population due to the expression of different alleles of a given gene
- *Primer:* Short single-stranded DNA sequences that are synthesized to correspond to the beginning and ending of the DNA stretch to be copied or identified.

Basic Molecular Biology

- DNA contains four nucleotides that are linked together (base pair) to form the double helix structure **(Figs. 53.1A to C)**.
- The nitrogenous bases are adenine, guanine, cytosine, and thymine. RNA contains uracil.
- Using DNA as a template, complementary single stranded mRNA is synthesized via transcription.
- There are long stretches of DNA that contain both non-coding sequences (introns) and coding sequences (exons). mRNA is processed in the nucleus to remove the non-coding areas. Then the mature mRNA is transported to cytoplasmic ribosomes for protein synthesis.
- Proteins are translated from mRNA by adding amino acid groups in a specific order determined by the codon sequence **(Fig. 53.1D)**.
- Twenty amino acids are specified by 64 codons (sets of 3 nucleotides).

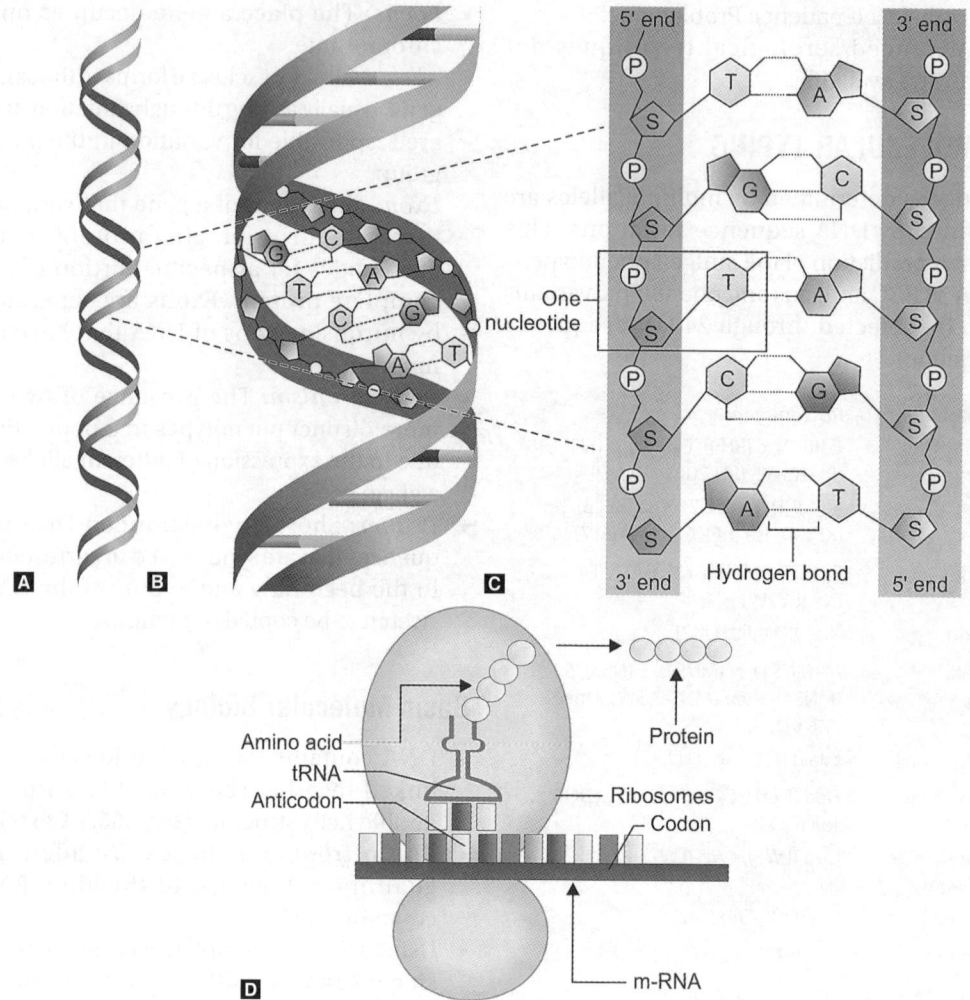

Figs. 53.1A to D: (A) DNA double helix; (B) Complementary base pairing; (C) Ladder configuration; (D) Translation.

- Each codon is matched with a specific anticodon on a smaller RNA form, the transfer RNA (tRNA).

  This is center dogma of molecular biology. Genes are composed of DNA which is Transcribed to RNA and translated into protein.

  DNA sequence variations occur naturally in the population.
- Many occur as only a single base difference (single nucleotide polymorphism, or SNP).
- There are approximately 10 million SNPs in the human genome. Some code for specific blood group antigens.
- Types of DNA sequence variations:
  - Point mutations substitute one nucleotide for another in the DNA.
  - Silent sequence variation. More than one codon (a functional part of the three-letter genetic code) codes for the same amino acid. Has no effect on the resultant protein.
  - Insertions add one or more extra-nucleotides into the DNA sequence.

- Deletions remove one or more nucleotides from the DNA sequence.
- Frame shift mutation causes a shift in the reading frame (insertion or deletion) and may lead to an altered protein.

Genes Detected By Molecular Typing

1. Promoter silencing mutation for Fyb (67T>C in FY), giving a Duffy-null phenotype (also known as GATA mutation). These patients will safely tolerate Fyb positive blood.
2. Silencing mutations for S-s-phenotype, predicting Uvar or Uneg antigen status (Intron 5 G>T and 230 C>T in GYPB) (**Fig. 53.2**).
3. RHCE point mutations 733C>G and 1006G>T, coding Leu245Val and Gly336Cys, predict the V and VS antigen phenotypes.
4. RhC based on three polymorphisms and the presence/absence of a 109bp insert in the RHCE gene, with indication of possible altered C antigen encoded by the (C)ces haplotype.
5. 265C>T in FY gene, predicting Fyx, with varying degrees of weakened Fyb antigen, which may not always react with serologic reagents.
6. Hemoglobin S marker (HgbS 173 A>T).

Molecular Typing

Polymerase Chain Reaction

The polymerase chain reaction (PCR) is a technique where in a single or a few copies of a piece of DNA segment are identified and amplified.
- PCR is used to amplify a specific allelic region of a DNA strand.
- With the human genome being completely decoded, the genes which encode most (or all) of the blood group systems.
- Any variation in the genetic coding can be picked up, though the physical manifestation of that variation may or may not be evident.

Molecular Biology Techniques for Blood Grouping

1. **SSP** (sequence-specific primer)-**PCR** = To detect specific sequences using primers against the targets of nucleotide sequences (Alleles) which are amplified.

   The procedure relies on the specificity of primer extension that is matched or mismatched with the template at its 3'end. A combination of 2 primers designed for each of 2 polymorphic sequence motifs in cis allows the identification of an allele or a group of alleles that are characterized by these 2 motifs. The presence or absence of the 2 motifs in cis is usually detected by gel electrophoresis, but other detection methods have been developed. The method is rapid and ideally suited for small numbers of samples. Because very few sequences are absolutely allele specific, SSP combine several primer to discriminate a particular allele unambiguously.

2. **SSOP** (sequence-specific oligonucleotide probes)-**PCR** = Amplification of DNA followed by attachment with sequence-specific oligonucleotide probe (**Fig. 53.2**).

   The procedure relies on the locus-specific amplification of the genomic DNA segment comprising the polymorphic sites of antigen alleles. Amplified DNA is then immobilized on a solid support, usually a nylon membrane, and then hybridized with a battery of sequence-specific oligonucleotide probes (SSOP) (direct hybridization). Fluorochromes are linked with the probes to allow their detection by chemiluminescence.

   Alternatively, SSO probes can be immobilized on a solid support, for example color-coded microspheres, and hybridized with labeled PCR product (reverse hybridization). The higher the number of probes the better the resolution level (**Fig. 53.2**).

3. **RT** (real time)-**PCR** = Amplify and simultaneously quantify a targeted gene in a DNA.

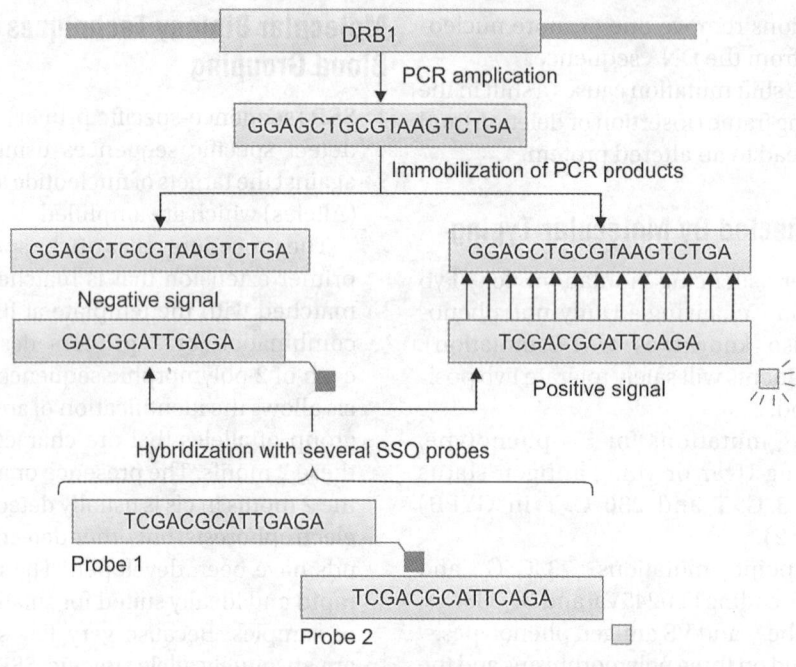

Fig. 53.2: PCR-SSOP.

As the name suggests, real time PCR saves time. The method allows for the direct detection of PCR product during the exponential phase of the reaction, combining amplification and detection in a single step.

4. **Microarray-PCR** = Microscopic DNA spots on a solid surface act as probes, thus this can accomplish many genetic tests in parallel.

DNA microarray is one such technology which enables the researchers to investigate and address issues which were once thought to be non-traceable. One can analyze the expression of many genes in a single reaction quickly and in an efficient manner. An array is an orderly arrangement of samples where matching of known and unknown DNA samples is done based on base pairing rules. An array experiment makes use of common assay systems such as microplates or standard blotting membranes. The sample spot sizes are typically less than 200 µ in diameter usually contain thousands of spots. Thousands of spotted samples known as probes (with known identity) are immobilized on a solid support (a microscope glass slides or silicon chips or nylon membrane). The spots can be DNA, cDNA, or oligonucleotides. These are used to determine complementary binding of the unknown sequences thus allowing parallel analysis for gene expression and gene discovery. An experiment with a single DNA chip can provide information on thousands of genes simultaneously. An orderly arrangement of the probes on the support is important as the location of each spot on the array is used for the identification of a gene.

5. **Sequencers** = Differentiates light signals originating from fluorochromes attached to nucleotides, and detects the sequence.

Genotyping by BeadChip involves multiplex PCR amplification of DNA followed by denaturation and hybridization to color-coded beads incorporating allele-specific probes

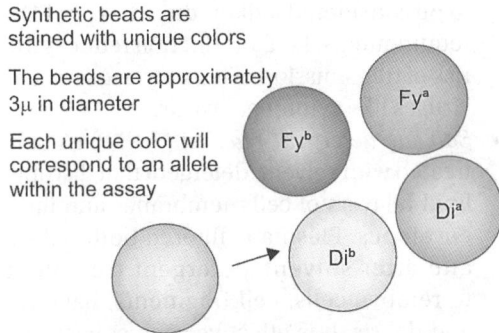

Synthetic beads are stained with unique colors

The beads are approximately 3μ in diameter

Each unique color will correspond to an allele within the assay

Fig. 53.3: Synthetic beads.

with variable 3' ends. When binding occurs between a complementary PCR product and probe, the probe elongates, producing a fluorescent signal. An image is taken with an automated array imaging system and the fluorescent signal intensities determined and correlated with the corresponding probes to provide the basis for genotype and predicted phenotype. The BeadChip assay genotypes up to 96 samples in five hours. The BeadChip microarray contains approximately 4000 beads comprising seven negative and positive reaction controls and 25–40 replicates per allele. Different BeadChip modules are available, with a focus on the range of blood group SNVs to be tested **(Fig. 53.3)**.

The human erythrocyte antigen (HEA) BeadChip genotypes 24 alleles encoding 38 antigens from the RHCE, KEL, FY, DO, LW, CO, SC, LU, DI, JK and MNS blood group systems. Additional chips are available (RHD BeadChip and RHCE BeadChip) for targeted red cell genotyping.

Applications in Transfusion Medicine

Detect blood group antigens in patients.
- Multiple/recently transfused patients blood grouping
- To distinguish an alloantibody from an autoantibody (e.g., anti-E)
- To identify alloantibody when a patient's RBCs type antigen-positive and a variant phenotype is suspected (e.g., anti-D in a D-positive)
- To detect weakly expressed antigens where the patient is unlikely to make antibodies to transfused antigen-positive RBCs
- Identify molecular basis of unusual serological results
- When antibody is weak or not available (e.g. anti-Doa, -Dob, -Jsa, -V/VS).

Detect Blood Group Antigens in Donors

- Mass screening to increase antigen-negative inventory (DNA Arrays)
- To find donors whose RBCs lack a high-prevalence antigen
- To resolve blood group discrepancies
- To detect genes that encode weak antigens
- Quality control of antisera
- To type donors for reagent RBCs for antibody screening cells and antibody identification panels, especially RhD zygosity.

Identify fetus at risk for hemolytic disease of the newborn (HDN)
- In prenatal setting to identify the fetus who is not at risk of HDN
- Should be considered when a mother's serum contains an IgG alloantibody that has been associated with HDN and the father's antigen status for the corresponding antigen is heterozygous
- A semi-invasive method such as amniocentesis can be used
- PCR using maternal plasma has also been used to find out the fetal blood group genotype. It is a routine procedure in many countries now.

In future molecular genotyping will completely replace today's serological methods as these are more accurate and time saving. It will be design a DNA based ABO blood typing protocol that does not require the use of blood.

■ PATHOGEN INACTIVATION METHODS

In the field of blood transfusion, blood safety is still a huge concern. A process designed to eliminate pathogens from transfusion product is Pathogen Inactivation (PI). In addition to strengthen donor screening, pathogen inactivation is one of the most important steps to ensure the blood safety. Pathogen inactivation is a technology that uses a variety of physical, chemical, or photochemical methods to remove or inactivate the blood-borne pathogens, such as viruses, bacteria, and parasites in blood components or products. These PI methods include—solvent/detergent(S/D), nanofiltration and photochemical inactivation such as using methylene blue (MB), psoralens, or riboflavin. PI has potential to decrease transmission of emerging infectious agents.

Essential Features of PI Method

- Must be efficacious to eliminate a broad spectrum of pathogens and prevent sepsis.
- Should cause minimal damage to the blood transfusion product.
- It must not compromise transfusion safety as assessed by in vivo assays and clinical outcomes.
- As an uncomplicated and cost-effective technology, it should be non-toxic, maintain functional cell integrity for transfusion purposes, and pass the stringent tests for bio-equivalency and bio-security.
- It should satisfy the main criteria of availability: being accessible, affordable, and safe, and demonstrate correct usage of the technology.

PI Methods

- *Leukoreduction*: It is based on filtration technique, to remove leukocytes from blood products. Filters remove leukocytes by pore size and charge exclusion. Filtration can be performed either in line as part of a blood collection kit or after collection with gravity based filters. Red blood cells, whole blood and apheresis derived platelets must contain $<5 \times 10^6$ leukocytes to be considered leukoreduced as per FDA requirements. Leukoreduction reduces the risk of transmission of leukocyte associated viruses like cytomegalovirus.
- *Solvent/detergent plasma (Sd)*: Plasma is treated with solvent/detergent that disrupts lipid bilayers of cell membranes and lipid envelopes. Plasma is filtered both before and after solvent/detergent treatment to remove cells, cell fragments, bacteria and debris. It is effective against bacteria, protozoa and enveloped viruses (including hepatitis B virus, hepatitis C virus and HIV). This method also reduces the risk of allergic transfusion reactions. It comprise of 1% tri-(N-butyl)-phosphate (TNBP) and 1% polyoxyethylene-p-t-octylphenol (Triton X-100). TNBP acts as an organic solvent which removes lipids from the membranes, while Triton X-100 is a non-ionic detergent which stabilizes TNBP and disrupts lipid bilayers for easier extraction of lipids. Plasma is treated for 1.5–4 hours at 30°C. Since solvent/detergent directly damages cell membranes, it cannot be used in cellular products (WBC, RBC and platelets).
- *INTERCEPT system*: In the INTERCEPT system, amotosalen—a synthetic psoralen compound, is added to the blood component followed by illumination with UVA light for 4–6 minutes on continuous agitation. Photoactivated amotosalen forms covalent bonds with nucleic acids and intercalates between nucleotide bases, preventing nucleic acid replication and blocking RNA from being transcribed. The INTERCEPT Blood system is used for the treatment of plasma. It can also be used for platelets, but potentially results in the loss of 10% of treated platelets. It is routinely used against bacteria, enveloped and non-enveloped viruses and protozoa. INTERCEPT blood system is less effective against some viruses and ineffective against prions and bacterial spores. Residual amotosalen and photoproducts are absorbed and removed

from transfusion product. UVA light is absorbed by hemoglobin, therefore, this PI cannot be applied for red blood cells.
- *Mirasol Pathogen Reduction Technology*: Riboflavin (vitamin B_2) is added to the blood component and exposed to UVA and UVB light. Riboflavin associates with nucleic acids and generates reactive oxygen intermediates, leading to irreversible modification and damage of nucleic acids. No need for removal of riboflavin after illumination. It is effective against both enveloped and non-enveloped viruses, protozoa, a broad range of bacteria and leukocytes. It has shown reduced efficacy against certain bacterial species such as *Staphylococcus aureus* and bacterial spores. It can be used for platelets as well.
- *Theraflex methylene blue (Theraflex MB)*: This is first PI method for plasma described in early 1990s. Methylene blue (MB) is a phenothiazine positively charged dye. It has high affinity for negatively charged compounds. When activated by visible light, a photodynamic reaction generates reactive oxygen species which target guanine and are responsible for the nucleic acid damage. After treatment, methylene blue and photoproducts are removed via filtration. It is effective in damage of enveloped and some non-enveloped viruses. It has also shown some efficacy against bacteria, including spore forming bacteria.

Note: Pathogen inactivation treatments for Whole Blood and RBCs still under research.

Limitations of Pathogen Inactivation

- Possible decreased effectiveness of blood product
- Leukoreduction can lead to red blood cell and platelet loss, which may not exceed 15% per FDA requirements
- Low to moderate loss of platelet function in vitro
- Not effective against spore-forming bacteria
- Variable effectiveness against non-enveloped viruses, depending on the virus strain and technology
- Not effective against prions
- No current technologies approved for use on red blood cells or whole blood, with various clinical trials underway
- Issues with UV light penetration of red blood cells
- Leads to increased costs of blood products with lack of well established reimbursement policies.

Erythropoietin Therapy

Despite impressive advances in the safety of the blood supply, the search for therapeutic alternatives to blood continues. Erythropoietin (along with iron, vitamin B_{12}, and folic acid) has been recommended as a specific medication "that should be used instead of blood transfusion if the clinical condition of the patient permits sufficient time for these agents to promote erythropoiesis. Therapy with recombinant human erythropoietin was first shown to correct the anemia caused by chronic renal failure in patients undergoing dialysis. Subsequently, erythropoietin was also approved for the treatment of chronic kidney disease and other anemias related to bone marrow suppression and/or failure, such as that due to radiation or chemotherapy treatment for cancer. It decreases the number of RBC transfusions in patients.

RECENT CROSSMATCH TECHNIQUES

Gel Column Agglutination

Gel column agglutination has gained popularity in recent years. It has the unique advantage of detecting mixed-field agglutination patterns, because the high-density media allows a clear separation between agglutinated and non-agglutinated cells, thus indicating the presence of a dual population of red blood cells.

Gel technology can be used for any immunohematology test that has hemagglutination at its endpoint: ABO-Rh typing, typing for other blood group systems, antibody screening and identification, compatibility testing—crossmatching, DAT/IAT, other Coombs phase test.

Advantages of Gel Technique

- Gel card technique is more suitable and less time consuming.
- The results are more stable can be recorded after long time.
- The test can be carried out with very small sample.

It has only one *disadvantage*, that this method is quite expensive as it requires special centrifuge, incubator and gel cards.

Gel Technique for Crossmatch

Principle

The serum and cell reaction takes place in a microtube consisting of a reaction chamber that narrows to become a column containing Sephadex gel and the specific reagent. Incubation takes place, followed by centrifugation under strictly controlled conditions. The serum and the unbound protein lack the weight necessary to be pulled from the reaction chamber to the Sephadex column and therefore do not enter the column. This eliminates the need for 'cell washing phase' as required in case of conventional techniques. During the centrifugation phase, the Sephadex gel matrix acts as a sieve. Agglutinated RBCs are too large to pass through the gel matrix, so they are trapped at various places within the gel, depending on the size of the agglutinates. A negative reaction is seen as a pellet of the cells at the bottom of the microtube. Grading of the reaction can be done according to the distribution of RBCs throughout the gel matrix.

Polyspecific antihuman globulin (AHG) reagents are used for compatibility tests and direct antiglobulin tests. The most important function of the polyspecific AHG reagent is to detect the presence of IgG. The importance of anticompliment in the AHG reagent is detectable since antibodies detectable only by their ability to bind complement are rather rare.

Material required: Gel card, incubator 37°C, centrifuge, micropipettes, suspension tubes.

Compatibility testing specimen: EDTA sample from donor and patient

Sample preparation for minor saline crossmatch: The minor crossmatch is the reaction between the donor serum or plasma and the recipient erythrocytes.

Prepare 5% of patients blood cells suspension in LISS (Low Ionic Strength Saline), by taking 0.5 mL LISS + 50 µL of whole blood or 25 µL of packed blood cells. Mix gently and use it for minor crossmatch.

Sample preparation for major saline crossmatch: Major saline Saline crossmatch is the reaction between the patients serum or plasma and the donors erythrocytes.

Procedure

- *Minor saline crossmatch*:
  - Label the tube as minor crossmatch with donor unit number
  - Using a Pasteur pipette add 3 drops of 5% patient's red cell suspension to the labeled tube
  - Using another Pasteur pipette add 3 drops of donor's serum to the same tube
  - Mix the tube well and centrifuge at 1000 RPM for 1 minute
  - Gently dislodge the cell button and observe for agglutination and hemolysis
  - If there is agglutination or hemolysis, indicates minor incompatibility
  - *Interpretation*: Agglutination or hemolysis indicates that the particular donor unit is incompatible
- *Major Coombs crossmatch*:
  - Identify the appropriate microtubes of the ID-Card with recipients and donor's name or number.

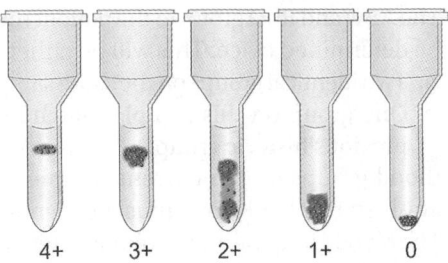

Fig. 53.5: Gel card reading.

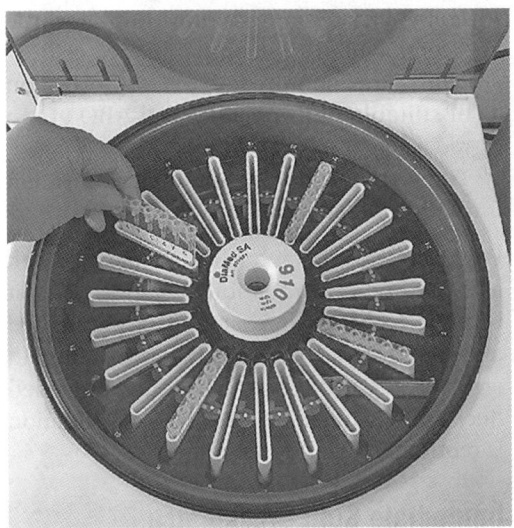

Fig. 53.4: Centrifuge for gel card.

- Remove the aluminum foil from as many microtubes are required by holding the card in the upright position. Pipette 50 µL of the donor red cell suspensions to the appropriate microtubes.
- Add 25 µL of the patient's plasma or serum to each microtube.
- Incubate the Card for 15 minutes at 37°C in the ID-Incubator.
- Centrifuge the Card for 10 minutes. Read and record the results **(Fig. 53.4)**.

A *negative reaction* indicates compatibility of the donor blood with recipient.

A *positive reaction* indicates incompatibility of the donor blood with the recipient, due to the presence of antibodies directed against antigens on the donor red cells.

Interpretation

- *Positive reaction*: Agglutinated red blood cells form a clear line on the surface of the matrix gel or get dispersed in the gel.
- *Negative reaction*: Unagglutinated red blood cells settle at the bottom of the microtube.

Reading and interpretation of results must be done after centrifugation process only. The reaction strength may be recorded as follows **(Fig. 53.5)**:

- G++++ *(G4+)*: Agglutinated red blood cells form a line at the top of the gel microtube.
- G+++ *(G3+)*: Most agglutinated red blood cells remain in the upper half of the gel microtube.
- G++ *(G2+)*: Agglutinated red blood cells are observed throughout the length of the microtube. A small button of red blood cells may also be visible at the bottom of the gel microtube.
- G+ *(G1+)*: Most agglutinated red blood cells remain in the lower half of the microtube. A button of cells may also be visible at the bottom of the gel microtube.
- G±: Most agglutinated red blood cells are in the lower third part of the gel microtube.
- *Negative*: Negative all the red blood cells pass through and form a compact button at the bottom of the gel microtube.

Electronic Crossmatch

Electronic crossmatch, is a type of major crossmatch done without the need for test tubes or contact between donor red cells and patient serum. The blood bank computer system compares ABO and Rh types of the donor and recipient for compatibility.

System Requirements

The Blood bank system for a patient to be suitable for electronic issue must meet the following criteria:

- The ABO and RhD group of the patient must be determined twice. This will be either:
  a. Two identical groups on the same sample
  b. One group on this sample matching a previous historic group
- Blood groups on the current sample and any historic blood group must be identical.
- The blood grouping and antibody screening on the latest sample must have been done using full automation.
- No editing of the ABO front group or RhD group must have occurred on the automated grouping system.
- The patient's serum/plasma must not contain or have ever been known to contain a clinically significant alloantibody reactive at 37°C.
- The following antibodies are not considered clinically significant: a. anti-Lea, b. anti-Leb, c. anti-HI, d. anti-H, e. anti-I, f. anti-P1 and g. HTLA antibodies (e.g., anti-Ch, anti-Rg, anti-Yka, etc.) which are no longer detectable.
- The latest sample must have a negative antibody screen.
- A facility to flag individual patients as unsuitable for electronic issue must be available. The patient's excluded will be:
  - Sickle cell disease patients—excluded for life
  - Post allo bone marrow/stem cell transplant patients who have received an ABO incompatible transplant—excluded for 1 year
  - Post solid organ transplant patients who have received an ABO incompatible transplant—excluded for 1 year
  - Patients with a positive direct antiglobulin test—exclude until DAT is negative
- The computer system must not allow the selection of ABO incompatible red cells.
- The system should demand authorization of suitable but non-identical ABO group red cells
- The system should demand authorization of RhD incompatibility.

Electronic crossmatch can only be accepted as a method of compatibility testing when it is properly designed, validated, implemented and monitored. It reduces the risk of human error through the use of software controlled decision making but high degree of validation is required to ensure accuracy.

Immediate Spin Crossmatch

Often abbreviated as "IS crossmatch," this is a type of serologic crossmatch performed by adding diluted red cells and patient serum/plasma to a test tube at room temperature, immediately centrifuging ("spinning"), and then examining visually for agglutination. This procedure is only used when a patient lacks evidence of "unexpected" (non-ABO) antibodies, both currently and historically (i.e., if a patient has evidence of a clinically significant antibody now or in the past, they are NOT eligible for an immediate spin crossmatch even if that antibody is no longer detectable).

Immediate spin crossmatch can save transfusion services lots of time, since an incubation and the AHG phase of testing are not required. This crossmatch really is designed for—detecting ABO incompatibility between donor red blood cells and recipient serum/plasma.

BLOOD DONOR QUESTIONNAIRE

Sr. No.   DATE (दिनांक) :

Name of the Donor (रक्तदाता का नाम) : _____

Address (पता) : _____

_____ Tel. No. (टेलिफोन नं.) _____

1. Age (उम्र) Sex (लिंग) (M/F) (स्त्री/पुरुष)   Wt (वजन)

2. Have you eaten anything in the last 4 hours ? Yes/No.
   क्या आपने पिछले चार घंटो में कुछ खाया है ? हां/ना.

3. Have you slept well last night ? Yes/No.
   क्या आप बीती रात को बराबर सोये थे ? हां/ना.

4. Have you taken aspirin in the last 3 days ? Yes/No.
   पिछले तीन दिनों में कोई दर्द-निवारक दवाई ली है ? हां/ना.

5. Are you taking any medicine at present ? Yes/No.
   क्या आपने हाल ही में कोई दवाई ली है ? हां/ना.

6. a) Have you donated blood in the last 3 months ? Yes/No.
   पिछले तीन महिनों में आपने रक्त-दान किया है ? हां/ना.

   b) Did you have any discomfort during prior blood donation ? Yes/No.
   क्या रक्त-दान के समय आपने असहज महसूस किया ? हां/ना.

7. a) Have you had jaundice in the last one year ? Yes/No.
   क्या आपको पिछले एक साल में पीलिया हुआ था ? हां/ना.

   b) Has your blood ever tested positive for HB_sAg ? Yes/No.
   क्या आपके रक्त परीक्षण में हेपटायटिस के किटाणु पाए गए ? हां/ना.

   c) Has any of your family members suffered from jaundice in the last 6 months ? Yes/No.
   क्या आपके परिवार के किसी व्यक्ति को पिछले छ: महिनों में पीलिया हुआ है ? हां/ना.

8. Have you had malaria or taken antimalarial drugs in the last 1 year ? Yes/No.
   क्या आपने पिछले एक साल में मलेरिया निवारक दवाई ली है ? हां/ना.

9. Have you any reason to believe you have been infected by the virus that causes AIDS ? Yes/No.
   क्या आपको ऐड्स के कोई भी लक्षण दिखाई देते हैं ? हां/ना.

   In the last 6 months have you had
   पिछले ६ महिनों से आपको यह बिमारियाँ हुई है ?

     Night Sweats (रात को पसीना आना) Diarrhoea (दस्त)
     Unexplained weight loss (बिना वजह वजन कम होना) Swollen glands (गांठ सुजन)
     Persistent fever (बारबार बुखार आना)

10. Have you had any of the following in the last 6 months ? Yes/No.
    पिछले ६ महिनों में आपको नीचे दी गई बिमारियाँ हुई है ? हां/ना.

      Typhoid (टाइफाइड) Measles (मीझलस्)
      Mumps (कनफडा) Chicken Pox (चिकन पोक्स)

11.	Have you been immunised or vaccinated in the last one month ? If yes, for what ? when ? (Cholera, Typhoid, Diphtheria, whooping cough, Tetanus, Hepatitis) पिछले एक महिने में आपने किसी तरह का टीका लिया है ? अगर 'हा' तो किसलिए और कब ? (कॉलरा, टाइफाइड, डिप्तेरिया, काली खांसी, टेटानस, हेपटायटीस)	Yes/No. हां/ना.
12.	Have you had any accident, operation or dental procedure in the last 6 months ? पिछले छ: महिनों में कोई दुर्घटना, शल्य चिकित्सा, दन्त चिकित्सा हुई है ?	Yes/No. हां/ना.
13.	Have you received any blood or blood components in the last 6 months ? क्या आपको पिछले ६ महिनो में खून चढाया है ?	Yes/No. हां/ना.
14.	Have you had a tattoo, acupuncture or ear piercing in the last 6 months ? पिछले छ: महिनो में क्या आपने टैटूय, अॅक्यूपंक्चर, कान छेद करवाया है ?	Yes/No. हां/ना.
15.	H/O Alcohol consumption in the last 24 hours. क्या आपने पिछले २४ घंटो में शराब पी है ?	Yes/No. हां/ना.
16.	H/O Dog bite & history of taking Rabies vaccination within a year. क्या आपको पिछले एक साल में कुत्ते ने काटा है या उसके लिये टिका लगवाया है ?	Yes/No. हां/ना.
17.	Have you had any of the following ? if yes, tick ( ) appropriate one. यदि आपको इसमेंसे कोई बिमारी हुई है तो उसके सामने टिक ( ) किजीए।	

        Allergy (अॅलर्जी)   Amoebiasis (पेट में किडा)   Asthma (दम)
        Bleeding tendency (स्त्री रक्तस्त्राव)   Cancer (कॅन्सर)   Cold/Cough (शर्दी/खांसी)
        Diabetes (मधुप्रमेह)   Fainting attack (चक्कर आना)   Epilepsy (मिरगी/आकडी)
        Fever (बुखार)   Gout (गाउट)   Gonorrhoea (गुप्तरोग)
        Heart disease (दिल की बिमारी)   Influenza (ईन्फ्लुएन्झा)   High B. P. (हाय बी.पी.)
        Kidney disease (गुर्दे की बिमारी)   Lung disease (फेफडों की बिमारी) Liver disease (Jaundice) (पीलिया)
        Skin disease (चर्मरोग)   Syphilis (गुप्तरोग)   Tuberculosis (टीबी)

18.	In case of women : (स्त्रियों के लिए)	
	Are you menstruating at present? क्या आपका महिना अभी चालू है ?	Yes/No. हां/ना.
	Are you pregnant / breast feeding ? क्या आप गर्भवती है ?	Yes/No. हां/ना.
	Have you a child less than one year of age ? क्या आपको एक साल से छोटा बच्चा है ?	Yes/No. हां/ना.
	Have you had an abortion in the last 6 months ? पिछले छ: महिनो में गर्भपात करवाया है ?	Yes/No. हां/ना.
19.	Have you read and understood all the information presented to you and have you answered all the question ? क्या आपको यह जानकारी पुरी तरह समझ में आई है और आपने सभी सवालों का जवाब दिया है ?	Yes/No. हां/ना.

Consent

I wish to Donate Voluntarily / as Replacement for my patient. _____
में अपनी मर्जी से रक्तदान करना चाहता हूँ / मरीज का नाम :-

Donar's Name (रक्तदाता का नाम)_____

Signature (सही) _____

Donar's blood group _____   Rh : _____

B. P. _____ mm Hg   Pulse _____ Temp _____

Hb _____ gms %   Site of Veni puncture _____

Signature of Medical Officer

CROSSMATCHING REPORT FORM

No. : _____   Date : _____

Patient's Name : _____   Age : _____ Sex : _____

Ref. by Dr. _____   Hospital : _____

Patient's Blood Group [　　　　]   Rh (D) : [　　　　]
                                         Factor

WHOLE BLOOD	[ ]		FRESH FROZEN PLASMA	[ ]
PACKED CELLS	[ ]		PLATELET CONCENTRATE	[ ]

FORWARD TYPING PATIENT'S CELLS				REVERSE TYPING PATIENT'S SERUM			INTERPRETATION			GROUP & RH		
Anti A	Anti B	Anti A, B	Anti D	Cells A_1	Cells B	Cells O + Bov	Auto Cont	Group	Rh	Du	Done By	Checked By	Date

COMPATIBILITY TEST (CROSSMATCHING)

Unit No.	Segment No.	GR+RH	X-Match Major			X-Match Minor			Serology						X Matched by			
			SAL	ALB	AHG	SAL	ALB	AHG	HBSAG	HCV	HIV 1+2	VDRL	MP	Antibody Screening	Done by Tech.	Checked by	Date	Time

EMERGENCY CROSSMATCH "QUICK SPIN"

Unit No.	Segment No.	GR+RH	X-Match Major SALINE	X-Match Minor SALINE	Serology						X Matched by			
					HBSAG	HCV	HIV 1+2	VDRL	MP	Antibody Screening	Done by Tech.*	Checked by	Date	Time
1														

_____   Time : _____   Date : _____
Receiver's Signature

Note : 1) Reservation of Cross matched unit will be kept reserved for 24 hours only.
       2) Blood or Blood Component once issued will not be taken back.
       3) Please send the relatives to Blood Bank for replacement of Blood.

_____
Signature

Index

Page numbers followed by *f* refer to figure, *fc* refer to flowchart, and *t* refer to table.

A

A antigens, production of 261
A blood group 259
AB blood group 260
ABO
  antibodies, characteristics
    of 260
  antigens, characteristics of 260
  blood group 260*t*
    selection of 304*t*
    system 259, 262, 275
  incompatibility 302
  system, biochemistry of 261
Absolute eosinophil count 143
Acanthocytes 175, 176*f*
Acetone 144
Acid-base balance 102
Acid-citrate dextrose 127, 129,
    287, 293
Acid-fast
  bacilli staining 93
  bacteria 95
Acidosis, acute 54
Acquired immunodeficiency
    syndrome 307
Actinomycosis 258
Activated partial thromboplastin
    time 186, 194, 197
Addison's disease 54
Adenine 287, 288, 313
Adenosine deaminase 73
Adenovirus 142
Adrenal corticotropic hormone 43
Adult stem cell 324
  transplant 324, 325
Agammaglobulinemia 258
  acquired 258
  congenital 258
Agglutination reaction 277*t*
  grading of 285
Agranulocyte 114
Albumin 81, 100
Albuminuria, causes of 81
Alkaline phosphatase 74, 75
Alkalosis 51
  metabolic 54
Allele 260, 265, 329

Allergic reactions 144, 295
Allergies 137
  seasonal 144
Alpha-fetoprotein 43, 44, 63
Alpha-thalassemia 167
Amastigote 216*f*
  stage 216
Amino acids 118
Ammonia 74
Ammonium 84
  biurate crystals 83*f*
  oxalate 287
Amniocentesis 301
Amniotic fluid 62, 63
  abnormal 63
  collection, procedure for 63
  findings, normal 63
Amylase 71, 74, 75
Amyloidosis 14, 17
Analyzers
  care of 101
  maintenance of 101
Anaphylactic reactions 295
Anemia 134, 200, 211, 301
  aplastic 166, 201
  autoimmune hemolytic 282
  diagnosis of 202
  drug-induced hemolytic 282
  hemolytic 150, 165*f*, 201
  hypochromic microcytic 201
  mild 300
  normochromic
    macrocytic 201
    microcytic 201, 201*f*
    normocytic 200
  pernicious 166, 201
  refractory normoblastic 166
  severe 300
  sideroblastic 166, 182, 202
  signs of 202
  symptoms of 202
  types of 201
Anti-A sera 276
Anti-B sera 276
Antibody 255
  antinuclear 160
  classes of 256

  monoclonal 274
  size of 257
  titration 284
Anticoagulant 129, 145–147, 288
  biological 130
  preparation of 286
  properties of 286
Antigens 43, 254
  binding 257
    sites, number of 257
  carcinoembryonic 43, 46, 74
  high frequency 254, 272
  low frequency 255, 272
  public 254, 272
Antiglobulin test, indirect 281
Antihuman globulin reagent 282
Antimalarial antibodies, detection
    of 215
Antinuclear cytoplasmic
    antibody 67
Antisera 273
  preparation of 273
  preservation of 273
  selection of 274
Anuria 54, 80
Anxiety 67
Apheresis 244, 290
  room 248
Apoptopic bodies 21, 21*f*
Apoptosis 14, 17, 18, 21, 21*f*, 21*t*
  embryological 18
  pathological 18
  physiological 18
Arachis hypogea 274
Arterial blood collection 122
Artery
  peripheral 304
  umbilical 304
Arthritis 137
  types of 77, 78
Ascaris 88
Asthma 137, 144, 258
Atrophy 10
  causes of 10
Auramine-rhodamine method 95
Autoimmune disease 27, 29, 144
Autoimmune disorders 137

Automated analyzers
  advantages of 234
  disadvantages of 234
Automation 98, 232, 235
Azoospermia 61

B

B antigens, production of 261
B blood group 260
Babesiosis 298, 309
Bacillus subtilis 41
Bacteria 74, 306
Bacterial contamination 296, 308
Balantidium coli cyst 89*f*
Band cell 119
Basophils 112, 113, 113*f*, 119, 140, 142, 181
B-cell 120
Bence-Jones proteinemia 258
Benedict's test 81
Beta-2-microglobulin 45
Beta-human chorionic
    gonadotropin 45
Beta-thalassemia major 165*f*
Bile
  pigments 82
  salts 82
Bilirubin 14, 16, 63, 64, 104
Biological safety cabinets 36
Biomedical wastes
  categories of 38*t*
  caution signs for 39*f*
  disposal of 39
  emission standards for 40*t*
  handling 36
  treatment of 39
Biopsy 179
  site of 180
  surgical 179
Biosafety laboratories, levels of 35
Blackwater fever 211
Bleeding 185
  external 134
  internal 134, 150
  time 190
Bloating, abdominal 75
Blood 88, 104, 111, 245
  agar 97
  anticoagulated 132, 138, 145
  artificial 325
  bank 239, 241, 251*t*, 257
    objectives of 245
    operation of 245, 249
    organization of 245, 246
    premises design 247
    recent advances in 323
    requirements for 247*t*
    spreading of 243

casts 84
cells 111, 112*t*, 209, 231
  counter machine 234, 234*f*
  counting of 131
  production of 117*fc*
clotting
  effect of 188
  significance of 187
coagulation 185, 187, 290
  disturbances of 187
collection 122, 128, 312
  proper 246
component
  centrifugation for 312
  isolation of 243
  preparation of 312
  transfusion 311
cultures 127
dilution of 137
donors 262
  instructions to 292
elements of 115*f*
film 162*f*
  examination of 162
  observation of 212
  thick 212
  thin 212, 213
fresh 165
function of 115
group 246, 259, 291, 291*t*, 329
  antigens 333
  discovery of 242
  importance of 262
  molecular biology techniques
    for 331
  system 264, 269
  technique of 275
  types of 269
loss of 286
pressure 288
proper preservation of 246
sample 131, 132, 135, 136, 143
  usage of 125*t*
smear
  preparation of 138
  staining of 139
specimen 148, 149, 151, 169, 172, 193
staining of 138
storage of 293
tests 67
transfusion 306
  autologous 290
  service 250
  technique 286, 294
type 259
volume of 291
Body fluid 59

Bombay blood group 272
Bone marrow 137, 178, 178*f*, 183, 220
  aspirate slides, staining of 180
  aspiration 220
  diseases 150
  disorders 137
  failure 134
  film, preparation of 180
  stem cells 324
Bovine albumin 284
Bowel disease 137
Breast cancer 46
Breath, shortness of 66
Bright red blood, streaks of 87
Bronchoscopy 92
Brown sputum 93
Brucellosis 142
Brugia malayi 224
Buffy coat smears, staining of 220
Bulbourethral glands 60

C

Calcification, pathological 14
Calcitonin 43, 46
Calcium
  amorphous 84
  carbonate 85
  chloride 195
  homeostasis, loss of 13
  oxalate 88
  serum 57
Calculus 88
Calibration 233
Cancer 144
  antigen-125 46
Candida albicans 97
Capillary blood 132, 138
  collection 122
Capillary tube 149
Carbohydrate metabolism 102
Carbon dioxide 111, 151
Card reader 149, 150*f*
Cardiac computed tomography 67
Cardiac magnetic resonance
  imaging 67
Cardiac tamponade 67
Casts 83
Catecholamines 43
Cat-scratch disease 29
Cell 83
  adaption 10
  animal 7
  condensation 21, 21*f*
  counter technology 230
  death 10, 14
    types of 17
  fragmentation 21, 21*f*
  function of 9

injury 13
  causes of 11
    general biochemical mechanisms of 13
    morphology of 12
    overview of 10
    types of 13, 14*fc*
  maturation stages 181*f*
  membrane 7
  normal distribution of 181*f*
  organelles 7
  pathology 10
  permanent 31
  pluripotential 116
  presence of 64
  swelling 21*f*
Cellular
  changes 18, 25
  components 311
  injury 11
  pathology 7
  swelling 13, 14
Central nervous system 223
Centrifugation 313, 320
Centrosomes 9
Cerebrospinal fluid 64
  cell counts 64
Chagas' disease 298, 309
Charcot-Leyden crystals 96
Chemical
  agents 12
  anticoagulants 129
  biochemistry 4
  examination 81, 88
  method 153
  pathology 4
  tests 65
  toxic substances 29
Chemiluminescent microparticle immunoassay technology 49
Chemistry tests 65
Chills 66, 75
Chloride, serum 55
Chocolate agar 97
Cholesterol 71
  effusions 69
Cholesterolosis 14, 15
Christmas disease 188
Chromogranin A 47
Chromosome 260
Chronic inflammation 24, 27*t*, 29
  causes of 27
  function of 29
Chronic inflammatory
  cells 27
  disease 142, 150
  response 27

Chyliform effusions 69
Chylothorax 69
Chylous urine 227
Circulatory system 161
Circumsporozoite protein 208
Citrate 129, 286, 287
  phosphate dextrose 129, 130, 287, 293, 313
Citric acid 287
Cleaning dispensing system 101
Clostridium perfringens 20
Clot retraction 190, 192
Coagulation
  factors 185
  mechanism of 186
Colony forming unit 116, 118, 119
Color 87
  reaction 173
  reagent 56
Colorimetric method 152
Commercial automated culture systems 97
Complete blood count 155, 202, 230
Compressor unit 53
Computer assisted semen analysis 62
Confusion 67
Connective tissue diseases 73
Continuous flow
  analyzers 99
  centrifugation 320
Convalescence 305
Cooley's anemia 202
Coomb's crossmatch 280
  major 336
Coomb's reaction 255
Coomb's serum 284
Coomb's test 202, 281
  indirect 281, 283
  positive 282
  direct 282*f*
  indirect 283*f*
Copper sulfate solution 153
Corrosive chemicals 22
Creatinine 63, 64
  serum 100
Crohn's disease 144
Cryopoor plasma 311
Cryoprecipitate 311, 312, 316
  issue of 317
Crystal 84, 88
Cushing's disease 144
Cushing's syndrome 4, 54
Cyanomethemoglobin 152
Cyst, concentration methods for 88
Cystine 84
Cytapheresis 319, 321

Cytochemistry 205
Cytogenetics 205
Cytokeratin fragment 47
Cytology 68, 72, 74
Cytomegalovirus 96, 142, 289, 298, 307
Cytopathology 4
Cytoplasm 8
Cytoskeleton 9

D

Dacryocytes 176, 176*f*
Deep vein thrombosis 188
Degmacytes 176, 176*f*
Dehydration 54, 80, 150
Denaturation 106
Dermatologic disorders 258
Dextrose 287, 288
Diabetes
  insipidus 54, 80
  mellitus 80
Diarrhea 54, 66
Differential leukocyte count 123, 230, 138
Direct antiglobulin test 281, 282
Disodium citrate 129
Disseminated intravascular coagulation 188
Distilled water 92, 131, 135, 144, 153, 287, 288
D-mannitol 288
Dolichos biflorus 262, 263, 273
Donor
  blood, processing of 249
  care of 292
  complex 248
  identification of 291
  rest room 248
  screening test 289
    development of 244
  selection 288
  proper 246
Down's syndrome 12, 64
Drabkin's solution 152
Drugs, coumarin group of 190
Dry gangrene 20
Ductless gland 120
Dukes method 190
Dysgammaglobulinemia 258
Dysproteinemia 258

E

Echinocytes 176, 176*f*
Echocardiography 67
Eczema 144, 258
Edward's syndrome 64
Electrical impedance 231
Electrocardiogram 67

Electrolyte 50
　classification of 50
　solution 231
Electrophoresis, bands of 108f
Elliptocyte 175
Elliptocytic red blood cells 175f
Embolism, pulmonary 188
Embryonic stem cell 323
Empyema 70
Endolimax nana cyst 89f
Endoplasmic reticulum 8, 12
Endotoxemia 24
Energy, loss of 13
Entamoeba
　coli cyst 89f
　hartmanni cyst 89f
　histolytica 90
　　cyst 89f
　polecki cyst 89f
Enzyme-linked immunosorbent assay 221
Eosin 144
Eosinophils 28, 112-114, 114f, 119, 140, 143, 144, 181
Epithelial casts 84
Epithelial cells 83
Epstein-Barr virus 298, 308
Erythroblastosis fetalis 282
Erythrocytapheresis 321
Erythrocytes 111, 113f, 116, 118, 182
　sedimentation rate 111, 130, 145, 161, 211
Erythrocytic cycle 208
Erythrocytopenia 134
Erythroid 118
　abnormal 182
Erythroleukemia 166
Erythropheresis 319
Erythropoiesis 116, 117
Erythropoietin
　deficiency 134
　level 202
　therapy 335
Ethylenediaminetetraacetic acid 124, 129, 132, 138, 172, 193, 288
Evacuated tube assembly system 127f
Exchange transfusion
　techniques 303, 304
　types of 304
Exercise 137
Exon 329
Eyes 161

F
Fanconi's syndrome 57
Fat necrosis 20
Fate 3

Fatigue 66, 199
Fatty acid crystals 88
Fatty casts 84
Febrile nonhemolytic transfusion reaction 294
Ferritin 202
Fetal hemoglobin 154, 164
Fever 24, 24f, 66, 75
　scarlet 144
Fibrin 47
Fibrinogen 47
Fibrinolysis 187
Fibroblasts 28
Fibrosis, pulmonary 134
Filariasis 206, 224
Fisher-race
　nomenclature 266
　system 266
Flame photometer 53
Flow cytometry 231
Fluorescence microscopy 94
Fluorescent
　dyes 219
　flow cytometry 231
　in situ hybridization 182, 205
Forensic pathology 5
Formalin 131
　citrate diluting fluid 131
Fouchet's test 82
Fragments 256
Fresh frozen plasma 311, 316-318
Frozen cells 314
Fuchs-Rosenthal chamber 144
Fungal infection 68, 91
Fungi 74

G
Gas gangrene 20
Gasometric method 153
Gastrin 43
Gastrointestinal system 161
Gaucher disease 179
Gel
　card
　　centrifuge for 337f
　　reading 337f
　column agglutination 335
　electrophoresis 107
　technique 336
　　advantages of 336
Gene 260, 329
Genetics 5
Genotype 261
Giant cell granuloma 29
Giemsa's stain 139, 140, 180, 212, 228
Glacial acetic acid 135
Gland 60
Glassware, cleaning of 252

Glomerulonephritis, 80
Glucose 65, 68, 71, 74, 75, 81, 103, 287, 288
　6-phosphate dehydrogenase deficiency 167
　test for 81
Glutamine 65
Glycerin 140
Glycerol 140
Glycosuria, causes of 82
Golgi bodies 9
Gomori's method 56
Gram staining 95
Gram-negative
　bacillus 29
　coccobacilli 96
　diplococcic 96
　rods 96
Gram-positive
　cocci 96
　diplococci 96
　yeast cells 96
Granular casts 83
Granulation tissue, ingrowth of 31
Granules
　basophilic 141
　eosinophilic 141
Granulocytes 113, 118, 231, 317
　apheresis 311
Granuloma
　epithelioid 28
　hypersensitivity 258
Guillian-Barre syndrome 321

H
H antigens, production of 261
Haemophilus influenzae 96, 97
Hair loss 161
Hay's fever 258
Hay's test 82
Haym's diluting fluid 131
Head defects 61
Health 3
　conditions 288
Heart 161
　disease, congenital 150
Heat and acid test 81
Heinz bodies 167, 168f, 177, 177f
Hemapheresis 319
Hematocrit 202
　reader 149
Hematology 5, 109
　analyzer 230, 232
　technology 230
Hematoxylin 228
Hemochromatosis 16
Hemocytometer 131, 132, 135, 136, 144

Index

Hemoglobin 151, 202, 288
  A 154
  A2 154
  concentration 158
  encapsulated 327
  estimation 151, 152f
  F 154
  S 155
  solutions 327
  structure of 154
Hemoglobinopathy 154
Hemolysis 128, 134, 165
  elevated liver enzymes, and low platelet count syndrome 317
  intravascular 54
Hemolytic disease 193, 269, 282, 299, 303, 333
Hemolytic reaction, delayed 297
Hemolytic transfusion reactions 270, 295
Hemoparasite 206
Hemophilia 188, 196
  A 188, 197
  B 188, 197
  C 197
  types of 197
Hemopoiesis 116, 120
Hemorrhage 188
Hemorrhagic disorders 189
  acquired 190
  screening tests of 190
Hemosiderin 14, 15
Hemosiderosis
  generalized 16
  localized 15
Hemostasis 187
Hemothorax 70
Heparin 130, 286, 287
  therapy of 190
Hepatitis 142, 298, 307
  A virus 307
  B 289
    virus 307
  C virus 307
  E 307
    virus 307
  G virus 308
  viruses 307
Herpes simplex virus 96
Hiccoughs 67
High security animal disease laboratory 36
Histidine-rich protein 214
Histopathology 4
Hodgkin's disease 179
Homeostasis 10
Hookworm 88

Hormones 43
Howell-Jolly body 177, 177f
Human
  cell, typical 8f
  chorionic gonadotropin 43
  herpes virus 6 298, 308
  immunodeficiency virus 137, 307
  T lymphotropic virus 298, 308
Hyaline casts 83
Hyalinosis 14, 17
Hybridomas 274
Hydrocele fluid 227
Hydrochloric acid 151
Hydrops fetalis 300, 301
Hydrothorax 70
Hyperbilirubinemia 300, 301
  severe 301, 303
Hypercalcemia 58
Hypercoagulation 187
Hypergammaglobulinemia, detection of 220
Hyperimmunization 258
Hyperparathyroidism 80
Hyperplasia 10, 11
  benign prostatic 49
  causes of 11
Hypersensitivity reactions 22
Hyperthyroidism 58, 142, 166
Hypertrophy 10
  causes of 10
Hypocoagulation 188
Hypogammaglobulinemia 258
Hypoprothrombinemia 188
Hyposplenism 167
Hypothyroidism 54, 142
Hypoxia 11

I

Iatrogenic effusions 70
Immunoglobulin 48
  A myeloma 258
  basic structure of 255
  clinical significance of 258
  D myelomas 258
  E myeloma 258
  G 258
    myeloma 258
  general functions of 257
  M 258
  production of 256
  serum 254
  synthesis of 258
Immunohematology 254
Immunological tests 229
Immunology 5
Incubation time 284
Indian Council of Medical Research 36

Indirect immunofluorescent antibody test 220
Infections 137, 142
  bacterial 24f, 290
  chronic 258
    granulomatous 258
    nonviral bacterial 29
  endogenous 306
  exogenous 306
  microbial 22
  parasitic 142, 309
  persistent 27
  severe 137
  viral 142
Inflammation 22
  acute 24, 26, 27t
  beneficial effects of 23
  causes of 22
  effects of 23
  goals of 22
  granulomatous chronic 28
  harmful effects of 23
  nongranulomatous chronic 29
  signs of 23
  systemic effects of 23
  types of 24, 30fc
Influenza 142
Infusion method 304
Inherited hemorrhagic disorders 189
Inner cell mass 323
Interferon gamma release assays 73
Intermittent flow centrifugation 320
International Council for Standardization in Hematology 235
Intracellular organisms 28
Intradermal test 229
Intraleukocytic malaria pigment 215
Iodine preparation 90
Iron deficiency anemia 201
Ischemia 11
Isotone 231
Isovolumetric exchange 304
Itchy skin 199
Ivy's method 190, 191

J

Jaswant Singh Battacharya stain 212
Jaundice 16, 300, 301, 303
  causes of 16
  hemolytic 16
  obstructive 16
Joints 161
  pain 75

K

Kala-azar 216, 218
Kaolin reagent 194
Karyolysis 18
Karyorrhexis 18
Kawamoto technique 219
Kell system 270
Kernicterus 301
Ketone 104
   bodies 82
Kidney 161
   failure 150
   function 102
   tumor 150
Killed vaccines 289
Klinefelter's syndrome 64
KRAS gene mutation analysis 48
Kupffer cells 218

L

Lactate dehydrogenase 48, 66, 74
Lambert-Eaton myasthenic
   syndrome 321
Langhans giant cells 28
Laser flow cytometry 231
Lecithin 63
Lee-White method 191
Leishman stain 139, 140, 193,
   212, 220
   crystals 139
   powder 139
Leishmania 206, 216
   donovani 220, 310
Leishmaniasis 298, 310
   cutaneous 219, 221
Leprosy 29
Leucine 84
Leukapheresis 319, 322
Leukemia 134, 137, 144, 150, 179
   182, 203
   acute 203, 205
      granulocytic 204
      lymphoblastic 204, 204*f*, 258
      lymphocytic 142, 203
      myelocytic 203, 204
   chronic 203, 205
      granulocytic 204
      lymphoblastic 204, 205*f*, 258
      lymphocytic 142, 204
      myelocytic 204
   juvenile chronic myeloid 166
Leukocyte 105, 113, 116, 311
   count 211
   poor red cells 314
Leukocytosis 23, 137
Leukopenia 137
Leukopoiesis 118
Leukoreduction 334
Lewis system 269

Lipids, intracellular accumulation
   of 13
Lipofuscin 14, 15
Liquid waste
   dispose of 41*t*
   standards for 41
Lithium heparin 127
Live vaccines 289
Liver 137, 203
   disease 167, 258
   disorder 193
   enlargement of 300
   failure 54, 190
   function 102
Locke solution 220
Locus 260, 329
Lung 161
   diseases 150
Lupus 137, 144
   erythematosus 160, 258
      bodies 162*f*
      cell 160
      types of 160
Lymph
   exudates of 227
   nodes 203
Lymphocytes 28, 66, 114, 114*f*, 140,
   141, 231
   large 112, 114
   small 112, 114
Lymphocytopenia 142
Lymphoid 120
   aplasia 258
   tissue, gut-associated 120
Lymphoma 137, 150, 182
Lymphoproliferative
   disorders 258
Lysosomes 8

M

Macrohematocrit 148
Macrophage 118, 120
Macroscopic examination 87
Magnesium 84
   phosphates 84, 85
Malabsorption syndromes 258
Malaria 206, 214*t*, 258, 298, 309
Malarial parasite
   differentiation of 210*t*
   tests for 212, 215
Malnutrition 54, 134, 258
Manual cell counting, limitations
   of 234
Mast cells 181
Masturbation 60
Mean cell
   hemoglobin 158
      concentration 159
   volume 158

Mean corpuscular
   hemoglobin 200
      concentration 200
   volume 200
Medical examination room 248
Megakaryocyte 118, 181
Melanin 14, 15
Membrane
   filtration 320
   lipid peroxidation of 13
Mercuric chloride 131
Metamyelocyte 119, 181
   neutrophilic 119
Metaplasia 10, 11
   causes of 11
Methyl alcohol 139, 140
Microbiology 5
Microembolization 296
Microfilaria 224, 224*f*, 227
   bancrofti 225*f*
   staining methods for 228
Microhematocrit 148, 149
   centrifuge 149
Microscope 131, 132, 135, 136
Microscopic examination 72, 82, 88,
   138, 139
Microscopy 20, 76
   advantages of 213
   disadvantages of 213
Microtrephine biopsy 179
Microwaving, standards of 41
Mirasol pathogen reduction
   technology 335
Mitochondria 9
Molecular
   biology 329
   pathology 6
   typing 329, 331
Molybdate reagent 56
Monoblast 119
Monocytes 112, 114, 114*f*, 119, 140,
   142, 231
Mononucleosis, infectious 258, 282
Moraxella catarrhalis 96
Morphology 4
Multiple plastic packs system 312
Multistix urinalysis strips 103
Muscle aches 66
Myasthenia gravis 321
Mycobacterium
   leprae 29
   tuberculosis 28, 93
Mycoplasmal infection 282
Myeloblasts 118, 119, 181
Myelocyte 181
   basophilic 119
   eosinophilic 119
   neutrophilic 119
Myelodysplasia 182

Myeloid 118
Myeloma, multiple 179, 182
Myeloproliferative disorders 142

N
Nausea 66, 75
N-cetylpyridinium chloride 92
Neck defects 61
Necrosis 14, 18, 21, 21*f*
    causes of 18
    coagulative 19
    fibrinoid 20
    gangrenous 20
    liquefactive 19
    morphological types of 19
Necrozoospermia 61
Needle 123, 126
    aspiration 179
Neocytes 315
Nephritis, salt losing 54
Nervous system 161
Nervousness 80
Neubauer chamber
    central square of 132*f*
    corner squares of 136*f*
Neutrophil 28, 112, 113, 113*f*, 118, 119, 140, 141
    nuclei of 141
    segmented 181
Neutrophilic bands 181
Nitrite 104
Noninvasive method 92
Novy-Macneal-Nicolle medium 220
Nuclear matrix protein 48
Nucleus 8

O
O blood group 260
Occult blood test 82, 88
O-cresolphthalein complexone method 57
Odor 87, 93
Oligosaccharides 261
Oligospermia
    mild 61
    severe 61
Oliguria 54, 80
    causes of 80
Oncogenes 43
Oncopathology 6
Organ transplant rejection 144
Osmosis 162
    across red blood cell plasma membrane 163
Osmotic fragility 162
    curves 165*f*
    test 163, 164
        procedures for 164*t*
Ova, concentration methods for 88

Ovalocytes 175, 175*f*
Oxalate 84, 129, 130, 286, 287
Oxygen 111
    deprivation 11
    therapeutics 326
    transportation of 151

P
P system 269
Packed cell volume 111, 130, 148, 198
Packed red blood cells 313
Pain
    abdominal 75
    chest 66
Palpitations 66
Paracentesis biochemistry 75
Paralysis, familial hyperkalemic 54
Parasites 86, 88
    lactate dehydrogenase 214
Patau's syndrome 64
Paternity testing 262
Pathogen inactivation
    limitations of 335
    methods 333
Pathogenesis 3, 19
Pathology 1, 3, 4
    branches of 4
    clinical 3, 5
    general 3, 5
    laboratory 33
        automation in 98
    nutritional 5
    oral and maxillofacial 6
    systemic 3
Perfluorocarbons 326
Pericardial effusion, diagnosis of 67
Pericardial fluid 65
    analysis 66, 67
    normal values of 65
    tests 68
Pericardiocentesis 67
    biochemistry 68
Pericarditis
    causes of 66
    chronic constrictive 67
    complications of 67
Peripheral blood
    smear 140, 219, 224*f*
    stem cell transplant 325
Peritoneal fluid 73
    normal values of 74
    tests 75
Perl's staining method 182
Peroxisomes 9
ph 104
Phagocytosis, process of 25*f*
Phenotype 261
Philadelphia chromosome 45

Phlebotomy 290
Phosphate crystals, triple 88
Phosphatidylcholine, saturated 64
Phosphatidylglycerol 63
Phosphorus
    serum 56
    standard 56
Phototherapy 303
PI methods 334
Picked-cell volume 158
Pigment accumulation 14
Pink sputum 93
Placental transfer 257
Plasma 114, 147
    cells 28
    components 311
    derivatives 311
    heavy spin 312
    membrane 13
    specific gravity 312
Plasmapheresis 319
Plasminogen activator inhibitor 49
Plasmodium 206, 208
    aldolase 214
    falciparum 215
    life cycle of 207*f*
    stage of 208
    vivax 215
Plastic bags, use of 243
Platelet 112, 114, 115*f*, 140, 141
    activation 187
    alloimmunization 297
    apheresis 311, 321*f*
    concentrate 311, 312, 318
    count 190, 193, 202
    pheresis 316, 318
    rich plasma 312
    specific gravity 312
    structure 121
    transfusion 315
        indications for 315
    yield, calculation of 316
Plateletpheresis 319, 321
Pleural effusion 70
Pleural fluid 69
    analysis 71
Pleurisy, tuberculous 72
Pneumocystis carinii pneumonia 91
Pneumonia 91, 93
Pneumothorax 70
Poikilocytosis 174
Polycarbonate membrane filtration 227
Polyclonal antibody 274
Polycythemia 196, 198, 303
    absolute 198
    primary 198
    secondary 198
    vera 134, 142, 150

Polymerase chain reaction 105, 205, 215, 221, 331
   advance 108
   analysis of 107
   applications of 108
   buffer 105
   mechanism 106*f*
Polymorphism 329
Polyspecific antihuman globulin 336
Polyuria 80
   causes of 80
Post-erythrocytic cycle 208
Post-kala-azar dermal leishmaniasis 218
Post-transfusion purpura 298
Potassium 52
   cyanide 153
   fericyanide 153
   oxalate 127, 287
   serum 51, 52
Pre-erythrocytic cycle 208
Pregnancy 134, 137, 166
   molar 166
Proerythroblast 117
Prolactin 43
Prolonged bleeding time 191
Promastigote 217*f*
Promonocyte 119
Promyelocyte 118, 119, 181
Prostate 60
   specific antigen 43, 48
Protein 65, 66, 74, 75, 104
   cross-linking 13
   extracellular accumulation of 14
   overexpression 48
   total 100
Prothrombin time 186, 190, 192
Protozoa 306
   infection 290
Pruritus 199
Pseudochylous effusions 69
Pulse 288
Pure red aplasia 166
Purpura 190, 195
Pus 88
   casts 84
Pyknosis 18
Pyothorax 70
Pyrexia 80

Q
Quantitative buffy coat
   test 212, 213, 214*f*
   tube 213*f*
Quarantine storage 248

R
Rabies 289
Radiation therapy 137
Rapid diagnostic tests 212, 214
   advantages of 215
   disadvantages of 215
Rapid malaria test 214, 215*f*
Reactive oxygen species 167
Recent crossmatch techniques 335
Red blood cell 72, 111, 112, 113*f*, 151, 154, 158, 163, 209, 231, 259, 318
   abnormal 171, 173
      morphology 177
   alloimmunization 297
   analysis 103
   anisochromic 174, 174*f*
   anisocytic 174, 174*f*
   count 202
   diluting fluid 131
   hyperchromic 173, 174*f*
   hypochromic 173, 173*f*
   indices 202
   macrocytic 174, 174*f*
   maturation, requirements for 118
   microcytic 174, 174*f*
   morphological analysis 103
   normal 172*f*, 173
      content of 176
      morphology 177
   nucleated 176
   pipette 131, 132*f*
   polychromic 174, 174*f*
   spherocytic 175*f*
   stomatocytic 175*f*
Red bone marrow 178
Red cell 140, 147, 312, 313
   antigens 254
      inheritance of 260
   concentrate 311
   count 76, 131
   indices 158
   saline washed 314
   specific gravity 312
   value, normal 151
Refreshment room 248
Refrigerated centrifuge 312
Refsum's disease 321
Renal diseases, chronic 166
Renal failure 80
Renal glomerular disease 54
Renal tubular damage 54
Respiratory disease, chronic 142
Reticulocyte 118, 169, 170*f*
   count 169, 202
Reverse transcriptase polymerase chain reaction test 106
Rhesus 264
   antibodies 265
   antigens 264
      characteristics of 265
   blood group 265
      system 243, 264
   blood typing 277
   factor 264
   nomenclature 266
   system inheritance 267
Rheumatoid arthritis 73, 258
Ribosomes 8
Ringer's lactate 326
Romanowsky stains 212
Rotary bead method 162
Rothera's mixture 82
Rothera's test 82
Routine test 40
RT-PCR 106

S
Sahli's acid hematin method 151, 152*f*
Saline
   adenine glucose mannitol 288
   normal 276
   wet mount examination 90
Saline/Saponin method 228
Salt poisoning 54
Sarcoidosis 58
Scar
   formation 31
   maturation of 31
Schilling test 202
Schistocytes 176, 176*f*
Schoenfeld and Llewellen's method, modified 55
Sedimentation 313
Semen 59
   analysis 62
Semi-automated analyzers 99, 100
Seminal fluid 59
Seminal vesicle 60
Serology
   disadvantages of 328
   tests 220
Serous fluid 65
Serum ascites albumin gradient 75
Serum glutamic
   oxaloacetic transaminase 100
   pyruvic transaminase 100
Serum prothrombin conversion accelerator deficiency 188
Serum-ascites albumin gradient 75
Shock, anaphylactic 258
Sickle cell 171, 175, 175*f*
   anemia 150, 165*f*, 202, 303
   laboratory diagnosis of 171

crisis 303
disease 171, 172, 172f
preparation 171
trait 171, 172
Sideroblast, detection of 182
Single blood volume exchange 304
Single donor plasma 311
Single nucleotide polymorphism 330
Single-stranded conformation polymorphism technique 221
Skin 161
  diseases, atopic 258
  wounds, healing of 32
Sleeping sickness 221
Slide method 276, 277
Slit skin smear 221
Smear
  observation of 139f
  preparation of 138f, 212
  staining of 138
  thick 212
  thin 212
Sodium 52
  chloride 92, 131, 288
    solution 169
  citrate 127, 169
  diet, high 54
  fluoride 127
  heparin 127
  phosphate 287
  serum 51
  sulfate 131
Special blood cell tests 160
Specific gravity 80, 104
  method 153
Specimen
  collection 34
  labeling 126
Sperm
  abnormal 62f
  concentration 61
  normal 61, 62f
Spherocyte 175
Spherocytosis, hereditary 165f
Sphingomyelin 63
Spleen 203
  diseases 137
  enlargement of 300
  role of 120
Splenectomy 167
Splenic aspiration 220
Spore testing 40
Sputum
  analysis 93
  bloody 93

culture 96
examination 91
microscopy 93
sample, collection of 92
Staphylococcus aureus 6, 335
Steatosis 14
Stem cell 323
  factor 45
Sterile collections 127
Stomatocytosis 175
Stool analysis 87
Streptococcus pneumoniae 93, 96, 97
Stress 137
Sulfosalicylic acid test 81
Supportive tests 221
Supravital staining 228
Syndrome inappropriate ADH secretion 54
Synovial fluid 76, 77
  characteristics of 78
  normal constituents of 77
Synthetic beads 333f
Syphilis 29, 282, 298, 309
Syringe 124
Systemic lupus erythematosus 73, 160, 321

T

Taenia 88
Tail defects 61
Target cells 175, 175f
T-cell 120
Tenderness, abdominal 75
Testes 60
Thalassemia 202
  major 166
  syndromes 154
Thawing 317
Theraflex methylene blue 335
Thoracentesis 70
Thrombapheresis 321
Thrombocytapheresis 321
Thrombocytes 112, 114, 116
Thrombocytopenia 188, 190
Thrombopoiesis 116, 120
Thrombosis 187
Thyroglobulin 49
Thyroid disorders 134
Tissue
  damage 137
  necrosis 23
  receptors 43
Total leukocyte count 123
Total red cell count 158
Total white cell count 135
Tourniquet test 190, 194

Toxicopathology 6
Toxoplasma gondii 309
Toxoplasmosis 142, 298, 309
Trachea, respiratory tract consists of 91
Transfusion
  medicine, applications in 333
  reactions 294
    delayed 297
    types of 294
  recipients 262
  transmitted diseases 298, 298t, 306
Treponema pallidum 27, 29, 290, 309
Trichloroacetic acid 56
Trichuris trichiura 88
Triglyceride 68, 71, 75
Trisodium citrate 129, 131, 287
Trisomy 64
Trypanosoma 206, 221
  brucei gambiense 221, 222f
  rhodesiense 224
Trypanosomiasis 258
TT virus 308
Tube method 276, 278
Tuberculosis 72, 91, 137, 142
Tubular necrosis, acute 54
Tumor 23, 137
  markers 42, 71
    limitations of 44
    list of 44
    testing of 49
    types of 42
    uses of 43
  necrosis factor 208
Türk's solution 135
Turner's syndrome 64
Tyrosine 84

U

Ulcerative colitis 144
Ulex europaeus 273
Ultrasound 301
Umbilical cord blood stem cell transplant 325
Urea nitrogen 100
Urinary phosphorus, high 57
Urinary tract infection 102
Urine
  analysis 79
  analyzer for 102
  calcium 57, 58
  casts observed in 84f
  cells observed in 83f
  chloride 55
  crystals observed in 85f

formation, complete absence
 of 80
inorganic phosphorus 57
output, low 75
phosphorus 56
potassium 54, 55
sodium 54
Urinometer 81*f*
Urinothorax 70
Urobilinogen 82, 104
Urokinase plasminogen activator 49

V

Vaccine, types of 289
Vacuoles 9
Vacuum
 blood collection system 126
 collection tubes 126
Vascular access device 122
Vasculitis 142
 autoimmune 321
Vasoconstriction 187
Vein
 peripheral 304
 umbilical 304

Venepuncture, procedure of 291
Venous blood collection 122, 123
Viruses 306 307
Visceral leshmaniasis 218, 219
Viscosity 93
Vitamin
 B_{12} 202
 D deficiency 57
 K
  deficiency 190, 193
Vomiting 54, 66, 75
von Willebrand's disease 188, 317

W

Waste
 autoclaving, standards for 40
 category 38, 39
 medical 40
 types of 38
Waxy casts 83
West Nile virus 298, 308
Westergren method 145, 146*f*
Westergren pipette 145
Westergren stand 145
Wet gangrene 20

White blood cell 72, 116, 230
 count 76, 202
 diluting fluid 135
 pipette 135, 136
 types of 113*fc*
Whole blood 313, 318
 coagulation time 190, 191
Wiener nomenclature 266
Wintrobe method 145, 146, 146*f*
Wintrobe pipette 146
Wintrobe stand 146
Wintrobe tube 146, 148
Wright's method 191, 191*f*
Wright's stain 139, 140, 180
 powder 140
Wuchereria bancrofti 206, 224

Y

Yellow bone marrow 179
Yersinia enterocolitica 296

Z

Ziehl-Neelsen
 staining method 93
 technique 93, 95